Donation

ONCOGENOMICS

ONCOGENOMICS
MOLECULAR APPROACHES TO CANCER

Edited By

Charles Brenner, Ph.D.
Departments of Genetics and Biochemistry
Norris Cotton Cancer Center
Dartmouth Medical School
Lebanon, New Hampshire

David Duggan, Ph.D.
Translational Genomics Research Institute
Phoenix, Arizona

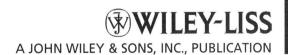
A JOHN WILEY & SONS, INC., PUBLICATION

Published by John Wiley & Sons, Inc., Hoboken, New Jersey.
Published simultaneously in Canada.

For general information on our other products and services please contact our Customer Care Department within the U.S. at 877-762-2974, outside the U.S. at 317-572-3993 or fax 317-572-4002.

Wiley also publishes its books in a variety of electronic formats. Some content that appears in print, however, may not be available in electronic format.

Library of Congress Cataloging-in-Publication Data

Oncogenomics : molecular approaches to cancer / edited by Charles
Brenner, David J. Duggan.
     P. ; cm.
Includes bibliographical references and index.
  ISBN 0-471-22592-4 (cloth : alk. paper)
  1. Cancer–Genetic aspects. 2. Cancer–Molecular aspects. 3.
Genomics. 4. Proteomics. 5. Oncogenes.
   [DNLM: 1. Neoplasms–genetics. 2. Neoplasms–therapy. 3. Gene
Therapy. QZ 200 05806 2004] I. Brenner, Charles. II. Duggan, David J.
  RC268.4.O49 2004
  616.99′4042–dc21

                                                  2003009480

Printed in the United States of America.

10 9 8 7 6 5 4 3 2 1

This book is dedicated to the patients.

CONTENTS

Section V CONCLUSION

CONTRIBUTORS

David Bearss, Montigen Pharmaceuticals, Salt Lake City, Utah

Patrick J. Biggs, The Wellcome Trust Sanger Institute, Hinxton, United Kingdom

Penelope E. Bonnen, Laboratory of Molecular Genetics, Rockefeller University, New York, New York

Anne-Lise Børresen-Dale, Department of Genetics, The Norwegian Radium Hospital, Oslo, Norway

David Botstein, Department of Molecular Biology, Princeton University, Princeton, New Jersey

Allan Bradley, The Wellcome Trust Sanger Institute, Hinxton, United Kingdom

Charles Brenner, Departments of Genetics and Biochemistry and Norris Cotton Cancer Center, Dartmouth Medical School, Lebanon, New Hampshire

Patrick O. Brown, Department of Biochemistry and Howard Hughes Medical Institute, Stanford University, Stanford, California

Arthur M. Buchberg, Department of Microbiology and Immunology, Kimmel Cancer Center, Thomas Jefferson University, Philadelphia, Pennsylvania

Julio E. Celis, Institute of Cancer Biology, The Danish Cancer Society, Copenhagen, Denmark

Yeun-Jun Chung, The Wellcome Trust Sanger Institute, Hinxton, United Kingdom

Mary B. Daly, Fox Chase Cancer Center, Philadelphia, Pennsylvania

David Duggan, Translational Genomics Research Institute, Phoenix, Arizona

Michael R. Emmert-Buck, Pathogenetics Unit, Laboratory of Pathology and Urologic Oncology Branch, National Cancer Institute, National Institutes of Health, Bethesda, Maryland

P. Andrew Futreal, Cancer Genome Project, The Wellcome Trust Sanger Institute, Hinxton, United Kingdom

Pavel Gromov, Institute of Cancer Biology, The Danish Cancer Society, Copenhagen, Denmark

Irina Gromova, Institute of Cancer Biology, The Danish Cancer Society, Copenhagen, Denmark

Haiyong Han, Department of Molecular and Cellular Biology, University of Arizona, Tucson, Arizona

Anne Kallioniemi, Laboratory of Cancer Genetics, Institute of Medical Technology, University of Tampere and Tampere University Hospital, Finland

Yong-son Kim, Cutaneous Biology Research Center, Havard Medical School, Massachusetts General Hospital, Charlestown, Massachusetts

Revati Koratkar, Department of Microbiology and Immunology, Kimmel Cancer Center, Thomas Jefferson University, Philadelphia, Pennsylvania

Per E. Lønning, Department of Medicine, Section of Oncology, Haukeland University Hospital, Bergen, Norway

Tia M. Maiolatesi, Departments of Genetics and Biochemistry and Norris Cotton Cancer Center, Lebanon, New Hampshire

Marina Markova, Department of Microbiology and Immunology, Kimmel Cancer Center, Thomas Jefferson University, Philadelphia, Pennsylvania

David L. Nelson, Department of Molecular and Human Genetics, Baylor College of Medicine, Houston, Texas

Paul Nghiem, Cutaneous Biology Research Center, Harvard Medical School, Massachusetts General Hospital, Charlestown, Massachusetts

Alicia Parlanti, Myriad Genetics, Salt Lake City, Utah

George C. Prendergast, Lankenau Institute for Medical Research and Department of Pathology, Anatomy and Cell Biology, Thomas Jefferson University, Philadelphia, Pennsylvania

Fritz Rank, Laboratory of Clinical Pathology, Diagnostic Center, Rigshospitalet, Copenhagen, Denmark

Stuart L. Schreiber, Department of Chemistry and Chemical Biology, Howard Hughes Medical Institute, Harvard University, Cambridge, Massachusetts

Karen A. Silverman, Department of Microbiology and Immunology, Kimmel Cancer Center, Thomas Jefferson University, Philadelphia, Pennsylvania

Linda D. Siracusa, Department of Microbiology and Immunology, Kimmel Cancer Center, Thomas Jefferson University, Philadelphia, Pennsylvania

Therese Sørlie, Department of Genetics, The Norwegian Radium Hospital, Oslo, Norway

Michael R. Stratton, Cancer Genome Project, The Wellcome Trust Sanger Institute, Hinxton, United Kingdom

Michael A. Tangrea, Pathogenetics Unit, Laboratory of Pathology and Urologic Oncology Branch, National Cancer Institute, National Institutes of Health, Bethesda, Maryland

Debrah M. Thompson, The Wellcome Trust Sanger Institute, Hinxton, United Kingdom

Louise van der Weyden, The Wellcome Trust Sanger Institute, Hinxton, United Kingdom

Andrew C. von Eschenbach, National Cancer Institute, National Institutes of Health, Bethesda, Maryland

Daniel D. Von Hoff, Departments of Medicine, Pathology and Molecular and Cellular Biology, Arizona Cancer Center, University of Arizona, Tucson, Arizona; Translational Genomics Research Institute, Phoenix, Arizona

John N. Weinstein, Genomics and Bioinformatics Group, Laboratory of Molecular Pharmacology, Center for Cancer Research, National Cancer Institute, National Institutes of Health, Bethesda, Maryland

Richard Wooster, Cancer Genome Project, The Wellcome Trust Sanger Institute, Hinxton, United Kingdom

PREFACE

The emergence of genomics has changed the way we need to think about cancer in radical ways. When the draft sequence of the human genome was published in 2001, we realized that no one had attempted to assemble the broad expertise to educate working scientists and clinicians, graduate and medical students, advanced practice nurses, genetic counselors, and health educators across all of the cancer-relevant disciplines that have been altered by genomics. We realized that a forward-looking book on cancer prevention, detection, classification, pharmacology, testing, and treatment would span the disciplines of very disparate readers so we would need to begin with an advanced introduction that would allow individuals to gain confidence with the entire scope of the work. The book would devote a number of chapters to molecular profiling of cancer-specific changes at the DNA, RNA, protein and tissue levels with the aims of identifying all of the mutations that occur in malignancies, classifying tumors into a manageable set of functionally different types, and correlating those types with drug sensitivities. The book would provide chapters by experts on model systems—model organisms and cellular and chemical genetic systems—that are increasingly essential for testing hypotheses and treatments. The book would include a section on molecularly targeted drugs to explore the successes, challenges and real-world complications of developing genotype-specific agents. Additionally, the book would feature someone highly experienced in oncology clinical testing to discuss the problems of conducting target-informed trials and a concluding chapter that would set out the expectations for future developments from an authoritative point of view.

Two years ago, bearing our wish-list of contributors ideally suited to write the sixteen chapters that would constitute *Oncogenomics*, this book's outline was shepherded through Wiley's internal and external review process by our able and enthusiastic project editor, Luna Han. Today, we are extremely pleased to present readers a volume written by this dream team of scientists and clinicians. Though we spent considerable effort quilting together their contributions into an enveloping work, the power of the book is clearly in the expertise and the breadth of our contributors. Readers are encouraged to visit the accompanying website, www.wiley.com/go/oncogenomics, for additional resources. Knowing our contributors, we are confident that students will find many of these investigators accessible to discuss experiments and to plan fellowships.

This brings us to the most powerful reason for expending the energy to create the first book on oncogenomics. Novel molecular approaches to cancer prevention, diagnosis, classification, and treatment need to be developed and championed by a new generation of scientists and clinicians who are more interdisciplinary than their mentors. It is our hope that this book will catalyze cross-training such that genomicists will think about pharmacology, model organism people with think about tumors, clinical oncologists will think about genetics, and all molecularly oriented people will think about cancer prevention.

Year 2004 cancer researchers and clinicians are necessarily wiser than we were in 2001. We are clearer in our understanding that federal and investment dollars will be limited. We know that not all targeted drugs will work as well as Gleevec. And we appreciate that the macro environment—smoking prevalence, healthcare delivery, etc.—will influence greatly the stages at which patients' tumors will be presented either in community hospitals or in academic health centers and that these factors limit the benefit that will be gleaned from oncogenomics. At the same time, successes breed successes and we are convinced that improvements in cancer outcomes from oncogenomics will lead to an improved environment for public and private healthcare investment, earlier and more extensive applications of molecular diagnostics, and earlier and more effective molecular cancer care.

ACKNOWLEDGMENTS

While taking the opportunity to thank our scientific contributors for producing state-of-the-art chapters for *Oncogenomics*, we also want to hold these individuals and groups out as models of scientific and clinical excellence, whose careers in academia and industry (and frequently both) bear emulation. As the leading figures in molecular profiling, model systems, targeted drugs, and clinical research and care, the book's contributors have been responsible for revolutionizing their fields. We expect that readers will appreciate the ways in which the contributors opened up their approaches to a wide audience without compromising intellectual precision.

We are grateful to Luna Han at Wiley for the vision to initiate this project and for entrusting it to us. We thank Kristen Hauser and Lisa Van Horn for moving the book through production and all of the people in the service and supply line for ably conducting their work.

David Duggan thanks mentors Thomas London, Kenneth Buetow, Eric Hoffman, Jeff Trent, and Dan Kastner for nurture and inspiration. Charlie Brenner thanks mentors the late Barry Kiefer, Tony Brake, Kunihiro Matsumoto, Bob Fuller, Greg Petsko and Dagmar Ringe for guidance and support, program project collaborators Kay Huebner and Carlo Croce for colleagueship and friendship, and Nancy Spock and Mark Israel for their vision. We thank our trainees for always asking the right questions and for the wonderful experience of working toward answers.

David thanks his wife, Debbie, and daughters, Jessica and Nicole for their support and tolerating quiet times. Charlie thanks his parents, Mort and Sandra Brenner, for support and encouragement and his wife, Loraine, and son, Freeman, for pleasurable distraction.

CHARLES BRENNER
DAVID DUGGAN

Lebanon, New Hampshire
Phoenix, Arizona
January 2004

Section I

INTRODUCTION

AT THE PRECARIOUS CUSP OF ONCOGENOMICS

Charles Brenner

Though "same as it ever was" and "nothing will ever be the same" are clichés, our lives as medical consumers, researchers, and providers are lived in between the clichés. Each day, new cases of cancer are detected by visual and tactile inspection. Each day, researchers consent patients for molecular analysis of tumor samples in the hope of molecular classification and pharmacogenomic profiling. Vast numbers of patients are treated with combinations of the same armaments of cytotoxic compounds that have long been available, while small but increasing numbers are treated with the first gene-based drugs such as Herceptin and Gleevec. The most informed patients seek information from resources made available by the National Cancer Institute and academic medical centers, fueling demand for experimental treatments unavailable from, and in some cases unknown by, community practitioners.

To introduce the first book on cancer genomics—a volume that spans molecular profiling, model systems to discover and validate drug targets, and molecularly targeted cancer pharmacology—an advanced introduction to cancer genetics and cancer pharmacology is provided. Additionally, some of the nontechnological roadblocks to the fruition of oncogenomics are considered. There is tremendous potential for improvements in cancer care to arise from advances in prevention, an improved environment for testing including insurance reimbursement of clinical trials, and hype-free reflection on the words of Hippocrates: "first, do no harm." The confluence of these streams—where

Oncogenomics: Molecular Approaches to Cancer, Edited by Charles Brenner and David Duggan
ISBN 0-471-22592-4 © 2004 John Wiley & Sons, Inc.

molecular sciences meet prevention and clinical testing in an environment free from unreasonable expectations—is the leading edge of oncogenomics.

WHAT IS ONCOGENOMICS?

Genetic Changes in Malignant Diseases

Cancer is not a single genetic disease but hundreds of diseases consisting of different combinations of genetic alterations. Several types of genetic alterations contribute to neoplastic transformation. Mutator genes that control the fidelity of genome mainte-nance and checkpoint genes responsible for quality control in cell division cycles are lost. Oncogenes are activated and tumor suppressor genes are lost.

To consider the types of alterations required to effect neoplastic transformation, it is useful to delineate several of the properties of normal cells. Normal cells cor-rect spontaneously occurring and induced mutations. Normal cells arrest their division cycles when progression would lead to damaged progeny or to mitotic catastrophes. Normal cells divide in harmony with their environments: those in stem cell popu-lations regenerate while terminally differentiated cells in epithelial layers slough off when they are worn out. Normal cells undergo programmed cell death in response to developmental signals and irreparable damage. Normal cells have tightly defined migratory potential.

We are accustomed to considering mutation and selection at the organism level. For example, we know that antibiotic-resistant microbes arise due to the existence of genetic heterogeneity and the survival of those with genes that confer resistance to the challenges to which the microbes are exposed. When the characteristics of normal cells are defined as we have defined them here (arrest, death, limits to migration), it is easy to appreciate that genetic changes leading to the initiation and progression of cancer are a selective process that results in loss of controls (i.e., failure to arrest, failure to die, unlimited migration). Inherited or acquired mutations in DNA repair genes generate the genetic diversity in somatic cells from which subsequent genetic selections occur. Losses of DNA repair genes do not directionally lead to oncogenic alterations: given the vast amount of noncoding DNA in any cell, more mutations are expected to be inconsequential than consequential. However, when a cell acquires the ability to divide more rapidly or evade apoptosis, it generates a clone of cells disencumbered from the rules that keep its neighbors in check. If the immune system does not eliminate such cells, they may survive to accumulate further genetic changes and become malignant.

Our Plastic Genomes: Sporadic versus Hereditary Cancers

I have just described genetic changes in neoplastic transformation in evolutionary terms—i.e., in terms of a population of *cells* within an individual that accumulate genetic differences in response to selective pressures. The more familiar Darwinian condition—i.e., populations of nonidentical *individuals* that exhibit different measures of fitness in different environments—is also at work in cancer biology. While all neoplastic diseases involve genetic alterations, most cancer is termed *sporadic*, while a minority of cases fall into what are termed *hereditary syndromes*, only some of which have a molecularly known basis.

In sporadic cases, we cannot see clear lines of descent, leading us to believe that the initiating genetic changes occurred within an individual's somatic cells. In cases that are classified as hereditary, we can see segregation of disease as a recessive or dominant trait with some measure of penetrance. It would be a mistake to create a sharp dichotomy between sporadic and hereditary cancer. Both the frequency and the consequences of sporadic events in terms of their expression as malignancies are clearly regulated by a variety of inherited factors. Additionally, while an inherited genetic change is *necessary* for a hereditary cancer syndrome, it is almost certainly *not sufficient* for malignancy. More insight into this assertion can be gleaned by considering the nature of genetic changes that occur in carcinogenesis.

It was stated at the outset that DNA repair and cell cycle checkpoint genes are lost in cancer, oncogenes are activated in cancer, and tumor suppressor genes are lost. By lowering the fidelity of DNA replication and cell division, losses in repair and checkpoint genes, produce some of the genetic variation from which transforming mutations are selected. Most of the genetic changes that occur in response to losses in fidelity are likely to be inconsequential and selectively neutral: these types of alterations are sometimes termed *bystander effects*. However, it is the alteration of oncogenes and tumor suppressor genes that contribute to the initiation and maintenance of the transformed phenotype.

Oncogenes

We say that oncogenes are *activated* in cancer because the genetic alterations are dominant and give rise to a gain of function at the gene level. An oncogene can become "switched on" by virtue of a single amino acid change, by translocation to a highly active promoter, by producing a constitutively active fusion protein, by producing a truncated protein product that is hyperactive, or by genetic amplification. All of these types of mutations are dominant with respect to the unaltered allele of the oncogene and can contribute to transformation in a heterozygous condition. These types of mutations are almost never inherited, probably because if every cell in the body contained an activating mutation in an oncogene, the embryo would not develop normally. Consequently, we know of no cancer syndromes in which there are adults who are germ-line heterozygous for activated oncogenes. The fact that oncogenes are switched on in cancer makes the oncoprotein products of oncogene mutations rational targets for genotype-specific cancer treatments, as discussed extensively in Chapters 10, 13, 14, and 15.

Tumor Suppressor Genes

Tumor suppressor genes, which become *lost* or *inactivated* in the development of cancer, are subject to cancer-associated mutations that are recessive at the gene level. These mutations occur both in sporadic cancer and in inherited cancer predisposition syndromes (Knudson, 1996). Whereas two "hits" are typically required to inactivate such genes in tumors that arise sporadically, if an individual is born heterozygous for such a loss, then only a single change is required in a cell to produce a preneoplastic lesion. The change can be an independent second mutation, an epigenetic change such as DNA methylation that reduces gene expression, or a gene conversion event that produces loss of heterozygosity at the locus. We consider such genetic and epigenetic changes to be *preneoplastic* because loss of (both copies of) a single tumor suppressor gene is not fully transforming: cancer is a multistage process involving multiple genetic changes.

The fact that tumor suppressor gene mutations are recessive at the gene and single-cell level and can be inherited in a heterozygous state through the germ line creates an additional fact about tumor suppressor gene mutations: when these mutations are followed through generations, they appear *dominant* at the level of the individual. The reason that a mutation that is loss-of-function at the gene level can be dominant at the organism level is that humans are multicellular organisms who live a long time, and given all of the cell divisions that occur in target tissues, it is not unlikely that a cell will suffer a second hit and produce the preneoplastic genotype. Cancer geneticists are careful to point out that individuals who carry such mutations are *dominantly predisposed* to get cancer: if the tumor suppressor mutations were dominant at the gene and single-cell levels, every cell that expresses the gene would be aberrant and the individuals could not develop normally. Because tumor suppressor gene mutations are recessive at the gene level, sufficient function is available to allow an individual to develop normally from a heterozygous embryo in order to produce the target organ tissue that may suffer loss of heterozygosity in one or more cells. As discussed in Chapters 10, 12, 13, and 15, cells with losses in checkpoint or tumor suppressor genes might have unique drug sensitivities that would allow them to be molecularly targeted, but—unlike activated oncoproteins—the tumor suppressor proteins themselves will not be cancer drug targets because these proteins are missing from the target tissue.

Penetrance

The final point that needs to be made in an introductory discussion of oncogenomics is that particular cancer-associated mutations bring with them a particular tumor spectrum and an approximate penetrance. For example, being born heterozygous for DNA mismatch repair gene *MSH2* is associated with hereditary nonpolyposis colorectal cancer (HNPCC; Fishel et al., 1993). This syndrome involves predisposition to malignant tumors in the colon, endometrial tissues, stomach, and other sites. While most colorectal cancer is not hereditary and mutations such as *MSH2-1906G→C* are rare in the general population, they are highly enriched among cancer patients in certain ethnic populations (Foulkes et al., 2002). Based on how deleterious the inherited mutation is, how likely a second hit in the *MSH2* gene is, and how many additional mutations are required to produce tumors (and other interacting genetic and environmental factors), individuals who inherit such a mutation have characteristic likelihoods of developing disease. These averaged likelihoods are termed *penetrance*. Because colon cancer is relatively common and involves many genetic changes subsequent to reduction of mismatch repair (Vogelstein and Kinzler, 1993), the background level of sporadic colon cancer is high and the penetrance of familial colon cancer is relatively low. A consistently updated resource on the relationship between *MSH2* mutations and HNPCC is maintained at Online Mendelian Inheritance in Man (www.ncbi.nlm.nih.gov:80/entrez/dispomim.cgi?id =120435).

In retinoblastoma, we encounter a rare tumor that is more typically hereditary and exhibits high penetrance. In high-penetrance retinoblastoma families, individuals are born heterozygous for a deleted *rb1* allele (Friend et al., 1987). During development of the retina, there is sufficient cell division to make loss of heterozygosity events likely during youth. Because an $rb1^-/rb1^-$ cell does not need a large number of further genetic changes to become malignant, individuals born as *rb1* heterozygotes are almost as likely to suffer bilateral or multifocal retinoblastoma (i.e., two independent tumors) as they are to escape disease. Thus, such mutations appear dominant in pedigrees with almost complete penetrance. McKusick and his colleagues maintain a comprehensive resource on the genetics and molecular cell biology of retinoblastoma at Online Mendelian Inheritance in Man (www.ncbi.nlm.nih.gov:80/entrez/dispomim.cgi?id =180200).

A NEW APPROACH

Toward a Molecular Oncology

From today's perspective, we know that tumors consist of specific genetic alterations and that cancers are treated with surgery, radiation, and chemotherapy. In the absence of molecular classifications, clinicians have been treating tumors with relatively nonspecific regimens for decades. Though these treatments were not developed specifically to target known genotypes, it has long been appreciated that some patients respond whereas others do not respond to the same treatments. As Von Hoff and co-workers from the Arizona Cancer Center point out in Chapter 15, the earliest molecular classifications of tumors, such as assays of estrogen receptor status for breast and cervical cancer, were followed by the first molecularly correlated and molecularly targeted treatments.

In the "same as it ever was" past, clinicians worked with nothing more than tumor site and size to design treatments. At the precarious cusp at which we find ourselves today, genetic counseling must play a key role in informing patients and family members of what can be done and why they may wish to play a role in well-designed studies. Every author has attempted to make chapters in this book accessible to a diverse target readership population that includes oncologists and oncology nurses, basic and population-based cancer scientists, science journalists, and genetic counselors. The contributors to this volume—all experts in the field of oncogenomics—never opted to dumb the material down in a way that would compromise scientific or medical precision, while thoroughly respecting the multidisciplinary nature of this book.

In the "nothing will ever be the same" future, it has been widely speculated that the molecular profiling technologies described in Chapters 2 through 9 will be used to determine tumor and patient genotypes and genotype-specific treatments will be available for many of the common tumor genotypes. The number of chapters devoted to profiling reflects the need at this early stage of oncogenomics to develop tools to classify the molecular nature of malignant diseases. Chapters 2, 3, and 4 focus on describing DNA changes in tumors, while Chapters 5 and 6 focus primarily on RNA expression changes. Chapter 7 focuses on known cancer cell lines, Chapter 8 focuses on microdissected tissue samples, and Chapter 9 focuses on proteomic analysis.

Cancer researchers seek not only to discover all of the genetic, epigenetic, and phenotypic changes in cancer but to turn these discoveries into molecular targets. Model systems are crucial for genetic and pharmacological validation of candidate diagnostic, preventive, and therapeutic targets. For cancer, model systems are either murine or nonmurine. We review the nonmurine approaches in Chapter 10, and devote Chapters 11 and 12 to complementary approaches to cancer modeling, gene discovery, and target validation in the mouse.

Basic cancer research culminates with drug development and clinical testing. Kinase-directed and Ras superfamily–directed compounds are reviewed in Chapters 13 and 14, respectively. The complexity of cancer as hundreds of different diseases makes clinical testing and clinical care extremely challenging. These issues are reviewed in Chapter 15. In the final chapter, National Cancer Institute Director Andrew C. von Eschenbach makes the case that application of resources to several bottlenecks along the drug development pipeline and exploitation of the fruits of oncogenomics can turn cancer into a manageable condition.

Molecular Profiling in Cancer: DNA, RNA, and Protein

In Chapter 2, Stratton and his co-workers describe the Wellcome Trust-Supported Cancer Genome Project (CGP) in its attempt to describe comprehensively every deletion and mutation that has occurred in a reference set of cancer-derived cell lines. This extremely high-tech effort is expected to significantly expand the number of oncogenes, tumor suppressor genes, and cancer-associated mutator and checkpoint genes. Moreover, CGP methods, over the long haul, may allow a patient's tumor to be comprehensively genotyped at high resolution.

In Chapter 3, Kallioniemi describes how the latest but relatively widely available microarray technologies can be used to detect DNA copy number changes and mRNA expression changes from patient samples. Though Kallioniemi's methods are not designed to detect single base mutations, they are designed such that they can be replicated in a skilled and well-equipped biomedical laboratory. With the proper training and patient consents, it is not difficult to picture 100 laboratories in the United States succeeding at genotyping via Kallioniemi's methods upon publication of this book. In contrast, it is difficult to conceive of five places in the world that could realistically take on base resolution whole-genome genotyping in the year 2003.

While Chapters 2 and 3 share the orientation of comparing tumor and normal cells, in Chapter 4, Bonnen and Nelson seek to discern genetic differences between individuals by virtue of identifying single nucleotide polymorphisms (SNPs) that correlate with alterations in cancer incidence. Goals of SNP projects are twofold. First, SNPs are important in cancer gene discovery. Second, SNP-based genotypes are expected to help oncologists stratify patients to improve clinical outcomes. These themes will recur in the Chapter 12 discussion of genetic modifier screens in the mouse.

Editing this volume on the 50th anniversary of the seminal Watson and Crick elucidation of the structure of DNA, we frequently reflected on how cancer biology and molecular biology have grown up together. While the "Central Dogma of Molecular Biology" seems quaintly simplistic in light of current awareness of DNA rearrangements, micro RNAs, RNA catalysis, and protein-based inheritance (among many other antidogmatic developments), the core concepts of gene expression are crucial to the molecular profiling approaches described in Chapters 5 through 9. The critical tool of Chapters 5 and 6 is the mRNA expression microarray whose patterns often reveal the underlying genotype without ever interrogating DNA.

In Chapter 5, Botstein and colleagues discovered a set of less than a thousand genes whose expression patterns allowed classification into five different subtypes of breast cancer. Considering that the clinical standard of diagnostic care is currently estrogen receptor positive versus negative, mechanistic dissection of breast cancer profiles and their correlations with treatment will be extremely important in oncogenomic care.

In Chapter 6, Daly and co-workers consider how much genomics has changed genetics. Dr. Daly's patients include those whose families have a high predisposition to breast cancer. Recent work has shown that microarray technologies (both for RNA changes and DNA changes) can add a great deal to traditional and molecular genetics in disease classification and risk assessment.

Just as Stratton focused on reference sets of cancer cell lines in Chapter 2, Weinstein, in Chapter 7, focuses on a set of 60 cancer cell lines that are a permanent resource for elucidating the relationships between genome, transcriptome, proteome, and drug sensitivity. Despite the tremendous power of analyses with distributed and well-classified cell lines, there is a need to develop tools to profile DNA, RNA, and protein samples from excised patients' tissues. In Chapter 8, Tangrea and Emmert-Buck describe the state of the art in tissue microanalysis. In Chapter 9, acknowledging the advantages and disadvantages of cell lines and tissues, Celis and co-workers reveal advanced methods to profile expressed proteins in cancer samples.

Model Systems

The chapters on molecular profiling create a dynamic tension regarding potential drug targets in cancer. Whereas the gene discovery efforts described in Chapters 2, 4, 5, 7, 8, and 9 will clearly expand the number of potential cancer targets, the pattern recognition goals of Chapters 3, 5, 6, 7, 8, and 9 imply that substantially fewer than a combinatorial number of genotypes are functionally similar. Essentially every cancer genotype or expression phenotype can be treated as a hypothesis—e.g., that pharmacological targeting of these genotypes and expression phenotypes will reduce cancer incidence or lead to death or redifferentiation of cancer cells. These hypotheses are tested in model systems. In Chapter 10, we review biochemical, cellular, fungal, fly, and fish approaches to validate potential cancer drug targets. In Chapter 11, Bradley and co-workers describe mostly reverse genetic approaches to analyze cancer genotypes in the mouse. By engineering mutations into mice that recapitulate human cancer genotypes, researchers can test human genetic hypotheses in the nearest practical experimental system.

In Chapter 12, Siracusa and co-workers use the mouse for forward genetic screens to find mutations that modify penetrance. It will not escape anyone's notice that the genetic approaches in Chapters 11 and 12 are eminently complementary, as well as complementary with pharmacological approaches. For example, identifying a second mutation that reduces cancer incidence can be followed up with a gene knockout experiment. Targeting an encoded protein with a drug might produce a similar effect pharmacologically.

We note in Chapter 10 that almost the entire history of pharmacology consisted of identifying the target and mechanism of action of compounds that had interesting effects on cells or organisms, while most pharmacology today is target oriented from the start. The combination of genetics and pharmacology has accelerated both successes and failures in cancer targeting. Although failure does not sound good, accelerating failure is important because resources are always limited and in need of prioritization. Moreover, failure to be an effective drug target does not mean failure to provide important insights into molecular, cellular, and organismal biology, all of which are essential for ultimate successes.

Molecularly Targeted Drug Development and Testing

The first two gene-based cancer drugs, Herceptin and Gleevec, are both targeted against oncoprotein kinases. Because many protein kinases are activated in different types of cancer and biochemical and cellular assays for these enzymes were straightforward to develop, it has been relatively easy to screen for compounds that inhibit oncoprotein kinase functions. In Chapter 13, Schreiber and colleagues describe ways to target protein kinases and study their modes of action using drugs. Just when we feel that the entire oncogenomic and pharmacological enterprise is fully logical and predictable, we read Prendergast's Chapter 14 on Ras superfamily–directed compounds. It has long been clear that *RAS* genes are activated in cancer and that Ras proteins need to be membrane localized by farnesyltransferase (FT) activity to be transforming. Moreover, FT was targeted for drug development and potent inhibitors (FTI) were developed that reduced anchorage-independent growth of many cancer cell lines. The problem is that cellular FTI activity does not correlate with *RAS* mutation status or with the kinetics of Ras processing inhibition. Thus, the lesson of Chapter 14 is that cell biology is often more complicated than can be anticipated based on genetics.

While it was surprising to discover unanticipated targets for FTIs late in the game, it is essential for as many failures or surprises to occur before drugs get to the clinic. The financial costs involved in clinical testing are such that a company's ability to raise funds and/or test other drugs may be jeopardized by clinical failures. The human costs can involve not only morbidity and mortality but loss of trust in the medical enterprise, which makes future testing more difficult. Clinical testing is performed in a complicated medical, regulatory, and economic environment that must be navigated by patients and their doctors. In Chapter 15, Von Hoff and colleagues steer us through the rocks with trial designs developed to convince clinicians of the utility of molecularly targeted therapeutics.

Presently, few patients are molecularly profiled and few cancer genotypes are known to be susceptible to molecularly targeted therapies. Living as we do between the "same as it ever was" past and the "nothing will ever be the same" future, we come to the first challenges of oncogenomics.

THE ROAD AHEAD

Challenge 1: Molecular Diagnostics Ahead of Molecularly Targeted Treatments

What we know about cancer genetics is substantially ahead of genotype-directed molecular pharmacology. The nature of molecular biology and molecular medicine is such that it will always be easier to determine tumor genotypes, gene expression, and protein expression patterns than to treat tumors genotype specifically. As described earlier, mutator, checkpoint, and tumor suppressor genes are lost in cancer while oncogenes are activated. Though the types of alterations that need to be detected are different from gene to gene, every genetic alteration can be detected by multiple methods. The considerations that determine widespread availability of oncogenomic diagnostics are matters of technology (i.e., whether the diagnostics will be based on DNA or cDNA sequencing, hybridization, or antibody methods), intellectual property, and economics.

Therapies will always be more complicated for a variety of reasons. First, though mutator genes are lost in cancer, it is not expected that restoring function will provide effective treatments: This would be akin to closing the barn door of mutagenesis after the horse of oncogenic mutations is out. Second, though restoring checkpoint and/or tumor suppressor genes has been accomplished in many laboratory-controlled experimental systems, cancer is a disease of escape, and there is no clinically established method to restore a gene to 100% of tumor cells that have a missing gene. As we have discussed, loss of mutator, checkpoint, or tumor suppressor genes might sensitize tumor cells to killing by drugs targeted to other proteins. Even for those oncoproteins that are validated as drug targets and known to be required for maintaining the malignant phenotype, there are few drugs available. Thus, widespread availability of diagnostics in advance of therapeutics runs the risk of offering only negative outcomes such as stress and discrimination.

Although genotype-specific therapies will not come overnight, molecular diagnostics may tell patients and clinicians which of the available therapies are unlikely to bring benefit and might be helpful in promoting lifestyle decisions that are preventive. The utility of molecular diagnostics in ruling out certain treatment regimens is a very significant piece of medicine. Because many of the available cancer chemotherapies involve unpleasant side effects and many individuals do not respond to particular agents, sparing costly and painful treatments to patients unlikely to respond provides a real benefit. It is apparent in these early days of oncogenomic medicine that to reduce ineffective treatments and to improve medical decision making is to "first, do no harm."

Challenge 2: Quality of Information in the Age of the Internet

Because patients make decisions that are irreversible, the quality of information available to physicians and their patients is crucial. In a study from the Rotterdam Family Cancer Clinic, 55% of women with *BRCA1* or *BRCA2* mutations chose to undergo bilateral mastectomies as opposed to frequent screening (Meijers-Heijboer et al., 2001). One cannot be confident of the precise risk reduction in breast cancer associated with radical mastectomy for such women, but figures as high as 90% reduction in risk have been calculated (Hartmann et al., 1999) and widely quoted. Confounding calculations of cancer risk is the fact that the original families used to identify *BRCA1* and *BRCA2* mutations exhibited high penetrance (Begg, 2002). Earlier we attributed penetrance to the severity of an inherited allele coupled to other interacting genetic and environmental factors. Indeed, in the latest study, which calculated the lifetime cancer risk of *BRCA1* and *BRCA2* mutation carriers to be 82%, pregnancy and physical activity were associated with later cancer onset (King et al., 2003).

No statement on cancer risk will be the final word—studies of breast cancer risk and risk reduction continue to be performed and debated in the literature. The problem is that patients who try to be informed are buffeted by the latest press releases. Press releases provide summaries of studies along with punchy and non-peer-reviewed quotes from study authors. Prophylactic mastectomy clearly reduces breast cancer risk: How much it reduces risk and what it costs in physical and psychological well-being vis-a-vis the procedure's psychological benefits and the procedure's alternatives are the questions. Because nearly all women that are not *BRCA1* or *BRCA2* mutation carriers appear to overestimate their lifetime cancer risks (Metcalfe and Narod, 2002), it is a concern that women may be choosing prophylactic mastectomy based on awareness of cancer among friends and family that is mostly sporadic and entirely unrelated to their own risk.

We live in an environment with a great deal of information available on the Internet and little regulation that would restrain or coordinate access to diagnostic and prognostic information with preventive or therapeutic options. Because a little knowledge can be a dangerous thing, we need to communicate clearly and carefully to the public and encourage bright people to be trained in genetic counseling.

Challenge 3: Community Commitment to and Financing of Clinical Testing

Recent experience with patients infected with HIV suggests that under the right confluence of circumstances a substantial proportion of affected individuals may be willing to volunteer for clinical trials of experimental treatments. However, because homosexual men who were disproportionately infected by HIV were amenable to community organization, and because HIV had essentially no treatment only a few years ago, the fast tracking and degree of community involvement in HIV drug testing may never be equaled in cancer clinical testing. Though the analogy strains on examination, we assert that the epidemic in cancer that most resembles HIV infection is that surrounding lung cancers in present and former smokers. With 150,000 new cases per year in the United States alone and 140,000 deaths per year, there are certainly enough cases to qualify as epidemic. Further, because the vast majority of airway cancer cases are due to the voluntary inhalation of tobacco carcinogens, there is a strong component of unsafe behavior in the etiology of the disease that must be fought prospectively by public health and education. Finally, because smoking is becoming prohibited inside public buildings, the smoking "lifestyle" has become ghettoized during the workweek to segregated spaces—a development that bears a slight resemblance to the demographic fact that many homosexual people live in enclaves. It is conceivable that, as more smokers' circles are affected by cancer diagnoses and deaths, this community will demand experimental treatments and rally to support clinical testing of cancer drugs.

One problem with genotype-specific medicine is that by limiting the target population for a drug to those with a particular genotype or molecular profile, rather than all of those with tumors in an organ site, it is conceded that only a subset of patients will benefit from new drugs. Though only a fraction of patients respond to the existing cancer chemotherapies, the less specific criteria for prescription provide profits to drug companies. And though much has been said about targeted therapeutics being a new and rational paradigm for drug development, available evidence suggests that research and development costs continue to rise. Thus, smaller and more directed markets and high development costs are likely to lead to high costs of treatment. Groups such as CaPCURE and the Susan B. Komen Foundation have organized effectively to fund early detection programs and research. Legislation that would require health insurers to cover health care costs in approved clinical trials could potentially relieve a major impediment to more rapid and conclusive clinical testing.

Challenge 4: Hype Harms

In general, scientists are raised to be cautious in making assertions and predictions. In general, businesspeople responsible for raising start-up capital for biotechnology ventures are substantially less reserved. Though this book is not the place for an analysis of the investment bubble that burst in March 2000, the fallout from oversold promises in networking and biotechnologies did more than hurt people financially. Though scientists are used to failure (we never compute lifetime batting averages on our hypotheses), patients, doctors, and investors have to be more risk adverse, and once bitten, they are twice shy.

The ethical standards that guide communications about clinical trials must be of the highest order. Drugs must be sufficiently tested preclinically prior to clinical testing and clinical trials must be designed in a manner that optimizes the analytical power behind them. In short, the collapse of the investment bubble of March 2000 and the economic climate that has followed has retaught us that we conduct our work with limited resources that must be prioritized. Of all our resources, the human ones that include the trust and support of the taxpaying, investing, and medical public are the most precious.

Balanced at the cusp of *Oncogenomics*, I invite the reader to turn the page.

REFERENCES

Begg, C. B. (2002). On the use of familial aggregation in population-based case probands for calculating penetrance. *J Natl Cancer Inst 94*, 1221–1226.

Fishel, R., Lescoe, M. K., Rao, M. R., Copeland, N. G., Jenkins, N. A., Garber, J., Kane, M., and Kolodner, R. (1993). The human mutator gene homolog MSH2 and its association with hereditary nonpolyposis colon cancer. *Cell 75*, 1027–1038.

Foulkes, W. D., Thiffault, I., Gruber, S. B., Horwitz, M., Hamel, N., Lee, C., Shia, J., Markowitz, A., Figer, A., Friedman, E., et al. (2002). The founder mutation MSH2*1906G → C is an important cause of hereditary nonpolyposis colorectal cancer in the Ashkenazi Jewish population. *Am J Hum Genet 71*, 1395–1412.

Friend, S. H., Horowitz, J. M., Gerber, M. R., Wang, X. F., Bogenmann, E., Li, F. P., and Weinberg, R. A. (1987). Deletions of a DNA sequence in retinoblastomas and mesenchymal tumors: Organization of the sequence and its encoded protein. *Proc Natl Acad Sci USA 84*, 9059–9063.

Hartmann, L. C., Schaid, D. J., Woods, J. E., Crotty, T. P., Myers, J. L., Arnold, P. G., Petty, P. M., Sellers, T. A., Johnson, J. L., McDonnell, S. K., et al. (1999). Efficacy of bilateral prophylactic mastectomy in women with a family history of breast cancer. *N Engl J Med 340*, 77–84.

King, M.- C., Marks, J. H., and Mandell, J. B. (2003). Breast and ovarian cancer risks due to inherited mutations in *BRCA1* and *BRCA2*, *Science 302*, 643–646.

Knudson, A. G. (1996). Hereditary cancer: Two hits revisited. *J Cancer Res Clin Oncol 122*, 135–140.

Meijers-Heijboer, H., van Geel, B., van Putten, W. L., Henzen-Logmans, S. C., Seynaeve, C., Menke-Pluymers, M. B., Bartels, C. C., Verhoog, L. C., van den Ouweland, A. M., Niermeijer, M. F., et al. (2001). Breast cancer after prophylactic bilateral mastectomy in women with a BRCA1 or BRCA2 mutation. *N Engl J Med 345*, 159–164.

Metcalfe, K. A., and Narod, S. A. (2002). Breast cancer risk perception among women who have undergone prophylactic bilateral mastectomy. *J Natl Cancer Inst 94*, 1564–1569.

Vogelstein, B., and Kinzler, K. W. (1993). The multistep nature of cancer. *Trends Genet 9*, 138–141.

Section II

MOLECULAR PROFILING IN CANCER: DNA, RNA, AND PROTEIN

2

GENOME-WIDE SEARCHES FOR MUTATIONS IN HUMAN CANCER

Michael R. Stratton, P. Andrew Futreal, and Richard Wooster

INTRODUCTION

All cancers arise due to the acquisition of mutations of a subset of critical genes. Describing the somatic genetic changes in each cancer and hence identifying the multiple mutated genes that contribute to the development of each human cancer is a central aim of cancer research. While there has been substantial progress in the identification of cancer genes, a large number probably remain to be identified. However, considerable problems exist in current approaches to cancer gene identification. In particular, it is not possible to map the genomic location of certain types of cancer genes, and of those that can be mapped, localization is often to a large and/or poorly defined region. The advent of the human genome sequence will substantially change the way that cancer genes are discovered. Systematic mutation screens of all genes will obviate the need for any prior physical or genetic localizing information. Therefore, cancer gene discovery will increasingly depend on high throughput detection of sequence variants/mutations. Ultimately we should envisage base-by-base descriptions of the status of cancer cell genomes.

THE GENETIC BASIS OF ONCOGENESIS

Approximately one in three individuals in Europe and North America develops one of the approximately 100 different classes of cancer, and it is the cause of death of

Oncogenomics: Molecular Approaches to Cancer, Edited by Charles Brenner and David Duggan
ISBN 0-471-22592-4 © 2004 John Wiley & Sons, Inc.

one in five (Higginson et al., 1992). Neoplasms evolve as a result of the acquisition of a series of fixed genetic abnormalities, each of which ultimately confers growth advantage upon the clone of cells in which it has occurred. As discussed in Chapter 1, the majority of such abnormalities are acquired through somatic mutation during the lifetime of the individual, but a proportion are transmitted through the germ line and may manifest as inherited susceptibility to cancer. The genes that are mutated and causally implicated in the development of human cancer have been divided into two major classes. Oncogenes contribute to cancer despite the presence of one or more normal alleles and their encoded proteins are usually activated. Tumor suppressor genes only contribute to oncogenesis when both alleles within the cancer cell (or all alleles within a multiploid cell) are mutated and their encoded proteins are usually inactivated. Although elaborations and exceptions to this simple classification exist, it remains useful from a genetic perspective.

Identification of the genes that are mutated in cancer is a central aim of cancer research. It forms the foundation for understanding the biological abnormalities within neoplastic cells, provides information on the function of gene products, and sheds light on more complex questions such as the relationships between genes and biochemical pathways. Current strategies for the development of new therapeutic and preventive agents in cancer are increasingly dependent on modulation of these critical molecular targets. Moreover, cancer classification and predictive or prognostic indices may increasingly be based on detection of abnormalities in cancer genes.

SUBSTANTIAL PROPORTION OF CANCER GENES TO BE DISCOVERED

Although there has been considerable progress in the identification of genes that are mutated in cancer, several lines of evidence indicate that there are many (probably the large majority) yet to be discovered. Studies of the age-dependent incidence of cancer suggest that five to seven low-frequency, random mutational events are required for the development of common adult cancers (reviewed in Miller, 1980). However, this type of analysis can only reflect rate-limiting steps and therefore may well underestimate the full set of genetic events present. Moreover, for most cases of most classes of cancer, even this number of abnormalities has not been detected. In addition, there are clearly differences between cancer types with respect to the genes that are mutated, and every cancer of a particular type does not acquire mutations in exactly the same set of genes (general review in Vogelstein and Kinzler, 2001).

Further evidence for the existence of currently unknown oncogenes derives from the observation that much more is understood of the genetic basis of some types of cancer than others (see Vogelstein and Kinzler, 2001, for review of the following information and references). For example, in colorectal and pancreatic cancers, several different mutated genes are recognized (although this is unlikely to represent the full complement). In colorectal cancers, 80% or more have small intragenic mutations (base substitutions or small insertions and deletions) of the *APC* gene, 10% have mutations of the beta-catenin gene, 50% have mutations of *ras* genes, 70% have mutations of the *p53* gene, 20% have mutations of the *TGF*-beta receptor, and 15% exhibit microsatellite instability indicative of mismatch repair gene abnormalities.

In pancreatic adenocarcinomas, 90% exhibit mutations of *ras* genes, 70% have mutations of the *p53* gene, 80% have mutations of *p16*, 40% have mutations of *APC*, and 50% have mutations of *DPC4/SMAD4*. Indeed, there are examples of pancreatic cancer with seven defined genetic events leading to the activation or inactivation of these genes (Rozenblum et al., 1997). Nevertheless, in these tumors there still remain a large number of loci on other chromosomes (defined by losses or gains of chromosomes) that are likely to harbor other tumor suppressor genes and oncogenes. By contrast, in other cancer types—for example breast or prostate cancer—mutations in only a small number of genes in a small proportion of cancers have been observed. In invasive ductal breast cancer, approximately 25% of cases have small intragenic mutations of *p53* with abnormalities in the *p16/Rb* pathway present in an ill-defined proportion, but mutations in other known genes have not been reported at more than 10% frequency. Similarly, in primary prostate cancer, no known gene shows intragenic mutations at greater than 25% frequency, although mutations of *p53*, *p16*, and *PTEN* become more common in metastatic disease.

Finally, in most tumor types, several loci believed to harbor cancer genes (usually on the basis of copy number analyses such as loss of heterozygosity or comparative genomic hybridization) have been reported for which the gene itself has not yet been isolated. Similarly, many cancer cell genomes show numerous structural chromosomal abnormalities, which, in the common epithelial neoplasms, are largely uncharacterized at the molecular level. As pointed out in Chapter 1, some of these changes may not contribute to oncogenesis and may be the consequences of defective DNA maintenance, it would be surprising if a proportion were not involved in neoplastic transformation. Indeed, an insight into the potential diversity of genes mutated in human cancer has been provided by the large number of different genes that are rearranged through chromosomal translocation in leukemias and lymphomas (Rabbitts, 1994, 1999; www.ncbi.nlm.nih.gov/CCAP/). Taken together, all these observations indicate that most somatic genetic abnormalities implicated in neoplastic transformation are yet to be discovered.

STRATEGIES FOR THE IDENTIFICATION OF CANCER GENES

In the past, identification of the mutated genes causally implicated in human neoplasia has depended on three major strategies:

1. The use of biological assays for transforming activity (e.g., the NIH3T3 transformation assay for the detection of activated *ras* genes)
2. Primary localization of the cancer gene to a small part of the genome by genetic linkage analysis for susceptibility genes, cytogenetics to detect somatic chromosomal rearrangements, and loss of heterozygosity analysis/comparative genomic hybridization to detect somatic chromosomal copy number changes followed by mutational analysis of the genes within the restricted region
3. The mutational analysis of candidate genes that recommend themselves on the basis of predicted or proven functions

By far the most successful of these strategies has been primary genomic localization followed by detailed mutational analysis of a restricted genomic region. However, cancer genes exist that cannot be physically or genetically mapped at all. For example, activating mutations in the *ras* family of genes, which are found at high frequency in many cancers, leave no clear genomic footprint that allows physical localization. Similarly, genes such as FGFR3 (point mutated in more than half of bladder cancers; Sibley et al., 2001) and beta catenin (point mutated in a wide range of cancers; Hajra and Fearon, 2002) could not have been identified by this approach.

Moreover, even genes that do yield localizing information can be problematic to identify because the defined interval is large and components of the mapping data are misleading. Many putative tumor suppressor loci mapped in cancer cells by loss of heterozygosity have failed to yield the critical target gene for this reason. In addition, because there is a level of random abnormality in cancer genomes, the significance of some alterations that actually are directed at cancer genes (e.g., regions of loss of heterozygosity or chromosomal rearrangements) can be missed in the noise of bystander effects. The inadequacy of current approaches to cancer gene identification has prompted us to propose global strategies to gene identification based on the availability of the human genome sequence.

IMPLICATIONS OF THE HUMAN GENOME SEQUENCE FOR CANCER GENE DISCOVERY

The draft sequence of the human genome was announced in June 2000 and published in February 2001 (Lander et al., 2001). The "finished" sequence, with 98% of euchromatic DNA sequenced to 99.99% accuracy was accomplished by 2003 (Collins, et al. 2003). Currently in process and reaching fruition through 2005 is annotation of the sequence such that most genes are identified and their intron-exon structures are determined. All this information will be in the public domain.

The availability of the annotated human genome sequence will obviously facilitate and empower all previously employed approaches to the identification of cancer genes. However, it also offers a new prospect for the identification of cancer genes (and

---

• Searches for copy number changes: conventional and array-based CGH

• Searches for rearrangements: SKY, MFISH

• Searches for small intragenic mutations

    • Heteroduplex analysis

    • High throughput PCR fragment resequencing

    • Oligonucleotide array resequencing

• Searches for all the above: whole subcloned genome resequencing

Box 2-1. Strategies to search for cancer genes and identify mutations in cancer genes given the reference human genome sequence.

indeed mutated genes underlying other diseases). There is now the possibility of using the template of the reference sequence in systematic genome-wide direct searches for sequence variants/mutations—that is, we potentially have the option of bypassing the step of primary positional localization so commonly used in the past. Instead, we can directly analyze all genes and ultimately provide a description of the status of the cancer cell genome base by base. Such an approach will allow the identification of somatically mutated cancer genes (and other human disease genes) for which no primary positional mapping information is available or which are mapped to very large or poorly defined regions (Box 2-1).

CLASSES OF SOMATIC MUTATION IN HUMAN CANCER GENES

From the perspective of strategies for detection, there are six major classes of genetic abnormality that occur within cancer cell genomes and are known to alter the biological functions of cancer genes.

1. Homozygous deletions: They may range in size from 1 bp to several megabases. Large deletions may include several genes other than the targeted cancer gene. In general, homozygous deletions would be expected to result in inactivation of tumor suppressor genes by removal of both alleles.

2. Small intragenic mutations: Single base substitutions and small deletions/insertions. This type of change may result in the activation of oncogenes or the inactivation of tumor suppressor genes.

3. Gene rearrangements (other than homozygous deletions): In their most common manifestation, they usually result in the activation of a target gene either by formation of a chimeric gene derived from two distinct coding sequences (and hence chimeric mRNA and protein) or by apposing a novel regulatory sequence adjacent to a gene. In these circumstances, the particular sequences/genes involved in the rearrangements are often consistently paired together, and the specific sequence pairings are often associated with a particular cancer type. Rearrangements, however, may also disrupt (and hence inactivate) tumor suppressor genes.

4. Increase in gene copy number (gene amplification): Increases in copy number of a gene within the cancer cell may vary from 1.5-fold (three copies as compared to two) to several thousand–fold. In the case of high copy number amplification, the region amplified is often of the order of several hundred thousand kilobases to a couple of megabases in size. Such high-level restricted amplifications are usually believed to be of a gene with wild-type sequence and result in a substantial increase of steady-state levels of wild-type mRNA and hence protein (although direct evaluation of the sequence of the critical target gene has not always been sought and occasionally the sequence of the amplified target may be abnormal—e.g., the epidermal growth factor (EGF) receptor in malignant gliomas; Wong et al., 1992). Lower copy number increases (1.5- to 4-fold) may extend over much larger distances sometimes including the whole chromosome. The significance of these extended low copy number increases is not fully understood. However, at least some may be preferentially increasing the copy number of alleles of genes that are activated by

point mutation—for example, activated *MET* in hereditary papillary carcinoma of the kidney (Zhuang et al., 1998).

5. Reduction in gene copy number (excluding homozygous deletion): There is some circumstantial evidence from animal studies that somatically acquired reduction in gene copy number from two to one in a cancer may be sufficient to provide clonal advantage (Kwabi-Addo et al., 2001). This has been invoked as an explanation for the many areas of loss of heterozygosity in human cancers in which a clearly mutated tumor suppressor gene has not yet been identified. However, there is little evidence in favor of this hypothesis from human cancers. Indeed, it is difficult to see what would constitute evidence other than complete exclusion of all other explanations of regions of loss of heterozygosity (LOH). Indeed, if there are key target genes that contribute to oncogenesis by this mechanism (known as haploinsufficiency), they may be difficult to identify.

6. Changes in methylation: Substantial changes in methylated status of CpG dinucleotides, both hypomethylation and hypermethylation, occur in human cancers. There is now strong evidence to suggest that some increases in methylation of CpG-rich regions immediately 5′ to genes (including the promoter) result in transcriptional suppression and functional inactivation. The role of hypomethylation changes is less well understood.

A particular tumor suppressor gene may be inactivated in different cancers by large homozygous deletions, small intragenic mutations, gene rearrangements, or promoter methylation. The extent to which each of these mechanisms contributes varies markedly between different genes and probably also between different cancer types. In contrast, a particular dominantly acting oncogene is typically activated by a single mechanism, either small intragenic mutations, rearrangements, or gene amplification. Although there are dominantly acting genes for which multiple mechanisms of activation are known, the different mechanisms are usually present in different tumor types. For example, activating rearrangements of the FGFR3 gene are found in multiple myeloma and activating point mutations of the same gene without rearrangement are found in bladder cancers (Chesi et al., 1997; Sibley et al., 2001).

GENOME-WIDE TECHNOLOGIES FOR SOMATIC MUTATION SCREENS

The diversity of classes of mutation that are present in human cancers poses a problem. In order to provide a complete description of the somatic genetic changes in human cancer, a genome-wide mutation detection platform would need to provide information about all these types of abnormalities. The only currently available unified approach to detect of all these somatic abnormalities (excluding changes in methylation) is construction of a genomic library from a cancer cell genome, isolation of large numbers of individual clones, and sequencing to obtain multiple-fold coverage at each base—that is, a strategy similar to that used in provision of the reference genome sequence. (Note that complete coverage of the genome by a series of overlapping PCR fragments designed to amplify the wild-type sequence would not achieve this goal because it would fail to detect regions of rearrangement and would poorly report regions of copy number change.)

In light of the substantial resources invested to obtain a single high-quality haploid normal human genome sequence by this approach, the exhaustive analysis of even a single multiploid cancer cell genome is impractical without the advent of a major technological advance in sequencing. There are a number of novel technologies in development for large-scale sequencing and resequencing that may increase the throughput and reduce the cost by several orders of magnitude (e.g., www.solexa.co.uk/). However, none of these technologies are fully developed or publicly available. Nevertheless, should one or more of them come to fruition, they may turn out to be the future methods of exhaustively analyzing cancer cell genomes for mutations.

In the meantime, each class of sequence abnormality previously listed lends itself to different strategies for detection. Therefore, an alternative would be to provide several different mutation screening platforms, each of which can detect one class of abnormality. We have employed this approach in the Cancer Genome Project (CGP), an initiative specifically designed to perform systematic genome-wide searches for mutations in cancer. CGP is located at the Wellcome Trust Sanger Institute, the genome center that generated one-third of the reference human genome sequence (Lander et al., 2001). Placement of CGP at a genome center acknowledged the fact that conducting genome-wide searches for sequence alterations would potentially require many millions of individual experiments.

It may be possible ultimately to perform these enormous experimental loads in parallel (i.e., many experiments conducted simultaneously). Indeed, some forms of mutation in cancer—for example, copy number changes—now lend themselves to multiparallel analyses in the form of arrays for comparative genomic hybridization. However, it is possible that some classes of genomic alteration—for example, small intragenic mutations—will require substantial new technology development before a platform for their detection in multiparallel format becomes available. For such abnormalities it may be necessary to conduct the requisite huge numbers of experiments in series, and this is precisely the expertise of a genome center, with its intrinsic robotics, informatics, and infrastructure.

Genome-Wide Approaches to the Detection of Homozygous Deletions

Representational Difference Analysis (RDA).   RDA is a strategy employing in-solution hybridization between the two genomes to be compared (in this case, a cancer genome and a normal genome; Lisitsyn et al., 1993). It has been used successfully by several groups and has yielded numerous homozygous deletions, some of which have led to the identification of tumor suppressor genes. However, RDA is a laborious technique that requires time-consuming evaluation of numerous false positives. Moreover, it is not always clear what the density of clone representation across the genome is in individual experiments and therefore the exhaustiveness of the search. Nevertheless, relatively small homozygous deletions have been detected by RDA (less than 100 kb) and therefore the representation may be quite dense in some experiments.

Comparative Genomic Hybridization by Arrays.   Conventional comparative genomic hybridization (CGH) using metaphase spreads does not have the resolution to detect most homozygous deletions. Recently, as described in Chapter 3, hybridization of whole cancer cell genomic DNA to a variety of types of arrays has been demonstrated to have the potential for detection of homozygous deletions. These include arrays of bacterial artificial chromosomes (BACs; Pinkel et al., 1998) and cDNAs (in the latter case, identical to those used in expression analysis; Pollack et al., 1999). The possibility of using arrays of short or long oligonucleotides is currently under evaluation in CGP. The resolution of these arrays depends on the density of the clones and their size. Currently, most of the BAC/cDNA arrays used for CGH have an average coverage of 1–2 clones per megabase and therefore will not reliably report homozygous deletions less than 500 kb in size, since these may fall between two adjacent probes. Moreover, the large size of BACs (150–250 kb) means that small homozygous deletions may result only in a reduction of signal intensity, even if the BAC covers them. However, these types of arrays may be usable with primary cancer tissues if contaminating normal cells are reduced to a minimum. Conversely, most other approaches will be somewhat sensitive to the presence of normal tissue and therefore are optimally used in conjunction with cancer cell lines.

Dense Coverage by Sequence Tagged Site–PCR. At the Cancer Genome Project, we have employed a set of approximately 5500 STS amplified by PCR to detect homozygous deletions in cancer cell lines. Success of amplification (and hence absence of a homozygous deletion) is detected by a TAQMAN-type assay and therefore does not require gel electrophoresis (Fig. 2-1). Because TAQMAN probes are expensive, we have used a generic probe for all 5500 STS that is complementary to a (CA)n repeat sequence present within each STS (which are designed from the genetically mapped set originally reported by Genethon; Dib et al., 1996). Note that for this usage the CA repeat need not be polymorphic and therefore the approach can use all of the approximately 50,000 CA repeats of greater than 10 repeat units present in the human genome. The probe density of this current set of STS is therefore similar to the BAC/cDNA arrays currently in use for this purpose. However, the small size of each STS (100–400 bp) means that most homozygous deletions will be easily detected if they fall over an STS in the series.

Genome-Wide Approaches to the Detection of Small Intragenic Mutations (base substitutions and small intragenic mutations)

High Throughput Direct Sequencing of PCR-Amplified Fragments. This approach is being used by a small number of groups for genome-wide detection of constitutional SNPs. While technically feasible in principle, the sequencing of large numbers of diverse PCR-amplified fragments presents different technical challenges to high-throughput clone sequencing. In particular, the quality of the sequence traces is more variable and the automatic detection of heterozygotic nucleotides can be problematic. These problems are exacerbated in cancer cell genomes, where the equimolar ratio of the two parental alleles cannot be guaranteed, hence making even greater demands on sequence quality and heterozygote detection.

Use of Mutation Screens. In the past, a number of mutation screening techniques have been used for the detection of sequence variants in both the research and diagnostic contexts. These include heteroduplex analysis (Ganguly et al., 1993, 1998), single-strand conformational analysis (Orita et al., 1989), denaturing gradient gel electrophoresis (Fodde and Losekoot, 1994), denaturing HPLC (Xiao and Oefner, 2001), the protein truncation test (Roest et al., 1993), mismatch cleavage (Saleeba

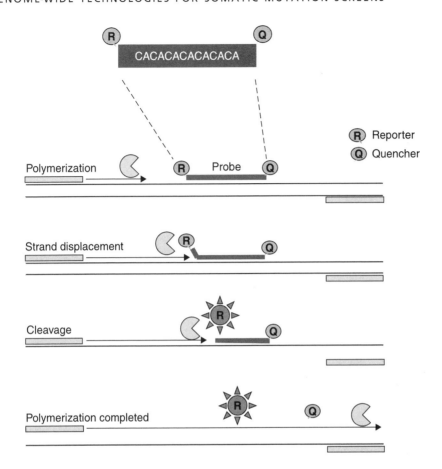

Figure 2-1. Use of a PCR based TAQMAN assay for the detection of homozygous deletions in cancer cell lines by the Cancer Genome Project. The assay can be carried out in microtiter plates and the presence of a homozygous deletion is indicated by the absence of a fluorescent signal. Use of a (CA)n repeat means that a single probe can be used for many thousands of loci in the genome that contain (polymorphic or non-polymorphic) (CA)n repeats. The assay requires high throughput PCR capacity and may now have been superceded by various forms of CGH array, but has yielded approximately 170 novel loci with homozygous deletions.

et al., 1992), and several others. The requirements in selecting one of these for a genome-wide survey include not only the usual criteria of high sensitivity and specificity but also the feasibility of carrying out the huge numbers of analyses envisaged and thus the ability of the technique to be transferred to high-throughput platforms. For these purposes, the technique needs to be as simple as possible with a minimum of processing steps between the PCR and readout. For this reason, CGP has chosen heteroduplex analysis as its main platform. This has been transferred from its usual application on slab polyacrylamide gels to the capillaries of the ABI3100 DNA sequencer.

Unfortunately, the 96 capillary ABI 3700, which was generally the workhorse for human genome sequencing, is not usable for heteroduplex analysis because it does not have the requisite temperature control. The recently launched 96 capillary ABI 3730 does, however, have the appropriate temperature regulation and is currently being evaluated. In our hands, heteroduplex analysis applied on the ABI3100 has a sensitivity of approximately 95% for single base substitutions and will detect virtually all small insertions and deletions. To facilitate the analysis of the large amounts of information that this platform can generate, we have developed software that will automatically compare the heteroduplex traces derived from cancers and from normal tissues. Traces that are identical are automatically stored in the database, while traces that are different in tumor and normal samples are brought to the attention of observers and are sent for sequencing (Fig. 2-2).

Mutational Screens of Genomic DNA or cDNA?.   CGP is applying a heteroduplex screen to genomic DNA extracted from cancer cells (see below). It has been suggested that it may be more parsimonious to apply genome-wide mutation screening platforms to cDNA synthesized from cancer cell mRNA. The underlying basis for this proposal is the assumption that most cancer-causing mutations are likely to be in the coding sequences of genes. However, there are a number of major problems associated with use of cDNA in this context. First, high-throughput PCR amplification from cDNA is more problematic than from genomic DNA because of widely varying numbers of each transcript in the cell (and key mutations can be in genes that are expressed at very low levels). Second, truncating mutations can cause nonsense-mediated RNA decay and hence the mutated allele in cDNA may be swamped by the wild type. Third, alternative splicing can cause complex patterns in which mutations can be missed. For these reasons, we have restricted our analyses to genomic DNA.

Use of Parallel Sequencing Arrays.   The development of arrays for resequencing has perhaps been slower than the development of arrays for expression analysis or comparative genomic hybridization (Lipshutz et al., 1999). Nevertheless, they still have enormous potential for large-scale detection of unknown sequence variants/mutations. One application has been by the Perlegen group using Affymetrix-type technology in the development of large chips or "wafers" for SNP detection (Patil et al., 2001). However, to our knowledge this technology is currently not available outside the companies that have developed it. Moreover, its ability to detect 90% of single base substitutions in a cancer genome, particularly when they are in heterozygous form, is unproven. Whatever the current virtues and limitations of this platform, however, this type of technological approach will be necessary if we are ultimately to search genome-wide for mutations in large numbers of cancers.

Genome-Wide Approaches to the Detection of Chromosomal Rearrangements

Conventional Cytogenetics and Fluorescence-Enhanced Karyotyping Approaches.   Of course, there have been genome-wide descriptions of chromosomal rearrangements in cancer cell genomes for several decades in the form of conventionally stained cancer cell metaphase spreads. This has yielded substantial information, particularly in the understanding of oncogenesis in leukemias, lymphomas, and sarcomas. Unfortunately, the complex nature of the structural rearrangements in many common epithelial cancer cell genomes has often made it difficult to distinguish the constituent

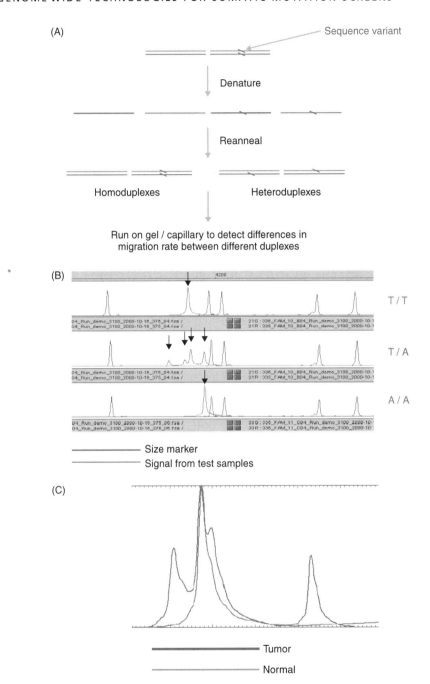

Figure 2-2. Principle of heteroduplex analysis for small intragenic mutation detection (A). Capillary based heteroduplex analysis on the ABI3100 as used at CGP (B). Note four peaks in heterozygous individual carrying both T and A alleles corresponding to each of the four duplexes seen in Fig 2A. (C) Automated calling of somatic mutations. Software has been developed to superimpose the heteroduplex trace from a tumor sample (dark line) onto the equivalent trace generated by normal DNA (light line) from the same individual. This platform is being used in genome-wide surveys for somatic mutations in cancer.

chromosomal contributions to marker chromosomes. More recently, fluorescence labeling of chromosome-specific probes in techniques such as spectral karyotyping (SKY) or multicolor fluorescence in situ hybridization (M-FISH) has allowed much clearer discrimination of the constituent chromosomes (for review, see Schrock and Padilla-Nash, 2000). However, these techniques still suffer from a lack of resolution, with breakpoints only resoluble to regions of tens of megabases in size.

To understand the importance of the complex patterns of chromosomal rearrangement present in common epithelial cancers, it would be informative to know the position of each breakpoint with much higher resolution, optimally down to the nucleotide at which the rearrangement has taken place. By comparing such a catalog of rearrangements (which may include 10–100 or more breakpoints for a single cancer sample) between numbers of cancers, it may become easier to work out whether all the breakpoints are random (and perhaps therefore simply genomic noise) or whether some (probably a minority) are recurrent in particular regions of the genome and hence perhaps involved in oncogenesis. If translocations are unbalanced (i.e., if one translocation derivative has been lost from the genome), the positions of breakpoints in cancer cell genomes can be discerned at much higher resolution using array CGH. However, the experience from the study of leukemias, lymphomas, and sarcomas is that it is precisely the balanced translocations that may be of interest (these are essentially invisible to CGH arrays because they do not result in copy number changes). Therefore, we probably need new technologies to achieve these aims.

High-Throughput FISH.   One possibility that CGP has investigated to a limited extent has been the use of the current mapped BAC resources in high-throughput FISH analyses. In principle, although this approach would require intact cells from the cancer or early cultures (which would likely limit the practicality of the approach), the analyses could be performed on interphase nuclei, which are considerably more numerous than metaphase nuclei and would not necessarily require the tumor to be cultured. One formulation of such an approach would be to hybridize two adjacent BACs (each labeled with a different color) from a currently constituted 3000-genome-wide BAC map used for a CGH array separated from each other by about a megabase in the genome. If the region between them had been rearranged/translocated in the tumor, signals from these probes would be more distant in interphase FISH of cancer cell nuclei than if the probes remained on a contiguous piece of DNA. The data accrual and analysis in these experiments could conceivably be automated. Subsequently, the adjacent pair of BACs would be investigated until 3000 pairs of BACs had been examined, providing coverage of the whole genome of a single cancer sample. Such high-throughput FISH analyses have not been previously contemplated and are certainly associated with many problems. Moreover, the approach would rely on the availability of cells of sufficient preservation to be used in the FISH analyses. Ultimately, a DNA-based approach that would be applicable to most cancer samples would be preferable.

End Sequencing of Large-Fragment Cancer Genomes.   One strategy that we have been considering and has been suggested by others (Colin Collins and Joe Gray, personal communication and presented at Oncogenomics 2002, Dublin) is to end sequence large numbers of fragments originating from cancer genomes (e.g., by constructing libraries from cancer cell genomic DNA), then align, in silico, pairs of end sequences to the reference genome. If pairs of end sequences align to the same genomic region, the DNA between them is probably normal. If the pair of end sequences from a fragment/clone align to different parts of the genome, it is likely that the DNA between the two sequences in the cancer has been rearranged (or that there is an artifact of library formation).

This strategy is attractive because it simply requires genomic DNA from the cancer. Moreover, the end sequences can be relatively short: 20 bp should be sufficient to align and map each sequence unambiguously if it is nonrepetitive. However, the shorter the cloning inserts in the library, the larger the number of end sequences that are required. For a BAC library of average insert size of 150 kb treated in this way, 20,000 pairs of end sequences would be required to obtain single-fold genome coverage. Multiple-fold clone coverage of the genome would be required to detect a high proportion of rearrangements in a diploid cancer genome, and for triploid and tetraploid cancer genomes the coverage would need to be even greater. Nevertheless, with further technical embellishments and perhaps improvements in sequencing technology, this strategy may be the practical basis of cataloging rearrangements in cancer cell genomes at high resolution in the future.

Genome-Wide Detection of Copy Number Changes Other Than Homozygous Deletions

Comparative Genomic Hybridization.   Conventional CGH using metaphases is now being superceded by array-based CGH (see Chapter 3 for the various types of array-based CGH). Using BAC clones, this approach is able reliably to detect relatively subtle changes in sequence copy number and can even be used on DNA extracted from paraffin-embedded sections (Barbara Weber, personal communication). As the arrays become denser, ultimately constituting a tiling path through the genome, they will detect a higher proportion of copy number changes that are restricted to relatively small DNA segments. This is probably now the method of choice for characterizing amplified regions.

Identification of the critical gene targeted by an amplicon can be problematic even if the amplicon is relatively small (e.g., an amplicon of 500 kb will include five genes on average), particularly if the amplified target gene sequence is wild type. It has been unusual for mapping information obtained by comparing the genomic extent of amplification in several cancers to unambiguously define the target. Therefore, a key step in the identification of the likely amplified target is evaluation of gene expression, particularly it is necessary to demonstrate that a candidate target gene within the region is expressed in the cancer, preferably at higher levels than other candidates within the amplicon. As shown in Chapter 3, the use of the same arrays for expression analysis and CGH is particularly convenient in this context. Even so, it can be difficult to obtain unambiguous genetic evidence that a particular gene within an amplicon is the critical target, and in many cases in the past this has been presumptive, based on knowledge of biological function of a particular gene. Indeed, it has been suggested that in some cases there may be more than one gene on an amplicon that is contributing to oncogenesis.

Copy Number Changes Detected by Loss of Heterozygosity.   Many limited or genome-wide LOH analyses of cancer genomes have been published since the first report of the approach in 1983 (Cavenee et al., 1983). Initially performed by Southern analyses using probes to polymorphic fragments of restriction digestion, currently LOH studies are usually conducted using polymorphic microsatellite markers or even more recently on single-nucleotide polymorphism arrays (Lindblad-Toh et al., 2000). Although these have usually depended on comparing normal and tumor cell DNA from the same individual, the advent of dense polymorphic marker maps has meant that LOH in cancers can be revealed by detection of large regions of contiguous marker homozygosity that are very unlikely to occur in constitutional DNA by chance. We use this approach at CGP on the large number of publicly available cancer cell lines for which no normal sample from the same individual exists. It should be recognized that LOH analyses and CGH analyses are complementary. Allele losses revealed by use of polymorphic markers may not be revealed by CGH if there has been loss and reduplication or if the LOH occurred by mitotic recombination. Similarly, subtle changes in relative copy number detected by CGH that leave both parental alleles in the cancer genome may not be detected by LOH.

As indicated, modest changes in copy number (both increases and decreases) are common in cancer cell genomes and can extend over very large distances. Assuming that there are key genes targeted by each of these changes, such genes may be very difficult to identify. In general, the identification of tumor suppressor genes by positional cloning methods has depended on the detection of a key homozygous deletion that has dramatically mapped the location of the gene. No tumor suppressor genes have yet been identified simply by mapping of reduction in copy number changes or LOH. Similarly, no activated genes have been identified by mapping of the overlap of modest copy number changes (two- to fourfold increases) that extend over very large chromosomal distances.

Genome-Wide Detection of Changes in Methylation

The methylation changes that occur within cancer cell genomes are complex. Although it would be of considerable interest to obtain detailed descriptions of the methylated status of CpG dinucleotides within cancer cell genomes, it is not yet clear how these patterns would be interpreted. Some acquisition of methylation is clearly associated with transcriptional repression of tumor suppressor genes and with loss of heterozygosity in the cancer. Presumably these changes contribute to the neoplastic phenotype. Equally, there would seem to be indirect evidence that some acquired methylation is unlikely to be causally implicated in oncogenesis, is not associated with LOH, and may be an epiphenomenon of the transformed phenotype. Indeed, the methylation status of some genes changes during normal aging and in response to other biological influences.

Analyses of the methylation status of small numbers of genes within cancer cell genomes have been generated by several techniques dependent on bisulfite conversion (for review, see Jones and Baylin, 2002). In this approach, unmethylated cytosine is converted to uracil by treatment with bisulfite while methylated cytosine is protected. In a different approach, use of methylation-sensitive restriction enzymes and two-dimensional electrophoresis (methylation-sensitive restriction landmark scanning) has generated overall estimates of the numbers of CpG islands that become methylated in various types of cancer (Costello et al., 2000; Smiraglia et al., 1999).

Early Results from Genome-Wide Searches for Mutations in Cancer

Numerous reports have been published of genome-wide copy number changes detected by LOH analyses and conventional CGH. Similarly, conventional cytogenetics, M-FISH, and SKY have yielded low-resolution perspectives on genomic rearrangement in human cancers. Most of this information was generated before the advent of the human genome sequence. Through the generation of extensive BAC contigs from which BAC clones were chosen for human genome sequencing, large numbers of well-mapped BACs have recently become available for the new generation of CGH analyses by array. The impact of the human genome sequence on the elucidation of the genetic basis of cancer is, however, just beginning. It will generate its effects through the sequence itself, as well as through the resources and the technologies that have been developed. The availability of this information and reagents will, in general, allow higher-resolution genome-wide mutational analyses. At the Cancer Genome Project, since its inception in 2000, we have focused on genome-wide searches for two of the classes of mutations: homozygous deletions and small intragenic mutations (base substitutions and small insertions and deletions).

Genome-Wide Search for Homozygous Deletions

Our search for homozygous deletions is based on the application of a map of 5500 STSs detected by PCR amplification and TAQMAN technology to a large series of immortal cancer cell lines. CGP has obtained over 1500 cancer cell lines of different types from public repositories and private resources, which will all ultimately be screened for homozygous deletions. These studies are still in progress. However, it is clear that a large number of homozygous deletions are detectable in cancer cell lines.

In the first 600 cancer cell lines studied, we have found over 170 homozygous deletions that do not correspond in their genomic locations to the known tumor suppressor genes or known fragile sites (unpublished data; fragile sites are prone to break in cancers and hence can manifest as homozygous deletions). Although some of these could be random breakages due to deficiencies of DNA maintenance in cancer cells, there are more than 20 loci at which two or more cancer cell lines exhibit a homozygous deletion in the same location (unpublished data). This clustering is unlikely to be due to chance and presumably has an underlying biological explanation: either the presence of a tumor suppressor gene or a fragile site. Therefore, there is considerable information of this type left to mine in human cancer. It is anticipated that some of these clustered homozygous deletions are targeted at currently unknown tumor suppressor genes. These will be revealed by examining all the genes within each homozygously deleted region for the inactivating mutations that are the trademark of tumor suppressor genes. The remainder of these regions may well be areas of genomic fragility that are undetectable by conventional approaches for revealing fragile sites. Thus, in addition to the human genome sequence being critical in understanding cancer, the unusual intracellular milieu in which cancer cell genomes are incubated will reveal important features of genome structure.

Genome-Wide Search for Small Intragenic Mutations

Using a serial STS-PCR approach, parallel array-based comparative genomic hybridization, or representational difference analysis, could have been implemented without the full human genome sequence. However, the systematic search for small intragenic mutations requires the complete annotated sequence of the genome and hence is one of the first initiatives directed at elucidation of the genetics of human disease that is completely dependent on the genome sequence itself.

The aim of the first phase of this project at CGP is to screen all coding exons and splice junctions of the genome by heteroduplex analysis for small intragenic mutations in a set of 48 cancers and 48 normal samples from the same individuals who developed the cancers. By comparing DNA from cancer and normal tissue, somatic mutations are read out and hence the analysis is not confounded by constitutional polymorphisms. The set of cancers is designed to include as great a diversity of cancer types as possible (in order to maximize the number of cancer genes detected) but is also focused on the common epithelial cancers in order to detect mutated genes that are associated with the highest mortality. In order to conduct this search, approximately 400,000 primer pairs will require design, testing, storage, and retrieval. Approximately 50 million PCRs and mutation screening assays will need to be performed, and the sequencing that follows the heteroduplex screen is anticipated at about 1 million sequencing reactions.

At the time of this writing, this genome-wide search is currently about 1% complete. In the course of developing the platform, we commenced mutation screening on a small scale and these early experiments led to the first cancer gene discovery. We focused on genes that were members of families previously known to be mutated in human cancer (particularly kinases) and genes that encoded members of signal transduction pathways in which one component was already known to be mutated in cancer. Among the latter was the RAS-RAF-MEK-ERK-MAP kinase pathway in which mutations of RAS genes had previously been identified in 10–20% of human cancer. As discussed in Chapters 13 and 14, RAS proteins recruit to the membrane and activate members of the RAF protein family: RAF-1, BRAF, and ARAF (of which RAF-1 has been by far the most extensively studied for its biology and biochemistry). The systematic mutational search revealed that BRAF on chromosome 7q is commonly mutated in human cancer (most notably malignant melanoma and colorectal carcinoma), while RAF-1 and ARAF are mutated infrequently or not at all (Davies et al., 2002). Although the set of genes in these early analyses was selected, the fact that mutations of a novel cancer gene were detected at such an early stage suggests that there are several more genes of this sort to be found through genome-wide searches.

Long-Term Aims of Systematic Genome-Wide Mutation Searches in Human Cancer

The major aim of systematic mutational searches is to identify the key cancer genes, hence to elucidate the biology of cancer and provide new targets for therapies and diagnostics. As discussed in Section IV, the advent of Gleevec, a drug selected to inhibit ABL kinase for the treatment of chronic myelogenous leukemia, was a paradigm shift that dramatically indicated how mutated proteins in cancer may serve as important targets for effective new therapies (Druker, 2002).

In addition, however, genome-wide searches for mutations will yield a wealth of information relating to the normal structure of the genome and particularly to the personal history of each cancer. Following such searches it will become possible to estimate the numbers of critical somatic mutations in each cancer. Current estimates based on epidemiological studies have indicated that five to seven rate-limiting events are required for the development of a common epithelial adult cancer. However, the biological substrates of these events have not been determined. Do these statistically defined rate-limiting events reflect all the mutations that contribute to oncogenesis in a single cancer or do they indicate a small subset of the changes that the cancer cell needs to acquire? The fact that there are well-studied cancer samples in which more than seven mutations have already been detected suggests that the number of mutations that contribute to each cancer may have been substantially underestimated.

Comparisons between individual cancers may then reveal differences in the numbers of mutations between cancers of a particular type and between cancers of different classes. In some instances, these differences may reflect the different biological requirements for different classes of cells to become symptomatic neoplasms. However, between cancers of the same type that presumably arise from similar progenitor cells, these differences may indicate that some cancers use one mechanism of mutation acquisition (e.g., leading to small intragenic mutations) while others use a different mechanism (e.g., predominantly leading to chromosome loss and gain). Such differences in mechanisms of genomic instability have already been proposed for colorectal cancer (Cahill et al., 1999).

In the course of a genome-wide screen, random somatic mutations that are not contributing to oncogenesis will also be detected. Because they will not have been biologically selected for clonal growth advantage, these bystander mutations will more faithfully report the pattern of mutations that the cancer genome has acquired during its history than the disease-causing mutations in cancer genes. The number and classes of these bystander mutations will yield information on mutagenic exposures or defects in DNA repair for individual cancers. Mutational spectra have previously been generated in cancer classes using reporter genes such as p53. Now the potential exists to provide detailed and statistically highly informative mutational spectra for individual cancers.

Finally, genome-wide searches for all the classes of mutation will begin to provide insights into the number of cancer genes. Are there a few cancer genes that are the targets of most of the cancer-causing mutations? Or are there a very large number of cancer genes, each of which is infrequently mutated and hence makes a limited contribution? The evidence from the study of leukemias, lymphomas, and sarcomas, in which a bewildering diversity of translocations has been identified, suggests that the latter picture may be closer to reality. Currently, summing all the known oncogenes and tumor suppressor genes, nearly 1% of genes in the human genome are involved in the causation of one cancer or another. It may eventually turn out that 5–10% or more of the genes in the human genome can contribute to oncogenesis.

REFERENCES

Cahill, D. P., Kinzler, K. W., Vogelstein, B., and Lengauer, C. (1999). Genetic instability and Darwinian selection in tumours. *Trends Cell Biol 9*, M57–60.

Cavenee, W. K., Dryja, T. P., Phillips, R. A., Benedict, W. F., Godbout, R., Gallie, B. L., Murphree, A. L., Strong L. C., and White, R. L. (1983). Expression of recessive alleles by chromosomal mechanisms in retinoblastoma. *Nature 305*, 779–784.

Chesi, M., Nardini, E., Brents, L. A., Schrock, E., Ried, T., Kuehl, W. M., and Bergsagel, P. L. (1997). Frequent translocation t(4;14)(p16.3;q32.3) in multiple myeloma is associated with increased expression and activating mutations of fibroblast growth factor receptor 3. *Nat Genet 16*, 260–264.

Collins, F. S., Morgan, M., and Patrihos, A. (2003). The human genome project: Lessons from large scale biology. *Science 300*, 286–290.

Costello, J. F., Fruhwald, M. C., Smiraglia, D. J., Rush, L. J., Robertson, G. P., Gao, X., Wright, F. A., Feramisco, J. D., Peltomaki, P., Lang, J. C., Schuller, D. E., Yu, L., Bloomfield, C. D.,

Caligiuri, M. A., Yates, A., Nishikawa, R., Su Huang, H., Petrelli, N. J., Zhang, X., O'Dorisio, M. S., Held, W. A., Cavenee, W. K., and Plass, C. (2000). Aberrant CpG-island methylation has non-random and tumour-type-specific patterns. *Nat Genet 24*, 132–138.

Cotton, R. G., Rodrigues, N. R., and Campbell, R. D. (1988). Reactivity of cytosine and thymine in single-base-pair mismatches with hydroxylamine and osmium tetroxide and its application to the study of mutations. *Proc Natl Acad Sci USA 85*, 4397–4401.

Davies, H., Bignell, G. R., Cox, C., Stephens, P., Edkins, S., Clegg, S., Teague, J., Woffendin, H., Garnett, M. J., Bottomley, W., Davis, N., Dicks, E., Ewing, R., Floyd, Y., Gray, K., Hall, S., Hawes, R., Hughes, J., Kosmidou, V., Menzies, A., Mould, C., Parker, A., Stevens, C., Watt, S., Hooper, S., Wilson, R., Jayatilake, H., Gusterson, B. A., Cooper, C., Shipley, J., Hargrave, D., Pritchard-Jones, K., Maitland, N., Chenevix-Trench, G., Riggins, G. J., Bigner, D. D., Palmieri, G., Cossu, A., Flanagan, A., Nicholson, A., Ho, J. W., Leung, S. Y., Yuen, S. T., Weber, B. L., Seigler, H. F., Darrow, T. L., Paterson, H., Marais, R., Marshall, C. J., Wooster, R., Stratton, M. R., and Futreal, P. A. (2002). Mutations of the BRAF gene in human cancer. *Nature 417*, 949–954.

Dib, C., Faure, S., Fizames, C., Samson, D., Drouot, N., Vignal, A., Millasseau, P., Marc, S., Hazan, J., Seboun, E., Lathrop, M., Gyapay, G., Morissette, J., and Weissenbach, J. (1996). A comprehensive genetic map of the human genome based on 5,264 microsatellites. *Nature 380*, 152–154.

Druker, B. J. (2002). Perspectives on the development of a molecularly targeted agent. *Cancer Cell 1*, 31–36.

Fodde, R., and Losekoot, M. (1994). Mutation detection by denaturing gradient gel electrophoresis (DGGE). *Hum Mutation 3*, 83–94.

Ganguly, A., Rock, M. J., and Prockop, D. J. (1993). Conformation-sensitive gel electrophoresis for rapid detection of single-base differences in double-stranded PCR products and DNA fragments: Evidence for solvent-induced bends in DNA heteroduplexes. *Proc Natl Acad Sci USA 90*, 10325–10329.

Ganguly, T., Dhulipala, R., Godmilow, L., and Ganguly, A. (1998). High throughput fluorescence-based conformation-sensitive gel electrophoresis (F-CSGE) identifies six unique BRCA2 mutations and an overall low incidence of BRCA2 mutations in high-risk BRCA1-negative breast cancer families. *Hum Genet 102*, 549–556.

Hajra, K. M., and Fearon, E. R. (2002). Cadherin and catenin alterations in human cancer. *Genes Chromosomes Cancer 34*, 255–268.

Higginson, J., Muir, C., and Munoz, N. (1992). Human cancer: Epidemiology and environmental causes. *Cambridge Monographs on Cancer Research*. Cambridge, UK.

Jones, P. A., and Baylin, S. B. (2002). The fundamental role of epigenetic events in cancer. *Nat Rev Genet 3*, 415–428.

Kinzler, K., and Vogelstein, B. (2001). *The Genetic Basis of Human Cancer*. McGraw Hill. New York.

Kwabi-Addo, B., Giri, D., Schmidt, K., Podsypanina, K., Parsons, R., Greenberg, N., and Ittmann, M. (2001). Haploinsufficiency of the Pten tumor suppressor gene promotes prostate cancer progression. *Proc Natl Acad Sci USA 98*, 11563–11568.

Lander, E. S., et al. (2001). Initial sequencing and analysis of the human genome. *Nature 409*, 860–921.

Lindblad-Toh, K., Tanenbaum, D. M., Daly, M. J., Winchester, E., Lui, W. O., Villapakkam, A., Stanton, S. E., Larsson, C., Hudson, T. J., Johnson, B. E., Lander, E. S., and Meyerson, M. (2000). Loss-of-heterozygosity analysis of small-cell lung carcinomas using single-nucleotide polymorphism arrays. *Nat Biotechnol 18*, 1001–1005.

Lipshutz, R. J., Fodor, S. P., Gingeras, T. R., and Lockhart, D. J. (1999). High density synthetic oligonucleotide arrays. *Nat Genet 21*(Suppl 1), 20–24.

Lisitsyn, N., Lisitsyn, N., and Wigler, M. (1993). Cloning the differences between two complex genomes. *Science 259*, 946–951.

Miller, D. G. (1980). On the nature of susceptibility to cancer. The presidential address. *Cancer 46*, 1307–1318.

Patil, N., Berno, A. J., Hinds, D. A., Barrett, W. A., Doshi, J. M., Hacker, C. R., Kautzer, C. R., Lee, D. H., Marjoribanks, C., McDonough, D. P., Nguyen, B. T., Norris, M. C., Sheehan, J. B., Shen, N., Stern, D., Stokowski, R. P., Thomas, D. J., Trulson, M. O., Vyas, K. R., Frazer, K. A., and Cox, D. R. (2001). Blocks of limited haplotype diversity revealed by high-resolution scanning of human chromosome 21. *Science 294*, 1719–1723.

Orita, M., Iwahana, H., Kanazawa, H., Hayashi, K., and Sekiya, T. (1989). Detection of polymorphisms of human DNA by gel electrophoresis as single-strand conformation polymorphisms. *Proc Natl Acad Sci USA 86*, 2766–2770.

Pinkel, D., Segraves, R., Sudar, D, Clark, S., Poole, I., Kowbel, D., Collins, C., Kuo, W. L., Chen, C., Zhai, Y., Dairkee, S. H., Ljung, B. M., Gray, J. W., and Albertson, D. G. (1998). High resolution analysis of DNA copy number variation using comparative genomic hybridization to microarrays. *Nat Genet 20*, 207–211.

Pollack, J. R., Perou, C. M., Alizadeh, A. A., Eisen, M. B., Pergamenschikov, A., Williams, C. F., Jeffrey, S. S., Botstein, D., and Brown, P. O. (1999). Genome-wide analysis of DNA copy-number changes using cDNA microarrays. *Nat Genet 23*, 41–46.

Rabbitts, T. H. (1994). Chromosomal translocations in human cancer. *Nature 372*, 143–149.

Rabbitts, T. H. (1999). Of methods and mapping. *Nat Med 5*, 24–25.

Roest, P. A, Roberts, R. G., Sugino, S., van Ommen, G. J., and den Dunnen, J. T. (1993). Protein truncation test (PTT) for rapid detection of translation-terminating mutations. *Hum Mol Genet 2*, 1719–1721.

Rozenblum, E., Schutte, M., Goggins, M., Hahn, S. A., Panzer, S., Zahurak, M., Goodman, S. N., Sohn, T. A., Hruban, R. H., Yeo, C. J., and Kern, S. E. (1997). Tumor-suppressive pathways in pancreatic carcinoma. *Cancer Res 57*, 1731–1734.

Saleeba, J. A., Ramus, S. J., and Cotton, R. G. (1992). Complete mutation detection using unlabeled chemical cleavage. *Hum Mutation 1*, 63–69.

Schrock, E., and Padilla-Nash, H. (2000). Spectral karyotyping and multicolor fluorescence in situ hybridization reveal new tumor-specific chromosomal aberrations. *Semin Hematol 37*, 334–347.

Sibley, K., Stern, P., and Knowles, M. A. (2001). Frequency of fibroblast growth factor receptor 3 mutations in sporadic tumours. *Oncogene 20*, 4416–4418.

Smiraglia, D. J., Fruhwald, M. C., Costello, J. F., McCormick, S. P., Dai, Z., Peltomaki, P., O'Dorisio, M. S., Cavenee, W. K., and Plass, C. (1999). A new tool for the rapid cloning of amplified and hypermethylated human DNA sequences from restriction landmark genome scanning gels. *Genomics 58*, 254–262.

Vogelstein, B., and Kinzler, K. W. (2001). Achilles' heel of Cancer. *Nature 412*, 865–866.

Wong, A. J., Ruppert, J. M., Bigner, S. H., Grzeschik, C. H., Humphrey, P. A., Bigner, D. S., and Vogelstein, B. (1992). Structural alterations of the epidermal growth factor receptor gene in human gliomas. *Proc Natl Acad Sci USA 89*, 2965–2969.

Xiao, W., and Oefner, P. J. (2001). Denaturing high-performance liquid chromatography: A review. *Hum Mutation 17*, 439–474.

Zhuang, Z., Park, W. S., Pack, S., Schmidt, L., Vortmeyer, A. O., Pak, E., Pham, T., Weil, R. J., Candidus, S., Lubensky, I. A., Linehan, W. M., Zbar, B., and Weirich, G. (1998). Trisomy 7-harbouring nonrandom duplication of the mutant MET allele in hereditary papillary renal carcinomas. *Nat Genet 20*, 66–69.

3

MOLECULAR CYTOGENETICS: INCREASING RESOLUTION USING ARRAY-BASED CGH

Anne Kallioniemi

INTRODUCTION

Genome-wide analysis of DNA copy number changes by comparative genomic hybridization (CGH) has revealed a spectrum of recurrent chromosomal alterations in cancer. Genes affected by these chromosomal alterations are likely to be primary mediators of cancer progression and therefore represent ideal diagnostic and therapeutic targets. However, identification of genes involved in chromosomal aberrations has been difficult, mostly due to the limited mapping resolution of CGH. The implementation of arrayed DNA fragments, such as large-insert genomic clones or cDNA clones, as hybridization targets has dramatically increased the resolution of CGH. Current high-throughput technologies allow genome-wide analyses of copy number changes with a single gene resolution and are likely to fundamentally increase our knowledge of gene copy number changes in cancer. This chapter provides an overview of the different array-based CGH approaches and their applications in cancer research.

Stepwise accumulation of genetic changes that affect the functions of critical genes, such as those controlling cell growth, differentiation, and cell death, is crucial for the development and progression of cancer. Identification of such genetic changes and the

Oncogenomics: Molecular Approaches to Cancer, Edited by Charles Brenner and David Duggan
ISBN 0-471-22592-4 © 2004 John Wiley & Sons, Inc.

involved genes offers a basis for understanding the pathogenesis of cancer and provides essential tools for improved clinical management of cancer, including better diagnostic and prognostic indicators as well as therapeutic targets.

In hematological malignancies, conventional cytogenetic analyses have pinpointed several recurrent chromosomal translocations that are routinely used for classification and clinical management (Rowley, 1999). In many cases, subsequent molecular cloning of the translocation breakpoints has revealed the identity of the genes that are affected by these translocations and the exact role that they play in the disease pathogenesis has been elucidated. In the case of common solid tumors, the cytogenetic analyses have been less successful, mainly due to technical difficulties and the more complex nature of the chromosomal aberrations. Techniques, such as comparative genomic hybridization (CGH), which allow the identification of DNA sequence copy number changes throughout the tumor genome, were developed to overcome these problems (Kallioniemi et al., 1992).

In CGH, differentially labeled tumor and normal reference DNA are hybridized to normal metaphase chromosomes. Differences in the tumor to normal fluorescence ratio along the metaphase chromosomes are quantitated and reflect changes in the DNA sequence copy number in the tumor genome. To date, thousands of tumor samples have been analyzed by CGH and the results illustrate that recurrent chromosomal aberrations, such as amplifications and deletions, are also frequent in solid tumors (Forozan et al., 1997; Knuutila et al., 1998). Similar to the translocations in hematological malignancies, the recurrent chromosomal aberrations observed in solid tumors are likely to highlight the locations of cancer-related genes. Genes that are affected by chromosomal aberrations in tumors may represent primary mediators of the clonal evolution of cancer as well.

Despite the wealth of information from CGH studies, identification of such genes has proved to be very challenging. Traditional positional cloning procedures, especially the positional candidate gene approach, have been used successfully on a few occasions to uncover cancer-related genes. For example, identification of the androgen receptor gene as the target for amplification in recurrent prostate cancer was based on the positional candidate approach (Visakorpi et al., 1995). In breast cancer, extensive positional cloning efforts have uncovered several putative target genes for the 20q amplification (Anzick et al., 1997; Sen et al., 1997; Collins et al., 1998). However, both the positional cloning techniques and the positional candidate approach are time-consuming and labor intensive and evidently inadequate for the identification of multiple cancer genes located at different chromosomal regions.

The difficulties in the identification of target genes for the recurrent chromosomal aberrations identified by CGH are partly due to the limited mapping resolution of this technique, which does not allow precise localization of the genetic aberrations (Kallioniemi et al., 1994; Bentz et al., 1998). The limited resolution (approximately 10 Mb) leads to a situation where most of the genetic aberrations discovered by this technique span a large segment of the genome, therefore providing a suboptimal starting point for gene identification studies. It is also evident that the smallest aberrations that would be highly informative for pinpointing the exact region of interest will be missed by CGH. A logical way to improve the resolution of CGH was to replace the metaphase chromosomes with alternative hybridization targets (Box 3-1). At the same time, the microarray platform was adapted for CGH analysis to allow high-throughput

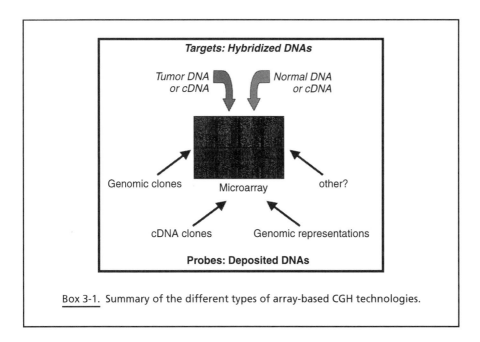

Box 3-1. Summary of the different types of array-based CGH technologies.

data collection. This chapter discusses the recent advances in the array-based copy number analyses and how these techniques have been applied in cancer research.

COPY NUMBER ANALYSIS BY CGH MICROARRAY

Large-Insert Clone Arrays

The first high-resolution CGH studies used arrayed large-insert genomic clones, such as cosmid, P1, PAC, and BAC clones, for copy number analyses (Solinas-Toldo et al., 1997; Pinkel et al., 1998). Solinas-Toldo et al. (1997) named this technique matrix-based CGH and used well-characterized tumor cell lines, such as those carrying *MYC* and *NMYC* amplifications, to establish the detection of high-level copy number increases. They also demonstrated reliable detection of low-level gains and losses using samples previously analyzed by chromosomal CGH (Solinas-Toldo et al., 1997). A fully automated procedure for matrix-based CGH that includes the generation of the DNA arrays, hybridization, data collection, and evaluation has been published (Wessendorf et al., 2002).

Pinkel and co-workers (1998) used genomic clone arrays to analyze cell populations with different numbers of X chromosomes and demonstrated that the fluorescence ratios obtained by CGH microarray were proportional to copy number. The array CGH technique was able reliably to detect previously known copy number increases, such as those involving the long-arm of chromosome 20 in breast cancer. In addition, a novel deletion at 20q was identified and subsequently verified using fluorescence in situ hybridization (Pinkel et al., 1998). These results demonstrated that the CGH microarray technique is suitable for the analysis of both increased and decreased copy number at the level of a single-copy difference (Pinkel et al., 1998). However, technical difficulties in the preparation of the BAC arrays, such as the low yield of DNA from BAC cultures and various problems in spotting of the high-molecular-weight DNA, hindered the utilization of this technology. In a subsequent modification, ligation-mediated PCR was used to generate representations of the BAC DNAs prior to spotting onto the microarrays (Snijders et al., 2001). This modification was also shown to allow for accurate detection not only of high-level copy number differences such as amplifications but also gains and homozygous as well as heterozygous deletions (Snijders et al., 2001).

CGH on cDNA Microarrays

cDNA microarrays were originally developed for high-throughput analysis of differential gene expression patterns (Schena et al., 1995; DeRisi et al., 1996). This technology has been widely applied for the study of expression changes both in normal cells and in various disease stages, such as genetic, metabolic, immunological, and degenerative diseases. In cancer research, cDNA microarray-based expression surveys have been successfully used—for example, for improved disease classification (Alizadeh et al., 2000; Bittner et al., 2000; Perou et al., 2000; Dhanasekaran et al., 2001; Hedenfalk et al., 2001; Khan et al., 2001) and is discussed extensively in Chapters 5 and 6.

Copy number analysis using cDNA microarrays was pioneered by Pollack and co-workers (1999). The greatest advantage of the use of cDNA clones as hybridization targets is that identical cDNA arrays can be applied for parallel expression and copy number analyses, thus providing means for rapid correlation between gene copy number and gene expression changes (Fig. 3-1). The paper by Pollack et al. (1999) illustrated that CGH on cDNA microarray can be used for reliable detection of both increased and decreased copy number. .

Analysis of established cell lines containing well-characterized copy number changes were used to demonstrate the detection of *ERBB2* and *MYC* amplifications and the homozygous deletion of the *TP53* gene. In addition, experiments using cell lines with different numbers of X chromosomes demonstrated that fluorescence ratios obtained by CGH on cDNA microarray were proportional to DNA copy number. The authors estimated that each array element provided approximately 85% sensitivity and 85% specificity for detection of single-copy deletion. A moving average analysis, where information from three adjacent clones was combined, improved the estimates of sensitivity and specificity to 98% (Pollack et al., 1999). Kauraniemi et al. (2001) performed a direct comparison between copy number ratios obtained by CGH on cDNA microarrays and actual gene copy numbers determined by fluorescence in situ hybridization. This comparison indicated 89% concordance between these two techniques and also confirmed the previous observation that ratio values obtained by CGH on cDNA microarrays underestimate the actual copy number increase (Kauraniemi et al., 2001).

Alternative Hybridization Targets

In addition to large-insert genomic clones and cDNA clones, other types of hybridization targets for copy number analysis have been attempted. For example, application of microarrays containing oligonucleotides has been tried (Baldocchi et al., 2001), but at this point it is not clear whether this approach will be successful. In contrast, genomic representations have been successfully used for microarray-based copy number analysis (Lucito et al., 2000). The advantage of this approach is that genomic representations

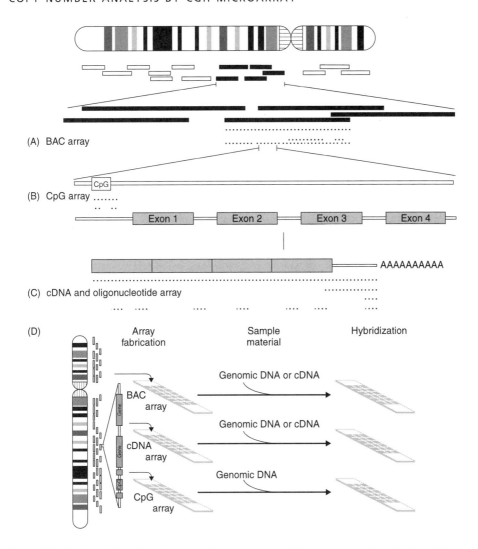

(A) BAC array

(B) CpG array

Exon 1   Exon 2   Exon 3   Exon 4

AAAAAAAAAA

(C) cDNA and oligonucleotide array

(D)   Array   Sample   Hybridization
          fabrication   material

          Genomic DNA or cDNA

BAC array

          Genomic DNA or cDNA

cDNA array

          Genomic DNA

CpG array

Figure 3-1. Probe choices for microarray-based analyses. Microarrays can be fabricated from a variety of genetic material. For example, (A) human genomic material contained in vectors such as bacterial artificial chromosomes (BACs) can be isolated in its entirety (larger dotted line) or PCR amplified using inter-Alu PCR (smaller dotted line). (B) CpG island arrays can be fabricated using clones derived from CpG islands (larger dotted line) or CpG-rich oligonucleotides (smaller dotted lines). (C) cDNA microarrays can be fabricated using full-length cDNAs (largest dotted line), 3′ expressed sequence tags (ESTs) (second largest dotted line), and oligonucleotides 70 nt (second smallest dotted line) or 25 nt in length (smallest dotted line). 3′ ESTs are most commonly found on cDNA microarrays while 25 nt oligomers are found on the more common oligo array by Affymetrix. (D) BAC, cDNA, and CpG island microarrays can be hybridized with genomic DNA to yield information on DNA copy number changes as well as methylation. cDNA microarrays can also be hybridized with cDNA to yield information on gene expression. Combined data from genomic DNA and cDNA hybridized to a cDNA microarray can be used to determine the association between genomic DNA amplification and gene expression changes. (Adapted from Jacobson and Duggan, 2002.)

offer reduced complexity as compared to the complete genome and therefore should provide improved hybridization kinetics (Lucito et al., 2000). In this variation of CGH microarray techniques, human genomic DNA is digested using a rare cutting restriction enzyme to produce a low-complexity representation (LCR). Cloned probes derived from the LCR are arrayed and these arrays are hybridized with LCRs of paired tumor and normal samples.

Because the genomic representations are sensitive to nucleotide polymorphisms at the restriction endonuclease sites, the tumor and normal samples should be derived from the same individual. This is a disadvantage because normal DNA is not always available, especially if archival tumor samples are studied. However, this feature also makes the technique suitable for detection of allelic loss, although the distinction between allelic loss and a deletion is difficult (Lucito et al., 2000). Moreover, genomic representations are currently not linked to physical or transcript maps and therefore the localization of the copy number changes remains challenging.

CGH MICROARRAY RESOLUTION

The mapping resolution of CGH microarray technology is dependent on several factors, including the total number of clones on the array, the local clone density, and the accuracy of the localization of the clones along the genome. Arrays containing approximately 3000 clones would provide an average resolution of 1 Mb, assuming

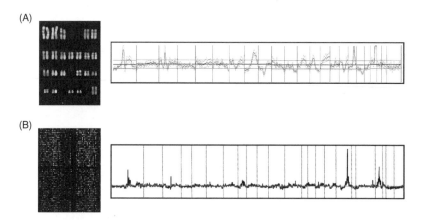

Figure 3-2. Increased resolution of CGH microarray. Genome-wide copy number analysis in MCF7 breast cancer cell line by chromosomal CGH analysis (A). The copy number ratio profile across the entire genome from 1p telomere to Xq telomere is shown along with ±1 SD. The heavy horizontal line indicates a ratio of 1.0; lighter, lower line, a ratio of 0.8; and lighter, upper line, a ratio of 1.2. (B) Genome-wide copy number analysis of MCF-7 by CGH on cDNA microarray (13,000 clones). The copy number ratios were plotted as a function of the position of the cDNA clones along the human genome. The horizontal line indicates a copy number ratio of 1.0. The resolution of chromosomal CGH analysis is about 10 Mb, whereas the 13,000 clone cDNA microarray provides an average resolution of 230 kb across the human genome. Chromosome boundaries are indicated with vertical lines. In CGH on cDNA microarray analysis, the length of each chromosome reflects the number of clones on the array, not the actual size of the chromosome.

T A B L E 3-1. Resolution of Cytogenetic Technologies

Technique	Resolution (kb)	Detectable Alterations Include
Karyotype	10,000–100,000	Large amplifications, deletions, and insertions; translocations; interband inversions; chromosomal copy number changes
CGH	3,000–10,000	Large amplifications, deletions, and insertions; chromosomal copy number changes
SKY/M-FISH	500–1,500	Large and small amplifications, deletions, and insertions; translocations; chromosomal copy number changes
FISH	50–100	Large and small amplifications, deletions, insertions, translocations, and chromosomal copy number changes minimally involving the 1–2 genes found within the FISH probe fragment
Array-based CGH[a]		
using BACs	100–200	Large and small amplifications, deletions, and insertions
using cDNAs	0.5–2	Individual gene amplifications, deletions, and insertions
(Molecular techniques)	0.001 (1 bp)	SNPs, small insertions and deletions

[a] These numbers represent theoretical limits. The actual limits of the technology are dependent on several factors including the total number of clones on the array, the local clone density, and the accuracy of the clone map location.
Source: From Jacobson and Duggan, 2002.

that the clones were evenly distributed across the human genome. This represents an approximately 10-fold increase in resolution as compared to chromosomal CGH (Fig. 3-2, Table 3-1). Even higher resolution can be easily obtained by increasing the number of clones or by using so-called targeted arrays containing clones from a specific region of interest.

In theory, a single gene resolution can be achieved by using cDNA clones as hybridization targets. However, as mentioned earlier, averaging of ratio data across neighboring clones is usually necessary to increase the sensitivity and specificity of the technique and leads to a slight decrease in resolution (Pollack et al., 1999). In the case of the large-insert clone arrays, the resolution is also dependent on the length of the clones and an approximately 40 kb resolution has been demonstrated using cosmid clones (Pinkel et al., 1998). However, subclone mapping resolution can be achieved by using sets of overlapping clones (Albertson et al., 2000). In this case, comparison of the copy number ratios between overlapping clones makes it possible to map copy number changes to a fraction of the length of the clone.

The availability of accurate mapping information is one of the key factors determining the resolution of CGH microarrays. In the case of cDNA microarrays, the earlier studies relied on radiation hybrid maps to obtain positional information for the cDNA clones (Pollack et al., 1999; Monni et al., 2001; Kauraniemi et al, 2001; Varis et al., 2002). However, the use of radiation hybrid maps can be problematic because their representativeness and resolution are limited. All cDNAs or transcribed sequences are not present in radiation hybrid maps and the order and position of genes within a particular chromosomal region is not necessarily correct. Precise mapping of cDNA clones is currently feasible by utilizing the sequence information available through the Human Genome Project (International Human Sequencing Consortium, 2001; Collins, 2003). Information on the annotation of the genomic sequence is directly available through several resources, such as the databases maintained at the University of California–Santa Cruz (www.genome.ucsc.edu) and the National Center for Biotechnology Information (www.ncbi.nlm.nih.gov/genome/guide/human).

Linking of the information between the genomic sequence and the cDNA sequence provides exact base pair localization of the genes on the array and therefore greatly improves the mapping resolution of CGH on cDNA microarrays (Hyman et al., 2002; Pollack et al., 2002). Usually, large-insert clone arrays have been constructed using clones with associated physical mapping information. Similar to cDNA clones, genomic sequence information can also be used to accurately localize large-insert clones along the genome either based on the sequence or STS content of the clones.

APPLICATIONS OF ARRAY-BASED CGH

The possible applications of array-based copy number analysis are numerous and include such areas, as cancer genetics and human genetics. In cancer research, CGH microarray technology has been most frequently used for the analysis of copy number changes involving selected sets of genes such as known oncogenes or specific sections of the genome where targeted analyses of previously discovered regions of copy number change have been performed. Genome-wide screening of copy number changes by CGH microarrays is also currently possible. In addition, this technology has recently been applied for disease classification in cancer.

Cancer Gene Discovery

Cancer Gene Arrays.   Several studies have utilized array-based CGH to evaluate copy number increases affecting a selected set of genes in cancer (Heiskanen et al., 2001; Hui et al., 2001; Takeo et al., 2001; Hui et al., 2002; Zhao et al., 2002). These studies have typically employed commercially available arrays (Vysis Inc., Downers Grove, IL) containing P1, PAC, and BAC clones representing oncogenes that have been previously shown to be frequently amplified in human tumors. For instance, a combination of chromosomal CGH and CGH microarrays was used to analyze glioblastomas (Hui et al., 2001), hepatocellular carcinomas (Takeo et al., 2001), as well as pulmonary artery intimal sarcomas and adrenocortical tumors (Zhao et al., 2002). The results from these studies indicate that CGH microarray was able to verify amplification of oncogenes that were located at regions of increased copy number detected by chromosomal CGH. Significantly, all genes from these chromosomal regions did not show increased copy number by array CGH, suggesting that this technique can be successfully used to exclude some of the positional candidate genes. In addition, amplification of oncogenes from regions with no copy number increase by chromosomal CGH was also observed in these studies, confirming the increased resolution of CGH microarray technique as compared to chromosomal CGH.

Heiskanen et al. (2001) used a commercially available oncogene microarray to screen for increased copy number in a breast cancer cell line known to harbor several high-level amplification sites by chromosomal CGH. CGH microarray analysis identified high-level amplification of the *FGFR2* gene and cDNA microarray-based expression analysis showed overexpression of this gene. Subsequent analysis of primary breast cancers using fluorescence in situ hybridization to tissue microarrays indicated that the *FGFR2* gene was amplified in a small subset of primary breast tumors.

Massion and co-workers (2002) used array CGH to evaluate the putative role of 348 known or suspected cancer genes in the development of non-small-cell lung cancer. They observed frequent copy number increases spanning a 30 Mb region at 3q22–q26 in squamous cell carcinomas and subsequently showed that the *PIK3CA* gene located in this region is amplified. In addition, the activity of the *PIK3CA* signaling was higher in tumors with amplification than in those without amplification, suggesting that this pathway is likely to be activated by the copy number increase in squamous cell carcinomas.

These studies illustrate how arrays containing selected sets of genes can be effectively used as a starting point for rapid evaluation of candidate cancer genes. However, it must be noted that the value of these studies is totally dependent on the selection of clones or genes included in the array. The same approach when applied on a genome-wide unselected scale could provide effective means to identify novel genes involved in copy number changes.

Targeted Region-Specific Microarrays. CGH microarrays have proved to be powerful tools for detailed characterization of specific regions of the genome that were previously shown to be involved in copy number aberrations by chromosomal CGH. For example, copy number increases affecting the long-arm of chromosome 20 in breast cancer have been studied in detail using large-insert clone arrays (Pinkel et al., 1998; Albertson et al., 2000). These studies relied on information obtained from previous positional cloning efforts to construct an array that covered the region of copy number increase at 20q. CGH microarray analysis provided detailed information on the structure of the 20q amplicon in breast cancer and two independent amplification peaks were identified. In addition, the results confirmed the location of the *ZNF217* gene at one of the amplification peaks and implicated the *CYP24* gene as a candidate oncogene involved in the 20q copy number increase in breast cancer (Albertson et al., 2000).

In a similar fashion, Fritz and co-workers (2002) utilized CGH microarrays containing a collection of clones derived from the long-arm of chromosome 12 for the analysis of copy number changes in dedifferentiated and pleomorphic liposarcomas (Fritz et al., 2002). The data revealed a noncontiguous amplification pattern at 12q where highly amplified clones were separated by clones with no copy number increase, presenting a high-resolution map of the structure of the 12q amplicon. As a result, CGH microarray analysis provided a useful starting point for the identification of the genes involved. However, positional candidate gene or positional cloning strategies are still needed to achieve this task.

Monni et al. (2001) constructed a chromosome 17–specific cDNA microarray using information on the radiation hybrid map (GeneMap'99, www.ncbi.nlm.nih.gov/genemap) and the human genomic sequence. This cDNA microarray contained a comprehensive collection of transcribed sequences from two specific areas of interest on chromosome 17: the 17q12-q21 and 17q23 regions. This region-specific microarray was applied to the analysis of both copy number and expression levels of chromosome 17–specific genes in breast (Monni et al., 2001; Kauraniemi et al., 2001) and gastric cancers (Varis et al., 2002). CGH microarray analyses resulted in precise localization and delineation of the boundaries of the chromosome 17 amplicons in these tumor types. More importantly, the parallel expression survey utilizing the same cDNA microarray allowed direct identification of genes that might represent putative amplification target genes because their expression levels were elevated due to increased copy number (Fig. 3-3).

These studies illustrate the power of the combination of copy number and expression analyses for rapid identification of genes involved in the copy number changes. They also illustrate a unique approach that provides means for systematic evaluation of gene copy number and gene expression levels of all transcripts from a specific chromosomal region. Construction of such full-representation targeted microarrays has been rather tedious and time-consuming. However, as argued in Chapter 2, the completion of the human genome sequence and especially the annotation of the genomic sequence will make such projects less demanding.

Clark and co-workers (2002) used an alternative strategy for identifying amplification target genes. In this approach, a cDNA library was prepared from a cancer specimen containing the amplicon of interest and a custom-made cDNA microarray was constructed using randomly selected clones from this library. Parallel copy number and expression analyses using DNA and RNA from the same cancer specimen were used to identify genes that were both amplified and overexpressed in this particular sample (Clark et al., 2002). This technique seems to be especially suitable for identifying amplification target genes because such genes are expected to be abundantly represented in the cDNA library.

The advantage of this approach is that it is not dependent on a preselected set of genes. It can reveal genes that are not present in standard cDNA microarrays or even targeted region-specific microarrays due to missing or erroneous mapping information. Although effective in identification of novel genes, this method is also time-consuming and labor intensive because cDNA libraries and cDNA microarrays need to be prepared individually from each specimen to be analyzed. Furthermore, the analysis leads to the identification of a set of anonymous cDNA clones, and further sequencing as well as sequence analysis is required to reveal the identity of these cDNA clones.

Genome-Wide CGH Microarrays. The studies reviewed here have utilized CGH microarray technology for the analysis of either selected sets of genes or specific regions of the genome. Based on the results obtained from these targeted analyses, it can be envisioned that arrays providing genome-wide coverage would be highly useful in cancer research. Large-insert clone arrays providing genome-wide coverage have been recently assembled. Snijders et al. (2001) constructed an array containing 2460 BAC and P1 clones across the human genome, providing an average resolution of approximately 1.4 Mb, and similar arrays have also been assembled for the mouse genome (Hodgson et al., 2001; Cai et al., 2002).

Genome-wide arrays in the cDNA format have been readily available because cDNA microarrays have been extensively used for genome-wide expression surveys (Alizadeh et al., 2000; Bittner et al., 2000; Perou et al., 2000; Dhanasekaran et al., 2001; Hedenfalk et al., 2001; Khan et al., 2001). The first genome-wide copy number survey by CGH on cDNA microarrays was published by Pollack and co-workers

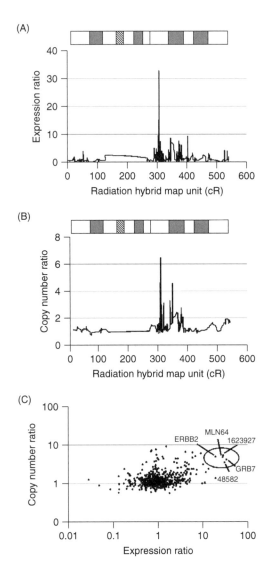

Figure 3-3. Region-specific microarrays. cDNA microarray-based analysis of (A) expression levels and (B) copy number changes of chromosome 17–specific genes in the BT-474 breast cancer cell line. The expression and copy number data are plotted as a function of the position of the cDNA clones (genes) in the radiation hybrid map. A moving average of three (a mean copy number of three adjacent clones) is shown for copy number data. (C) The copy number ratio as a function of the expression ratio in the BT-474 breast cancer cell line. The oval indicates a set of genes that are both highly amplified and overexpressed. (*Source:* From Kauraniemi et al., 2001.)

(1999). Their analysis on breast cancer confirmed previous data on copy number changes with higher resolution, and parallel expression analysis using the same array provided candidate target genes for the copy number changes.

    The combination of genome-wide copy number and expression surveys has recently revealed that copy number changes play a major role in determining gene expression

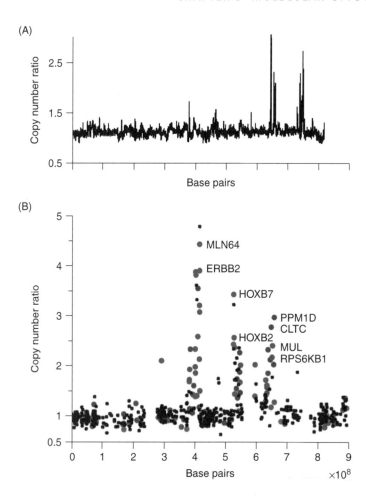

Figure 3-4. Identification of putative cancer genes. (A) Genome-wide copy number analysis in the BT-474 breast cancer cell line using CGH on cDNA microarrays containing 13,000 clones. The copy number ratios were plotted as a function of the position of the cDNA clones along the human genome from the p-telomere of chromosome 1 to the q-telomere of chromosome X. A moving average of 10 adjacent clones is shown. (B) Copy number and expression analysis of chromosome 17–specific genes in the BT-474 breast cancer cell line by cDNA microarrays. The copy number ratios were plotted as a function of the position of the cDNA clones along chromosome 17. Individual data points are labeled by color coding according to cDNA expression levels. Red dots indicate overexpressed genes (upper 7% of expression ratios) in BT-474 cells and green dots underexpressed genes (lowest 7% of expression ratios). The rest of the genes are shown in black. Several highly amplified and overexpressed genes, including the *HOXB7* gene, are indicated. (C) Clinical validation of *HOXB7* amplification in breast cancer. Kaplan-Meier analysis of breast cancer–specific survival for patients with or without *HOXB7* amplification. See insert for color representation of this figure.

APPLICATIONS OF ARRAY-BASED CGH

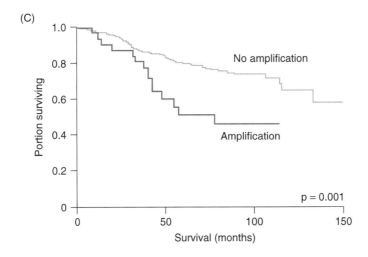

Figure 3-4. (*continued*)

patterns in breast cancer (Hyman et al., 2002; Pollack et al., 2002). These studies demonstrated that up to 62% of genes with increased copy number show elevated expression, indicating that gene copy number aberrations have a substantial impact on gene expression levels (Fig. 3-4) and therefore are likely to have an essential role in the development and progression of cancer. In addition, Hyman et al. (2002) used a statistical approach to identify a specific set of 270 genes whose expression levels were directly attributable to copy number increase and thus are expected to represent candidate amplification target genes. One of these genes, *HOXB7*, which had not been previously implicated in breast cancer, was also shown to be amplified in about 10% of primary breast tumors, and this amplification was associated with poor patient survival (Fig. 3-4C). These results demonstrate the power of genome-wide cDNA microarray-based copy number and expression surveys for rapid identification of putative novel cancer genes.

Disease Classification by CGH Microarray

CGH microarrays containing specific sets of genes are likely to be highly valuable in routine clinical setting. In an early demonstration, Wilhelm et al. (2002) applied CGH microarrays for the analysis of copy number changes in four different subtypes of renal cell cancer as well as normal kidney samples. Copy number information derived from 24 clones was used to accurately classify 33 of the 34 malignant tumors into correct histological subtypes. As expected, the benign neoplasms, which showed no copy number changes, and normal kidney samples were grouped together (Wilhelm et al., 2002).

Similarly, Fritz and co-workers (2002) utilized CGH microarrays for classification of liposarcomas. Microarrays containing a collection of clones derived from chromosome 12q as well as those representing known oncogenes were applied to the analysis of copy number changes in dedifferentiated and pleomorphic liposarcomas. The CGH microarray copy number data allowed clustering of the liposarcoma samples into correct histological subtypes and a small subset of clones were identified as potential class discriminators. The class prediction algorithm was further validated using two blinded samples (Fritz et al., 2002). Interestingly, clustering of the same set of samples using expression profiles did not provide as good a separation between the different liposarcoma subtypes, indicating that the copy number information was able to provide more accurate discrimination than the expression profile. However, the number of genes included in the expression analysis was rather small. Taken together, these results indicate that CGH microarrays have clear clinical value and can be successfully applied for improved diagnosis and disease classification.

It can also be envisioned that CGH microarrays could be applied for rapid analysis of copy number patterns that have been shown to be associated with patient outcome or treatment response. However, the selection of clones included in such arrays is critical for their clinical utility and is likely to differ from one tumor type to another. Large-scale studies with genome-wide coverage in various tumor types are therefore needed before appropriate clone sets can be defined.

Other Applications of CGH Microarrays

While the main focus of this chapter has been on the use of CGH microarrays in the analysis of copy number changes in cancer, it is worth mentioning that the applications of this technology can be extended beyond cancer research. CGH microarrays can also be utilized for the analysis of congenital genetic aberrations. For example, Bruder et al. (2001) used CGH microarrays to examine the frequency and extent of deletions of constitutional DNA from neurofibromatosis patients. A comprehensive analysis of a 7 Mb region at the NF2 locus on chromosome 22q revealed deletions in 15% of cases, ranging in size from 40 kb to 6.6 Mb (Bruder et al., 2001). This study also demonstrated detection of an approximately 100 kb homozygous deletion in a meningioma sample, thus illustrating the applicability of CGH microarrays for screening of homozygous deletions in tumors (Bruder et al., 2001). Veltman and co-workers (2002) analyzed patients with known subtelomeric chromosome rearrangements and showed that CGH microarrays could accurately detect all previously known aberrations. Furthermore, CGH microarray analysis identified additional previously unsuspected telomere rearrangements. These studies illustrate the potential utility of CGH microarrays in clinical genetics.

CGH on cDNA microarrays has also been applied for mapping of genes in somatic cell radiation hybrids (Lin et al., 2002). Hamster CHO cells deficient for hypoxanthine:guanine phosphoribosyl transferase (HPRT) were fused with irradiated normal human fibroblasts. After selection, DNA from the rescued cells (without the mutant phenotype) and nonrescued or wild-type cells were differentially labeled and hybridized to a cDNA microarray. The results showed increased fluorescence ratios at chromosome Xq26, the location of the HPRT gene, with no change in the fluorescence ratios elsewhere in the genome, thus illustrating the applicability of this technology for efficient positional cloning of disease genes.

CONCLUSIONS

Microarray technologies can provide increased resolution over the current CGH standards as well as insights into specific mechanisms of tumorigenesis. The increased resolution and sensitivity provided by microarray technologies will allow for more precise definition of abnormalities. Furthermore, by combining universal PCR amplification with microarray technology, it is quite possible to make analyses based on extremely small biopsies or even single cells (Klein et al., 1999). A single sample might also be sufficient to screen for a panel of potential diseases.

Identification of recurrent chromosomal aberrations in cancer provides a starting point for positional cloning of genes that are likely to have a crucial role in the development and progression of cancer and therefore represent ideal clinical and therapeutic targets. Implementation of high-throughput array-based technologies for genome-wide analysis of copy number changes by comparative genomic hybridization has greatly improved the resolution and accuracy by which the copy number aberrations can be localized along the human genome. Furthermore, the combination of copy number and expression analyses on cDNA microarrays has made it possible to rapidly identify genes that are affected by copy number alterations. These technical advances have enhanced our knowledge of copy number alterations in human tumors and will surely accelerate the identification of putative target genes involved in chromosomal aberrations in cancer.

Microarrays are poised to become an important part of disease diagnosis and discovery. To date, microarray-based technologies have been successfully used in cancer research, for analysis of copy number change (Pinkel et al., 1998; Albertson et al., 2000) and high-resolution analysis of regions previously known to have copy number changes (Monni et al., 2001; Kauraniemi et al., 2001). These technologies will not replace existing cytogenetic technologies, at least not in their entirety. As with conventional CGH, chromosomal rearrangements like reciprocal translocations or inversions are not detectable with microarray-based technologies. Their implementation, however, will greatly improve the resolution to which cytogenetic alterations, especially copy number changes, can be localized to the human genome.

REFERENCES

Albertson, D. G., Ylstra, B., Segraves, R., Collins, C., Dairkee, S. H., Kowbel, D., Kuo, W. L., Gray, J. W., and Pinkel, D. (2000). Quantitative mapping of amplicon structure by array CGH identifies CYP24 as a candidate oncogene. *Nat Genet 25*, 144–146.

Alizadeh, A. A., Eisen, M. B., Davis, R. E., Ma, C., Lossos, I. S., Rosenwald, A., Boldrick, J. C., Sabet, H., Tran, T., Yu, X., Powell, J. I., Yang, L., Marti, G. E., Moore, T., Hudson, J., Jr., Lu, L., Lewis, D. B., Tibshirani, R., Sherlock, G., Chan, W. C., Greiner, T. C., Weisenburger, D. D., Armitage, J. O., Warnke, R., Levy, R., Wilson, W., Grever, M. R., Byrd, J. C., Botstein, D., Brown, P. O., and Staudt, L. M. (2000). Distinct types of diffuse large B-cell lymphoma identified by gene expression profiling. *Nature 403*, 503–511.

Anzick, S. L., Kononen, J., Walker, R. L., Azorsa, D. O., Tanner, M. M., Guan, X. Y., Sauter, G., Kallioniemi, O. P., Trent, J. M., and Meltzer, P. S. (1997). AIB1, a steroid receptor coactivator amplified in breast and ovarian cancer. *Science 277*, 965–968.

Baldocchi, R., Glynne, R., Kowbel, D., Tom, E., Collins, C., Mack, D., and Gary, J. (2001). Hybridization to oligonucleotide arrays for the assessment of gene copy number. *Nat Genet 27*, 41.

Bentz, M., Plesch, A., Stilgenbauer, S., Dohner, H., and Lichter, P. (1998). Minimal sizes of deletions detected by comparative genomic hybridization. *Genes Chrom Cancer 21*, 172–175.

Bittner, M., Meltzer, P., Chen, Y., Jiang, Y., Seftor, E., Hendrix, M., Radmacher, M., Simon, R., Yakhini, Z., Ben-Dor, A., Sampas, N., Dougherty, E., Wang, E., Marincola, F.,

Gooden, C., Lueders, J., Glatfelter, A., Pollock, P., Carpten, J., Gillanders, E., Leja, D., Dietrich, K., Beaudry, C., Berens, M., Alberts, D., and Sondak, V. (2000). Molecular classification of cutaneous malignant melanoma by gene expression profiling. *Nature 406*, 536–540.

Bruder, C. E., Hirvela, C., Tapia-Paez, I., Fransson, I., Segraves, R., Hamilton, G., Zhang, X. X., Evans, D. G., Wallace, A. J., Baser, M. E., Zucman-Rossi, J., Hergersberg, M., Boltshauser, E., Papi, L., Rouleau, G. A., Poptodorov, G., Jordanova, A., Rask-Andersen, H., Kluwe, L., Mautner, V., Sainio, M., Hung, G., Mathiesen, T., Moller, C., Pulst, S. M., Harder, H., Heiberg, A., Honda, M., Niimura, M., Sahlen, S., Blennow, E., Albertson, D. G., Pinkel, D., and Dumanski, J. P. (2001). High resolution deletion analysis of constitutional DNA from neurofibromatosis type 2 (NF2) patients using microarray CGH. *Hum Mol Genet 10*, 271–282.

Cai, W. W., Mao, J. H., Chow, C. W., Damani, S., Balmain, A., and Bradley, A. (2002). Genome-wide detection of chromosomal imbalances in tumors using BAC microarrays. *Nat Biotechnol 20*, 393–396.

Clark, J., Edwards, S., John, M., Flohr, P., Gordon, T., Maillard, K., Giddings, I., Brown, C., Bagherzadeh, A., Campbell, C., Shipley, J., Wooster, R., and Cooper, C. S. (2002). Identification of amplified and expressed genes in breast cancer by comparative hybridization onto microarrays of randomly selected cDNA clones. *Genes Chrom Cancer 34*, 104–114.

Collins, C., Rommens, J. M., Kowbel, D., Godfrey, T., Tanner, M., Hwang, S. I., Polikoff, D., Nonet, G., Cochran, J., Myambo, K., Jay, K. E., Froula, J., Cloutier, T., Kuo, W. L., Yaswen, P., Dairkee, S., Giovanola, J., Hutchinson, G. B., Isola, J., Kallioniemi, O. P., Palazzolo, M., Martin, C., Ericsson, C., Pinkel, D., Albertson, D., Li, W. B., and Gray, J. W. (1998). Positional cloning of ZNF217 and NABC1: genes amplified at 20q13.2 and overexpressed in breast carcinoma. *Proc Natl Acad Sci USA 95*, 8703–8708.

Collins, F. S., Morgan, M., and Patrihos, A. (2003). The human genome project: Lessons from large scale biology. *Science 300*, 286–290.

DeRisi, J., Penland, L., Brown, P. O., Bittner, M. L., Meltzer, P. S., Ray, M., Chen, Y., Su, Y. A., and Trent, J. M. (1996). Use of a cDNA microarray to analyze gene expression patterns in human cancer. *Nat Genet 14*, 457–460.

Dhanasekaran, S. M., Barrette, T. R., Ghosh, D., Shah, R., Varambally, S., Kurachi, K., Pienta, K. J., Rubin, M. A., and Chinnaiyan, A. M. (2001). Delineation of prognostic biomarkers in prostate cancer. *Nature 412*, 822–826.

Forozan, F., Karhu, R., Kononen, J., Kallioniemi, A., and Kallioniemi, O. P. (1997). Genomic screening by comparative genomic hybridization. *Trends Genet 13*, 405–409.

Fritz, B., Schubert, F., Wrobel, G., Schwaenen, C., Wessendorf, S., Nessling, M., Korz, C., Rieker, R. J., Montgomery, K., Kucherlapati, R., Mechtersheimer, G., Eils, R., Joos, S., and Lichter, P. (2002). Microarray-based copy number and expression profiling in dedifferentiated and pleomorphic liposarcoma. *Cancer Res 62*, 2993–2998.

Hedenfalk, I., Duggan, D., Chen, Y., Radmacher, M., Bittner, M., Simon, R., Meltzer, P., Gusterson, B., Esteller, M., Kallioniemi, O. P., Wilfond, B., Borg, A., and Trent, J. (2001). Gene-expression profiles in hereditary breast cancer. *N Engl J Med 344*, 539–548.

Heiskanen, M., Kononen, J., Barlund, M., Torhorst, J., Sauter, G., Kallioniemi, A., and Kallioniemi, O. (2001). CGH, cDNA and tissue microarray analyses implicate FGFR2 amplification in a small subset of breast tumors. *Anal Cell Pathol 22*, 229–234.

Hodgson, G., Hager, J. H., Volik, S., Hariono, S., Wernick, M., Moore, D., Nowak, N., Albertson, D. G., Pinkel, D., Collins, C., Hanahan, D., and Gray, J. W. (2001). Genome scanning with array CGH delineates regional alterations in mouse islet carcinomas. *Nat Genet 29*, 459–464.

Hui, A. B., Lo, K. W., Yin, X. L., Poon, W. S., and Ng, H. K. (2001). Detection of multiple gene amplifications in glioblastoma multiforme using array-based comparative genomic hybridization. *Lab Invest 81*, 717–723.

Hui, A. B., Lo, K. W., Teo, P. M., To, K. F., and Huang, D. P. (2002). Genome wide detection of oncogene amplifications in nasopharyngeal carcinoma by array based comparative genomic hybridization. *Int J Oncol 20*, 467–473.

Hyman, E., Kauraniemi, P., Hautaniemi, S., Wolf, M., Mousses, S., Rozenblum, E., Ringnér, M., Sauter, G., Monni, O., Elkahloun, A., Kallioniemi, O.-P., and Kallioniemi, A. (2002). Impact of DNA amplification on gene expression patterns in breast cancer. *Cancer Res 62*, 6240–6245.

International Human Sequencing Consortium (2001). Initial sequence and analysis of the human genome. *Nature 409*, 860–921.

Jacobson, C., and Duggan, D. (2002). Increasing cytogenetic resolution using array technologies. *Applied Cytogenetics 28*, 128–133.

Kallioniemi, A., Kallioniemi, O. P., Sudar, D., Rutovitz, D., Gray, J. W., Waldman, F. M., and Pinkel, D. (1992). Comparative genomic hybridization for molecular cytogenetic analysis of solid tumors. *Science 258*, 818–821.

Kallioniemi, O. P., Kallioniemi, A., Piper, J., Isola, J., Waldman, F., Gray, J. W., and Pinkel, D. (1994). Optimizing comparative genomic hybridization for analysis of DNA sequence copy number changes in solid tumors. *Genes Chrom Cancer 10*, 231–243.

Kauraniemi, P., Bärlund, M., Monni, O., and Kallioniemi, A. (2001). New amplified and highly expressed genes discovered in the ERBB2 amplicon in breast cancer by cDNA microarrays. *Cancer Res 61*, 8235–8240.

Khan, J., Wei, J. S., Ringnér, M., Saal, L. H., Ladanyi, M., Westermann, F., Berthold, F., Schwab, M., Antonescu, C. R., Peterson, C., and Meltzer, P. S. (2001). Classification and diagnostic prediction of cancers using gene expression profiling and artificial neural networks. *Nat Med 7*, 673–679.

Klein, C. A., Schmidt-Kittler, O., Schardt, J. A., Pantel, K., Speicher, M. R., and Riethmuller, G. (1999). Comparative genomic hybridization, loss of heterozygosity, and DNA sequence analysis of single cells. *Proc Natl Acad Sci USA 96*, 4494–4499.

Knuutila, S., Bjorkqvist, A. M., Autio, K., Tarkkanen, M., Wolf, M., Monni, O., Szymanska, J., Larramendy, M. L., Tapper, J., Pere, H., El-Rifai, W., Hemmer, S., Wasenius, V. M., Vidgren, V., and Zhu, Y. (1998). DNA copy number amplifications in human neoplasms: Review of comparative genomic hybridization studies. *Am J Pathol 152*, 1107–1123.

Lin, J. Y., Pollack, J. R., Chou, F. L., Rees, C. A., Christian, A. T., Bedford, J. S., Brown, P. O., and Ginsberg, M. H. (2002). Physical mapping of genes in somatic cell radiation hybrids by comparative genomic hybridization to cDNA microarrays. *Genome Biol 3*, research 0026.1–0026.7.

Lucito, R., West, J., Reiner, A., Alexander, J., Esposito, D., Mishra, B., Powers, S., Norton, L., and Wigler, M. (2000). Detecting gene copy number fluctuations in tumor cells by microarray analysis of genomic representations. *Genome Res 10*, 1726–1736.

Massion, P. P., Kuo, W.-L., Stokoe, D., Olshen, A. B., Treseler, P. A., Chin, K., Chen, C., Polikoff, D., Jain, A. N., Pinkel, D., Albertson, D. G., Jablons, D. M., and Gray, J. W. (2002). Genomic copy number analysis of non-small cell lung cancer using array comparative genomic hybridization: Implications of the phosphatidylinositol 3-kinase pathway. *Cancer Res 62*, 3636–3640.

Monni, O., Bärlund, M., Mousses, S., Kononen, J., Sauter, G., Heiskanen, M., Chen, Y., Bittner, M., and Kallioniemi, A. (2001). Comprehensive copy number and gene expression profiling of the 17q23 amplicon in human breast cancer. *Proc Natl Acad Sci USA 98*, 5711–5716.

Perou, C. M., Sorlie, T., Eisen, M. B., van de Rijn, M., Jeffrey, S. S., Rees, C. A., Pollack, J. R., Ross, D. T., Johnsen, H., Akslen, L. A., Fluge, O., Pergamenschikov, A., Williams, C.,

Zhu, S. X., Lonning, P. E., Borresen-Dale, A. L., Brown, P. O., and Botstein, D. (2000). Molecular portraits of human breast tumors. *Nature 406*, 747–752.

Pinkel, D., Segraves, R., Sudar, D., Clark, S., Poole, I., Kowbel, D., Collins, C., Kuo, W. L., Chen, C., Zhai, Y., Dairkee, S. H., Ljung, B. M., Gray, J. W., and Albertson, D. G. (1998). High resolution analysis of DNA copy number variation using comparative genomic hybridization to microarrays. *Nat Genet 20*, 207–211.

Pollack, J. R., Perou, C. M., Alizadeh, A. A., Eisen, M. B., Pergamenschikov, A., Williams, C. F., Jeffrey, S. S., Botstein, D., and Brown, P. O. (1999). Genome-wide analysis of DNA copy-number changes using cDNA microarrays. *Nat Genet 23*, 41–46.

Pollack, J. R., Sorlie, T., Perou, C. M., Rees, C. A., Jeffrey, S. S., Lonning, P. E., Tibshirani, R., Botstein, D., Borresen-Dale, A.-L., and Brown, P. O. (2002). Microarray analysis reveals a major direct role of DNA copy number alteration in the transcriptional program of human breast tumors. *Proc Natl Acad Sci USA 99*, 12963–12968.

Rowley, J. (1999). The role of chromosome translocations in leukemogenesis. *Semin Hematol 36*, 59–72.

Schena, M., Shalon, D., Davis, R. W., and Brown, P. O. (1995). Quantitative monitoring of gene expression patterns with a complimentary DNA microarray. *Science 270*, 467–470.

Sen, S., Zhou, H., and White, R. A. (1997). A putative serine/threonine kinase encoding gene BTAK on chromosome 20q13 is amplified and overexpressed in human breast cancer cell lines. *Oncogene 14*, 2195–2200.

Snijders, A. M., Nowak, N., Segraves, R., Blackwood, S., Brown, N., Conroy, J., Hamilton, G., Hindle, A. K., Huey, B., Kimura, K., Law, S., Myambo, K., Palmer, J., Ylstra, B., Yue, J. P., Gray, J. W., Jain, A. N., Pinkel, D., and Albertson, D. G. (2001). Assembly of microarrays for genome-wide measurement of DNA copy number. *Nat Genet 29*, 263–264.

Solinas-Toldo, S., Lampel, S., Stilgenbauer, S., Nickolenko, J., Benner, A., Dohner, H., Cremer, T., and Lichter, P. (1997). Matrix-based comparative genomic hybridization: Biochips to screen for genomic imbalances. *Genes Chrom Cancer 20*, 399–407.

Takeo, S., Arai, H., Kusano, N., Harada, T., Furuya, T., Kawauchi, S., Oga, A., Hirano, T., Yoshida, T., Okita, K., and Sasaki, K. (2001). Examination of oncogene amplification by genomic DNA microarray in hepatocellular carcinomas: Comparison with comparative genomic hybridization analysis. *Cancer Genet Cytogenet 130*, 127–132.

Varis, A., Wolf, M., Monni, O., Vakkari, M. L., Kokkola, A., Moskaluk, C., Frierson, H., Powell, S. M., Knuutila, S., Kallioniemi, A., and El-Rifai, W. (2002). Targets of gene amplification and overexpression at 17q in gastric cancer. *Cancer Res 62*, 2625–2629.

Veltman, J. A., Schoenmakers, E. F., Eussen, B. H., Janssen, I., Merkx, G., van Cleef, B., van Ravenswaaij, C. M., Brunner, H. G., Smeets, D., and van Kessel, A. G. (2002). High-throughput analysis of subtelomeric chromosome rearrangements by use of array-based comparative genomic hybridization. *Am J Hum Genet 70*, 1269–1276.

Visakorpi, T., Hyytinen, E., Koivisto, P., Tanner, M., Keinanen, R., Palmberg, C., Palotie, A., Tammela, T., Isola, J., and Kallioniemi, O. P. (1995). in vivo amplification of the androgen receptor gene and progression of human prostate cancer. *Nat Genet 9*, 401–406.

Wessendorf, S., Fritz, B., Wrobel, G., Nessling, M., Lampel, S., Goettel, D., Kuepper, M., Joos, S., Hopman, T., Kokocinski, F., Dohner, H., Bentz, M., Schwaenen, C., and Lichter, P. (2002). Automated screening for genomic imbalances using matrix-based comparative genomic hybridization. *Lab Invest 82*, 47–60.

Wilhelm, M., Veltman, J. A., Olshen, A. B., Jain, A. N., Moore, D. H., Presti, J. C., Kovacs, G., and Waldman, F. M. (2002). Array-based comparative genomic hybridization for the differential diagnosis of renal cell cancer. *Cancer Res 62*, 957–960.

Zhao, J., Roth, J., Bode-Lesniewska, B., Pfaltz, M., Heitz, P. U., and Komminoth, P. (2002). Combined comparative genomic hybridization and genomic microarray for detection of gene amplifications in pulmonary artery intimal sarcomas and adrenocortical tumors. *Genes Chrom Cancer 34*, 48–57.

WEB RESOURCES

www.ncbi.nlm.nih.gov/sky/
www.helsinki.fi/~lgl_www/CMG.html
www.amba.charite.de/cgh/index.html
www.genome-www.stanford.edu/aCGH/
www.nature.com/ng/journal/v29/n3/suppinfo/ng754_S1.html

4

SNPs AND FUNCTIONAL POLYMORPHISMS IN CANCER

Penelope E. Bonnen and David L. Nelson

INTRODUCTION

Identification and description of the genetic contribution to the etiology of common complex disease remains one of the great challenges of modern medical genetics. It is widely accepted that common diseases such as cancer, mental illness, and heart disease have underlying genetic components that combine with environmental and stochastic factors. It has been hypothesized that the genetic component in cases without clear evidence of Mendelian inheritance might consist of relatively common alleles with moderate to low penetrance. To detect such lower-penetrance alleles requires approaches with greater statistical power than those that have been effective in detecting high-penetrance mutations. Genomic approaches to discovering these low-penetrance alleles include population-based association studies and genome-wide linkage scans. In this chapter we discuss genomic approaches to the identification of functional variants that contribute to cancer susceptibility.

It has been proposed that polymorphisms in the human genome may lead to functional variants of genes that predispose risk for cases of complex diseases (Collins et al., 1997; Lander, 1996). To provide a framework for studies that seek to identify such alleles, it is advantageous to understand the characteristics of disease alleles, such as allele frequency, number, and penetrance. Approximately 1% of the total cancer

Oncogenomics: Molecular Approaches to Cancer, Edited by Charles Brenner and David Duggan
ISBN 0-471-22592-4 © 2004 John Wiley & Sons, Inc.

cases are recognized to derive from heritable cancer syndromes. The germ-line mutations that cause many such syndromes have been identified (reviewed in Fearon, 1997). These heritable syndromes are generally caused by a diverse spectrum of numerous, generally infrequent mutations that confer nearly complete penetrance.

Traditional linkage studies have been used with great success to locate the high-penetrance mutations that cause these types of cancers. For example, linkage was used to identify *BRCA1* and *BRCA2* as causative loci in early-onset familial breast cancer. These two genes harbor more than 200 mutations that cause breast cancer, each exhibiting high penetrance and segregating at a low frequency ($<0.01\%$) in the population. However, more often cancer is observed with familial clustering that does not exhibit an obvious Mendelian pattern of inheritance.

Comprehensive studies of the genetics of familial breast cancer using different methods (population-based case control, family-based studies, and statistical modeling) agreed that strong evidence exists for loci other than the known early-onset genes *BRCA1* and *BRCA2* to contribute to familial breast cancer incidence (Antoniou et al., 2002; Ford et al., 1998; Peto et al., 1999). These studies concluded that the majority of non-*BRCA1/2* familial aggregation breast cancer cases must result from multiple low-penetrance alleles at other loci or other undiscovered high-penetrance alleles. Some of these cases may be caused by previously undetected highly penetrant mutations such as the larger genomic rearrangements that have been found at *BRCA1* (Payne et al., 2000; Unger et al., 2000). However, as discussed in Chapter 1, lower-penetrance alleles likely play an important role in these as well as apparently sporadic cancer cases. As discussed by Brenner, all cancer involves multiple genetic changes in the soma. Thus, the distinction between hereditary and sporadic cancer will evolve as our ability to identify and more fully describe risk bearing alleles increases.

The pursuit of a better understanding of the genetics of complex diseases has led some to propose the common disease/common variant (CDCV) hypothesis (Chakravarti, 1999; Lander, 1996). CDCV draws on population and disease genetics to provide a description of the allele distribution for complex disease. CDCV posits that many cases of commonly occurring diseases, such as specific cancers, are caused by a small number of commonly occurring alleles segregating in the population (Reich and Lander, 2001). Due to the later age of onset of many cancers, disease-causing alleles do not measurably decrease reproductive fitness and as a result are not subject to strong purifying selection. In addition, alleles that contribute to complex disease appear to have incomplete penetrance. These factors may allow these alleles to rise to a higher frequency in the population than Mendelian disease-causing alleles.

One alternative possibility to the CDCV hypothesis is that there could be many rare disease-conferring alleles in the population, each with high penetrance. However, this would predict a higher familial risk than is observed in most cases of common disease (Risch, 1990). The familial relative risk for many common cancers is only two times the sporadic background. Furthermore, Pharoah et al. conducted a study to determine if cancer risk could be predicted for an individual using a polygenic model with common genetic variation (Pharoah et al., 2002). Using data from a population-based series of individuals with breast cancer, they were able to group individuals into low- and high-risk categories. They predicted that high-risk individuals could account for 88% of affected individuals if all risk alleles were identified. This suggested that common genetic polymorphisms could account for the majority of breast cancer cases. Because fewer than 10% of breast cancer cases can be attributed to known inherited mutations, this polygenic inherited view would place a great value on identifying common human polymorphisms for clinical applications (Pharoah et al., 2002).

Some are skeptical of the CDCV hypothesis, citing a lack of success in identifying such alleles in prior studies. Critics point out that recombination, repeat mutation, and gene conversion are factors that may render common disease alleles difficult or impossible to detect due to the disruption of linkage they cause between causal variants and the markers used to find them (Weiss and Clark, 2002). While the number and frequency of disease-causing alleles for common cancers is not known, it is certain that malignancies are multigenic and consist of alleles that exhibit incomplete penetrance. The decreased penetrance and the potential for multiple loci to act in concert make the task of isolating these alleles more difficult than monogenic or monoallelic forms of disease. Models and estimates based on empirical data suggest that haplotypes can be followed to discover alleles contributing to complex diseases (Pritchard and Cox, 2002; Reich and Lander, 2001). These methods rely on the use of single nucleotide polymorphisms (SNPs) as markers that segregate with risk and as potentially causative variants. Various aspects of such an approach are discussed in the remainder of this chapter.

STRATEGY FOR DISCOVERY OF FUNCTIONAL POLYMORPHISMS

Linkage analysis and positional cloning have been used to great effect to find genetic causes of disease. With monogenic diseases, linkage analysis has been used to map the genomic locations of causative genes to within 100–1000 kb (reviewed in Risch, 2000). This required multigenerational families with multiple affected individuals, high penetrance of the disease, and Mendelian segregation of the disease gene with the disease. Positional cloning was then employed to identify the genes within the genomic region and ultimately to identify the causative mutations. Linkage analysis benefits from a low false positive rate (Rao et al., 1978). This is due in large part to its application to Mendelian single-gene disorders. Linkage analysis has demonstrated less utility for detecting genetic contributions to non-Mendelian traits.

Association studies are favored for identifying alleles that contribute to complex disease because of the increased statistical sensitivity they provide over family-based linkage studies. Linkage analysis does not have the statistical power or sensitivity for the task of teasing out a genetic contribution when it is subtle or when several genes may be working together (Risch and Merikangas, 1996). Risch and Merikangas showed that for moderate relative risk, $RR \leq 2$, and intermediate allele frequencies, $0.05 \geq p \geq 0.50$, successful linkage analysis would require prohibitively large sample sizes. Alternatively, given the same parameters (for RR and p), association studies offered sufficient power with reasonable sample sizes.

When designing association studies it is important to be aware of the factors that can influence outcome. False positive results and inconsistency in replication of results in what superficially appear to be similar studies can be due to many factors. Some of these include inadequate statistical power, differential selection criteria for case and control individuals, and failure to take into account multiple tests. Larger sample sizes increase the power of a study. Replica studies also provide stronger support for results. Combining data from multiple independent studies is known as meta-analysis. Meta-analyses allow for reanalysis of data with consistent criteria for cases and controls and also increase power through increasing sample size.

Population structure has also been hypothesized to affect study outcome. Population stratification due to individuals having mixed genetic backgrounds or admixture can produce false positive association of unlinked markers. Molecular and statistical methods of addressing this issue are reviewed by Pritchard and Donnelly (2001). Computer programs have also been developed that can be used to test for population structure (Pritchard et al., 2000). Another influential factor in study outcome is variation in linkage disequilibrium between populations, which is addressed later in this chapter. We also discuss examples of association studies that have identified cancer risk alleles and illustrate some of the aspects of successful association study design.

One of the earliest examples of successful association of a polymorphism and cancer is the HRAS1 minisatellite. The HRAS1 minisatellite, located 1 kb downstream of the *H-ras1* gene, has four common alleles and multiple rare alleles. These rare alleles were demonstrated to confer increased risk for cancer by an investigation that included an association study and a meta-analysis (Krontiris et al., 1993). This investigation was a replica study based on a previous finding with a smaller study population (Krontiris et al., 1985). Researchers conducted a case-control association study with 326 controls and 368 patients with various cancer types including bladder, non-Hodgkin's lymphoma, breast, and prostate. Analysis of the combined cancer patient group showed that individuals possessing one rare HRAS1 allele were at increased risk for cancer (odds ratio = 1.83, *p*-value = 0.002). Analyses of individual patient groups also showed increased risk for specific cancers including bladder (odds ratio = 2.18), breast (odds ratio = 2.29), colorectal (odds ratio = 2.84), and acute leukemia (odds ratio = 2.82).

A meta-analysis of 23 independent studies was also completed as part of the same investigation and confirmed increased cancer risk with odds ratio = 1.93 and *p*-value = 0.001. The cancer risk conferred by individual rare HRAS1 alleles is relatively small; as such, this was one of the first successful demonstrations of the use of association studies to identify low-penetrance risk alleles for cancer. Despite the low penetrance of these alleles, the attributable risk they confer is considerable (0.09) due to their moderate frequency in the population (combined frequency of rare HRAS1 alleles is 0.06; Krontiris et al., 1993). This is likely one of the contributing factors to the success in identifying the risk associated with these low-penetrance alleles and illustrates the principal idea of the CDCV hypothesis.

The HRAS1 minisatellite has also been shown to increase risk of ovarian cancer in individuals with *BRCA1* mutations (Phelan et al., 1996). In a study of more than 300 *BRCA1* mutation carriers, those who had ovarian cancer were more likely to have a rare HRAS1 allele than *BRCA1* carriers who did not have ovarian cancer (odds ratio = 2.85, *p*-value = 0.002). The risk for ovarian cancer was 2.11 greater for individuals with one or two rare HRAS1 alleles and *BRCA1* mutation than those with *BRCA1* mutation alone. The same study examined if *BRCA1* carrier risk for breast cancer was increased by the HRAS1 rare allele and found no evidence for association. This study presented the first identification of a modifier locus of an inherited cancer syndrome.

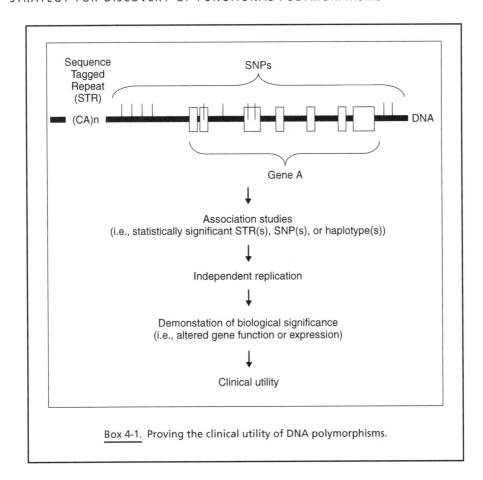

Box 4-1. Proving the clinical utility of DNA polymorphisms.

For more information on the use of murine systems to explore such genetic interactions, interested readers are referred to Chapters 11 and 12.

The underlying biological reason for the association between the HRAS1 minisatellite and cancer is not clear. It has been hypothesized that the minisatellite may influence transcriptional regulation of HRAS1 and other nearby genes. Members of the rel/NF-kappa B family of transcriptional regulatory proteins bind to the HRAS1 minisatellite (Trepicchio and Krontiris, 1992). A later study observed allelic variation in regulatory activity as well as promoter and cell-type specificity (Green and Krontiris, 1993). These findings provide evidence for a potential biological basis for the association between the HRAS1 minisatellite and cancer. However, it is also possible that the HRAS1 minisatellite is not itself a causative factor but instead is in linkage disequilibrium with some causative factor.

In the search for variation in the human genome leading to functional alleles that influence disease risk, another type of polymorphism in the human genome—single nucleotide polymorphism (SNP)—has come into favor. The means by which a SNP can affect gene function is more transparent than for a minisatellite. A SNP may cause a change in amino acid sequence or protein truncation. In addition to effecting changes at the level of protein composition, SNPs in regulatory regions can cause changes in gene expression. Many studies now focus on identifying SNPs that cause functional differences in gene function, as well as using SNPs as markers to identify functional alleles (Box 4-1).

THE UTILITY OF SNPs

Along with the shift from linkage to association studies, marker preference has moved from short tandem repeats (STRs) to SNPs. The high level of polymorphism in STRs makes them ideal for linkage studies where distinguishing alleles among the chromosomes segregating within a family is vital. However, this high variability derives from high mutability, which can have a confounding effect on population-based studies. SNPs are biallelic markers with a lower mutation rate than STRs, which is an advantage for association studies. The lower mutation rate and the presence of only two alleles in nearly all cases also renders SNPs less informative than STRs; however, using multiple SNPs, often in the form of haplotypes, can make up for this lack of power. In contrast to STRs, which may not be numerous enough for association-based approaches (Gray et al., 2000), there appears to be no shortage of SNPs in the genome. Figures for SNP density range from 1/300 to 1/1000 bp. Finally, SNPs are more amenable to high-throughput genotyping than STRs.

Efficient and effective SNP identification and genotyping are crucial for execution of large-scale studies. SNP discovery is primarily carried out through two methods: resequencing of multiple chromosomes and data mining. Consequently, due to the large interest in SNP-based studies, a concerted effort has been made by both private and public groups to identify candidate SNPs throughout the genome. This has produced an explosion of entries in the public database, dbSNP, maintained by the National Center for Biotechnology Information (ncbi.nlm.nih.gov/SNP/index.html). dbSNP holds several million human entries. As a data repository, dbSNP holds many entries that have yet to be confirmed as SNPs, as well as entries that are not unique. More than one-half million entries have been validated as actual, unique SNPs.

The Human Genome Variation Database (HGVBase) is another repository for SNPs. HGVBase contains fewer entries than dbSNP but is more highly curated (hgvbase.cgb.ki.se). There are also numerous polymorphism/mutation databases with a gene- or disease-centric focus. The National Cancer Institute's Cancer Genome Anatomy Project Genetic Annotation Initiative (CGAP-GAI) has documented thousands of SNPs in cancer-related genes. These are accessible through their searchable database (lpgws.nci.nih.gov).

Due to the tremendous number of SNPs, or candidate SNPs, currently publicly available, SNP identification has become increasingly focused on screening known or suspected SNPs to acquire those with the appropriate genomic location and information content. It was shown that SNPs with rarer allele frequency ≥ 0.20 provide greater power for association studies (Kruglyak, 1997). SNP allele frequencies vary between populations, and it is imperative to utilize SNPs that have the appropriate frequency in the study population (Cargill et al., 1999; Goddard et al., 2000; Halushka et al., 1999; Lai et al., 1998; Nickerson et al., 1998). This section discusses studies that used SNPs in the human genome to discover commonly occurring functional alleles that increase cancer risk. Table 4-1 summarizes these alleles and the evidence for their association with cancer.

TABLE 4-1. Commonly Occurring Functional Alleles in Cancer

Allele	Allele Frequency	Effect	Odds Ratio	Evidence for Association				
				Association Study	Replica Study	Family Study/ Segregation Analysis	Meta-analysis	Functional Study
HRAS1 minisatellite rare alleles	0.06[a]	Increase risk of breast, bladder, colorectal cancers	OR = 1.83	Yes[e]	Yes[e]	—	Yes[e]	Yes[f,g]
HRAS1 minisatellite rare alleles	0.06[a]	Modifier of ovarian cancer risk in BRCA1 mutation	OR = 2.85	Yes[h]	—	—	—	Yes[f,g]
APC(I1307K)— missense	0.06[b]	Increase risk of colorectal cancer	OR = 1.5–1.7	Yes[i,k]	Yes[i,k]	Yes[i]	—	Yes[i,j]
BRCA2(N372H)— missense	0.22–0.29[c]	Increase risk of breast cancer	OR = 1.31	Yes[l]	Yes[l]	—	—	—
CHEK2 1100delC— truncating	0.01[d]	Increase risk of breast cancer in non-BRCA	OR = 2.27	Yes[m,n]	Yes[m,n]	Yes[m,n]	—	Yes[n,o,p]

OR = odds ratio.
[a] Frequency of all rare alleles combined.
[b] Frequency in Ashkenazim.
[c] Frequency in Northern European populations.
[d] Frequency in Northern European and North American populations.
[e] Krontiris et al., 1993.
[f] Trepicchio and Krontiris, 1992.
[g] Green and Krontiris 1993.
[h] Phelan et al., 1996.
[i] Laken et al., 1997.
[j] Gryfe et al., 1998.
[k] Gryfe et al., 1999.
[l] Healey et al., 2000.
[m] Meijers–Heijboer et al., 2002.
[n] Vahteristo et al., 2002.
[o] Wu et al., 2001.
[p] Lee et al., 2001.

The familial cancer syndrome, familial adenomatous polyposis (FAP), is caused by truncating mutations in *APC*. During the course of screening a colorectal cancer patient who had a positive family history of colorectal cancer for truncating mutations, investigators identified a SNP (3920T-A) in the *APC* gene. The single base change from T-A is not a truncating mutation and does not directly alter gene function. Rather it creates a mononucleotide repeat (A_8) that is hypermutable compared to the wild-type *APC* sequence (A_3TA_4; Gryfe et al., 1998; Laken et al., 1997). Additional individuals were screened for the presence of this SNP. It was found at a frequency of 6–7% in Ashkenazi Jews and was not observed in a non-Jewish population (Laken et al., 1997; Woodage et al., 1998). Case-control association studies found the variant increased risk of colorectal cancer in Ashkenazi Jews, conferring a relative risk of 1.5–1.7 (Gryfe et al., 1999; Laken et al., 1997). The risk associated with this allele is relatively low as is consistent with a low-penetrance allele. However, it is clinically relevant due to the relatively high frequency of this allele in the Ashkenazi Jewish population.

Investigators found evidence for a common polymorphism in *BRCA2* (N372H) to increase the risk for breast cancer (Healey et al., 2000). Researchers conducted a series of five population-based case-control studies. The rarer allele frequency of BRCA2(N372H) was ≥ 0.22 in all five populations, each of which was Northern European. Individuals who were homozygous for the rarer allele showed a 1.3-fold greater risk for breast cancer than individuals who were homozygous for the common allele. This study provides especially strong evidence for association due to the large population sample sizes and numerous replica studies. BRCA2(N372H) shows potential to have functional consequences. BRCA2(N372H) causes the substitution of an amino acid located in a region of the protein that has been shown to interact with transcriptional coactivator protein, P/CAF (Fuks et al., 1998). However, it is not known whether the BRCA2(N372H) polymorphism disrupts this interaction. Conclusive evidence for whether BRCA2(N372H) is a causative variant or in linkage disequilibrium with some causative functional variant has yet to be determined.

Another example of a low-penetrance allele that increases the risk for breast cancer is CHEK2 1100delC. This allele is found at a frequency of 0.01 in healthy individuals. Investigators conducted association studies with CHEK2 1100delC and found an elevated breast cancer risk in persons with a family history of breast cancer (Meijers-Heijboer et al., 2002; Vahteristo et al., 2002). The CHEK2-Breast Cancer Consortium found CHEK2 1100delC at a frequency of 0.05 in 718 breast cancer families that did not possess BRCA1/2 mutations (Meijers-Heijboer et al., 2002). The same study showed that CHEK2 1100delC did not increase penetrance of breast cancer in BRCA1/2 mutation carriers. Vahteristo et al. observed CHEK2 1100delC at a frequency of 0.03 in 358 patients from breast cancer families (odds ratio = 2.27, p-value = 0.021; Vahteristo et al., 2002). Both studies examined segregation of the CHEK2 1100delC mutation through breast cancer families (Meijers-Heijboer et al., 2002; Vahteristo et al., 2002). Vahteristo et al. (2002) described one family in which the four affected individuals all possessed the mutation along with four unaffected individuals. This family demonstrated segregation of the mutation with breast cancer with incomplete penetrance. CHEK2 1100delC leads to truncation of the encoded CHEK2 protein and has been shown to abolish the kinase activity of CHEK2 (Lee et al., 2001; Wu et al., 2001), making this allele a likely candidate for cancer predisposition.

These studies are representative examples of SNPs that may lead to low-penetrance functional variants that influence cancer risk. Despite these successes, it has been difficult to ascribe associations for low-penetrance alleles with certitude. One example is the *ATM* gene, which is responsible for the disease ataxia telangiectasia. There has been great debate as to whether individuals heterozygous for *ATM* mutations are at increased risk for breast cancer (Gatti et al., 1999; Morrell et al., 1990; Stankovic et al., 1998; Swift et al., 1987, 1991). Studies have been carried out with two basic approaches. One is to screen breast cancer cases and controls to assess directly the presence of *ATM* mutations. The other is to count breast cancer incidence among *ATM* obligate carriers. Studies of obligate carriers have indicated increased breast cancer risk for individuals heterozygous for mutations in *ATM* (Athma et al., 1996; Olsen et al., 2001; Swift et al., 1991). Population genetic-based screening studies generally have not agreed, however (Bay et al., 1998; FitzGerald et al., 1997; Vorechovsky et al., 1996).

The breast cancer risk conferred by *ATM* in studies of obligate carriers is relatively low. The lack of finding in population screening studies could be in part due to a lack of sensitivity of screening methods such as the protein truncation test (PTT). PTT and other methods such as sequencing and single strand conformational polymorphism (SSCP) are predominantly focused on detecting changes in coding regions, leaving out the possibility of mutations in noncoding regions. The combination of a low-penetrance allele with a lack of sensitivity in mutation detection could lead to a false negative result in an association study. This illustrates some of the difficulties in taking a direct/screening approach to finding causative variants that lead to low-penetrance-risk alleles.

HAPLOTYPES: LEVERAGING UP STUDY POWER

An additional consideration in developing an approach to detection of functional variants is the use of single markers versus haplotypes. Studies have shown that utilization of multiple markers in association studies provides greater statistical power than do individual markers (Johnson et al., 2001). As a result, haplotypes should be an excellent tool for seeking low-penetrance alleles where a more sensitive approach is critical. Haplotype association with disease by the linkage disequilibrium (LD) approach has been used successfully for identifying genomic regions containing loci responsible for disease phenotypes (MacDonald et al., 1992; Yu et al., 1996). The same principle can be applied by using haplotypes of biallelic markers to detect disease association. Using several SNPs distributed across 100–200 kb should result in increased statistical sensitivity over studies executed with fewer loci. This was demonstrated by findings at the β2-adrenergic receptor gene ($\beta 2AR$) where individual SNP data predicted no association for individual $\beta 2AR$ polymorphisms and broncodilator response to β-agonists in asthmatics (Drysdale et al., 2000). However, one haplotype was associated with greater physiologic response ($P = 0.007$), and cells transfected with the haplotype showed $\beta 2AR$ mRNA levels 50% greater than cells transfected with a nonassociating haplotype.

An additional advantage to employing haplotypes is that they can span a large genomic region that includes coding and noncoding regions. It has been shown that polymorphisms in noncoding regions can have functional consequences, so it is valuable to extend searches for functional variants to these regions. Haplotypes also can detect different types of mutations ranging from SNPs to larger genomic rearrangements. This is in contrast to other screening methods that target particular types of mutations. For example, PTT detects only protein truncating mutations, and excludes missense alterations and changes in levels of expression.

Other screening methods, such as conformation-sensitive gel electrophoresis, can be used to detect single base changes in coding or noncoding regions but not large rearrangements. Detecting large genomic rearrangements such as those that have been found at the *BRCA1* locus requires Southern blot analysis (Payne et al., 2000; Petrij-Bosch et al., 1997; Unger et al., 2000). Haplotypes can be used to detect all of the aforementioned mutations with equal sensitivity. Another strength of the haplotype approach is the ability to use purely epidemiological populations, as opposed to family-based collections, to detect chromosomal backgrounds that confer risk for disease.

THE IMPORTANCE OF CHARACTERIZING LD AND HAPLOTYPE DIVERSITY

Linkage disequilibrium (LD) occurs when alleles at different loci are found within an individual more often than would be predicted by chance (Risch, 2000). Characterizing LD is especially important for haplotype-based association studies where multiple markers are used in concert to detect associations. For a haplotype to represent a genetic region, some amount of LD must exist between markers. Moreover, the haplotype is used not only to represent a genetic region/allele but more pertinently as a surrogate for the actual causative variant. Without LD, the markers cannot be used as a surrogate. The extent of LD in a particular region influences the marker density needed to represent the region. Equally important, interruptions in LD can be exploited for mapping a causative variant from its location on a haplotype. A thorough characterization of the structure of LD, both peaks and valleys, across the region of interest is a necessary companion to the successful pursuit of LD-based studies.

Our understanding of the distribution of LD in the genome has evolved as empirical data have accumulated. Analysis of the beta-globin gene cluster was one of the initial illustrations of the complexity of the structure of LD. Regions 5′ (35 kb) and 3′ (19 kb) to the beta-globin structural gene were found to have high LD with little measurable LD between these two clusters (9 kb; Chakravarti et al., 1984). The lack of LD observed at *LPL* (Clark et al., 1998) and *TP53* (Bonnen et al., 2002) is similar to the central region in the beta-globin study. Empirical data from *BRCA1* and *ATM* and others show regions of LD > 100 kb (Abecasis et al., 2001; Bonnen et al., 2000; Collins et al., 1999; Liu and Barker, 1999; Peterson et al., 1995; Taillon-Miller et al., 2000; Thorstenson et al., 2001). It has been suggested that the genome consists of blocks of LD (30–100 kb) interrupted by short (1–2 kb) hot spots of recombination (Daly et al., 2001; Jeffreys et al., 2001). A block-like structure has been observed in several studies of different regions of the genome (Bonnen et al., 2002; Daly et al., 2001; Gabriel et al., 2002; Johnson et al., 2001; Patil et al., 2001; Reich et al., 2001; Taillon-Miller et al., 2000).

An additional feature of the LD structure is that just as there are regions of extended LD, there are lengthy regions without measurable LD. The *TP53* locus shows no LD across as much as ∼90 kb, which is considerably more than the expected 1–2 kb for a recombination hot spot (Bonnen et al., 2002). A similar finding of an expansive region of little LD in two separate regions of Xq25 (129 kb and 308 kb) adds to the evidence that genome-wide LD patterns remain a complex issue that may only be resolved when a genome-wide map of LD is available (Taillon-Miller et al., 2000).

LD structure and intensity varies throughout the genome. Correspondingly, the number of common haplotypes at each locus varies widely, reflecting the variation in LD patterns and intensity at the genomic locations (Bonnen et al., 2002). The seemingly substantial differences in numbers of haplotypes and LD patterns between loci highlight the importance of characterizing each locus of interest prior to association studies. This diversity also underscores the inefficiency of applying a standard marker density genome-wide for association studies or genome scans. More importantly, it points to an inability to estimate a priori the LD for a particular region; instead, LD must be characterized for each region of interest. LD pattern and intensity also varies between human populations and extends this argument for needing to characterize haplotypes and LD in each study population as well as locus (Bonnen et al., 2000, 2002; Goddard et al., 2000; Kidd et al., 2000; Reich et al., 2001; Trikka et al., 2002). Exploitation of such differences between populations has been suggested to have significant potential for identification of alleles contributing to common disease (Reich et al., 2001; Todd et al., 1989). Figure 4-1 shows the LD patterns and intensity at five unlinked cancer loci in four ethnic populations and illustrates the variation in LD between genomic regions and populations.

One of the most salient findings of recent haplotype studies is that there are a small number of haplotypes that are shared among all populations, and these haplotypes account for a very high percentage of the total chromosomes segregating in a population (Bonnen et al., 2002; Daly et al., 2001; Gabriel et al., 2002; Patil et al., 2001; Trikka et al., 2002). For example, Bonnen et al. genotyped 295 individuals from 4 different ethnic populations for 14 SNPs that span the *ATM* locus (140 kb) and found that 6 haplotypes accounted for 91% of the total chromosomes (Bonnen et al., 2000). This high degree of sharing has been observed even in regions with little LD (Bonnen et al., 2002). These findings show that commonly occurring polymorphisms can be used to mark a few distinct versions of chromosomes (haplotypes) that are present across the human population. Because these haplotypes are present in all populations, they are likely the oldest haplotypes. It is important to note that these shared haplotypes do not have the same frequencies in all populations. A haplotype that is present in all populations may have a frequency of 0.02 in one population and 0.30 in another. This again points to the importance of characterizing haplotype frequencies in the particular populations used for association studies.

The above findings are promising for SNP haplotype-based association studies. For such studies in search of a commonly occurring functional variant, the commonly occurring haplotypes are the most pertinent tool. These findings demonstrate that SNPs can be used to mark a few distinct versions of chromosomes (haplotypes) that are present in the human population at a high frequency. This points toward the possibility that haplotype-based association studies could be executed with relatively small numbers of markers, thereby minimizing costs. This low-haplotype diversity combined with the block structure of LD led to the possibility of using "haplotype tag" SNPs for association studies (Johnson et al., 2001). Haplotype tag SNPs are the minimal number of SNPs required to define the common haplotypes for an LD block. This study demonstrated haplotype tag SNPs could be utilized to comprehensively represent the commonly occurring haplotypes in a population.

For association studies in search of a commonly occurring functional variant, the commonly occurring haplotypes are the most pertinent, and too many haplotypes can lead to a loss of power and information. Conversely, regions of extreme LD such as

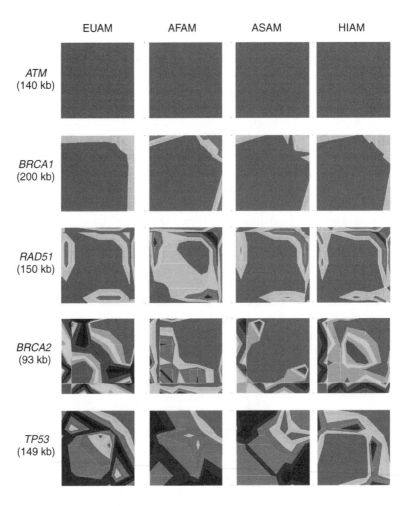

Figure 4-1. A comparison of the linkage disequilibrium (LD) for five widely studied cancer susceptibility genes: *ATM, BRCA1, BRCA2, RAD51,* and *TP53.* Unphased SNP genotype data were generated for markers that encompassed ~150 kb per locus. LD was assessed at each locus in four populations: African American (AFAM), Asian American (ASAM), Hispanic American (HIAM), and European American (EUAM). LD was measured for the five loci in all populations using the statistic |D′| in a pairwise manner across markers. GOLD (Abecasis and Cookson, 2000) generates these plots through interpolation of the resulting triangular matrices. |D′| ranges from 1 to 0, with 1 showing in red and 0 in dark blue. The intensity of LD across the chromosome from 5′ to 3′ is illustrated by following the diagonal of each plot from the bottom left to top right. LD pattern and intensity varies between genomic locations and populations. See insert for color representation of this figure.

BRCA1 show such a small number of haplotypes that a haplotype-based study for this region may suffer from a lack of discrimination. Therefore, it may be useful for some studies to refine haplotypes by breaking the commonly occurring ones into subgroups through the addition of either population-specific or lower-frequency markers, especially in regions of high LD.

An international consortium of public and private groups has collaborated to generate a haplotype map of the genome. Similar to the Human Genome Project, it is thought that this second-generation genome map will greatly facilitate genetic studies—in particular, those in search of risk alleles for common disease. This project, termed HapMap, seeks to identify and genotype common SNPs in ~200 individuals from African, Asian, and American populations. From these genotype data, haplotype, LD, and recombination maps will be generated, providing a genome-wide resource for associating SNPs with disease. One expected outcome from the effort will be a set of SNPs appropriate for each genomic region and population.

CONFIRMING ASSOCIATIONS AND FUNCTIONAL POLYMORPHISMS

Distinguishing between a neutral polymorphism and one that has a functional consequence is no easy task. Polymorphisms that show association may be causative variants or they may be in linkage disequilibrium with a causative variant. None of the methods described previously provide conclusive evidence for causation. In this section, we discuss four criteria that contribute to establishing a polymorphism as functional: statistical significance, replication of results in an independent sample, biological relevance, and demonstration of alteration of gene function or regulation.

Association studies suffer from a higher false positive rate than family-based linkage studies. Statistical significance and replication of results in an independent sample are critical. One way to minimize the chance of false positive results is to apply a more stringent level of significance. A widely used criterion for statistical significance of an association is a P-value ≤ 0.05. However, utilization of a more stringent P-value might preclude some false associations. Additionally, larger sample sizes provide greater statistical power. Some have suggested sample sizes in the thousands as being necessary for detection of true associations for complex disease (Dahlman et al., 2002). Independent replica studies are also key to substantiating a true association.

A gene for which an association is found should have biological relevance to the phenotype. For cancer, such candidate genes are those that are known or suspected to act in a cancer-related pathway. These pathways include DNA repair, cell cycle, proliferation, apoptosis and cell migration. The CHEK21100delC association with breast cancer is an excellent example of this principle (Meijers-Heijboer et al., 2002; Vahteristo et al., 2002). CHEK2 is a checkpoint kinase that is involved in response to ionizing radiation-induced DNA damage. Mutations in *CHEK2* have been found in individuals with Li-Fraumeni who do not have *TP53* mutations, providing evidence that mutations in this gene can lead to cancer (Bell et al., 1999). These data lend credence to the case that the CHEK21100delC allele increases the risk for breast cancer.

Demonstration of alteration of gene function or regulation is the ultimate goal for definition of functional alleles. To understand how polymorphism in the human genome affects risk for disease, the way in which polymorphism affects gene function and expression must be examined. Yan et al. made a step in this direction when they developed an assay to quantitate the relative expression of two different alleles of a coding SNP (Yan et al., 2002). Common SNPs were identified in 13 different genes, some of which were candidate cancer genes. The SNPs were genotyped in 96 individuals and expression levels of each allele were measured in heterozygotes. Differences in expression levels were observed for 6 out of 13 genes studied. The combination of genotype and gene expression data is potentially very valuable as a means of linking genotype with phenotype. This study demonstrated that polymorphism at the genomic level can lead to functional differences in genes, moving us a step closer to understanding how variation in the human genome contributes to disease.

SUMMARY AND PERSPECTIVES

In this chapter, we discussed genomic approaches to identification of functional variants that contribute to cancer susceptibility. Based on the CDCV hypothesis, the goal of these studies is to assess the common variants of a gene for association with disease. Haplotype-based association studies are expected to provide greater statistical power to identify lower-penetrance alleles. Our ability to define distinct haplotype blocks and to comprehensively characterize the majority of haplotype diversity through commonly occurring SNPs bodes well for association studies for common complex diseases. The HapMap seeks to provide a framework for such studies by providing a genome-wide catalog of high-frequency SNPs in multiple populations that could provide a launching pad for genome-wide LD and haplotype-based studies. Following the rigorous standards outlined here, utilization of the haplotype approach with association studies will hopefully result in identification of alleles that influence the risk for cancer, the ultimate assessment of which lies in functional analysis.

Identification of loci and alleles associated with increased risk can be expected to be swiftly followed by characterization of the responsible functional variants. These in turn will form a new set of candidates for screening the general population to forecast risk. It is not difficult to imagine future efforts to customize screening and health management based on genetic risk to prevent cancer occurrence.

REFERENCES

Abecasis, G. R., and Cookson, W. O. (2000). GOLD-graphical overview of linkage disequilibrium. *Bioinformatics 16*, 182–183.

Abecasis, G. R., Noguchi, E., Heinzmann, A., Traherne, J. A., Bhattacharyya, S., Leaves, N. I., Anderson, G. G., Zhang, Y., Lench, N. J., Carey, A., Cardon, L. R., Moffatt, M. F., and Cookson, W. O. (2001). Extent and distribution of linkage disequilibrium in three genomic regions. *Am J Hum Genet 68*, 191–197.

Antoniou, A. C., Pharoah, P. D., McMullan, G., Day, N. E., Stratton, M. R., Peto, J., Ponder, B. J., and Easton, D. F. (2002). A comprehensive model for familial breast cancer incorporating BRCA1, BRCA2 and other genes. *Br J Cancer 86*, 76–83.

Athma, P., Rappaport, R., and Swift, M. (1996). Molecular genotyping shows that ataxia-telangiectasia heterozygotes are predisposed to breast cancer. *Cancer Genet Cytogenet 92*, 130–134.

Bay, J. O., Grancho, M., Pernin, D., Presneau, N., Rio, P., Tchirkov, A., Uhrhammer, N., Verrelle, P., Gatti, R. A., and Bignon, Y. J. (1998). No evidence for constitutional ATM mutation in breast/gastric cancer families. *Int J Oncol 12*, 1385–1390.

Bell, D. W., Varley, J. M., Szydlo, T. E., Kang, D. H., Wahrer, D. C., Shannon, K. E., Lubratovich, M., Verselis, S. J., Isselbacher, K. J., Fraumeni, J. F., Birch, J. M., Li, F. P., Garber, J. E., and Haber, D. A. (1999). Heterozygous germ line hCHK2 mutations in Li-Fraumeni syndrome. *Science 286*, 2528–2531.

Bonnen, P. E., Story, M. D., Ashorn, C. L., Buchholz, T. A., Weil, M. M., and Nelson, D. L. (2000). Haplotypes at ATM identify coding-sequence variation and indicate a region of extensive linkage disequilibrium. *Am J Hum Genet 67*, 1437–1451.

Bonnen, P. E., Wang, P. J., Kimmel, M., Chakraborty, R., and Nelson, D. L. (2002). Haplotype and linkage disequilibrium architecture for human cancer-associated genes. *Genome Res 12*, 1846–1853.

Cargill, M., Altshuler, D., Ireland, J., Sklar, P., Ardlie, K., Patil, N., Shaw, N., Lane, C. R., Lim, E. P., Kalyanaraman, N., Nemesh, J., Ziaugra, L., Friedland, L., Rolfe, A., Warrington, J., Lipshutz, R., Daley, G. Q., and Lander, E. S. (1999). Characterization of single-nucleotide polymorphisms in coding regions of human genes [published erratum appears in Nat Genet 1999 Nov;23(3):373]. *Nat Genet 22*, 231–238.

Chakravarti, A. (1999). Population genetics—making sense out of sequence. *Nat Genet 21*, 56–60.

Chakravarti, A., Buetow, K. H., Antonarakis, S. E., Waber, P. G., Boehm, C. D., and Kazazian, H. H. (1984). Nonuniform recombination within the human beta-globin gene cluster. *Am J Hum Genet 36*, 1239–1258.

Clark, A. G., Weiss, K. M., Nickerson, D. A., Taylor, S. L., Buchanan, A., Stengard, J., Salomaa, V., Vartiainen, E., Perola, M., Boerwinkle, E., and Sing, C. F. (1998). Haplotype structure and population genetic inferences from nucleotide-sequence variation in human lipoprotein lipase. *Am J Hum Genet 63*, 595–612.

Collins, A., Lonjou, C., and Morton, N. E. (1999). Genetic epidemiology of single-nucleotide polymorphisms [see comments]. *Proc Natl Acad Sci USA 96*, 15173–15177.

Collins, F. S., Guyer, M. S., and Charkravarti, A. (1997). Variations on a theme: Cataloging human DNA sequence variation. *Science 278*, 1580–1581.

Dahlman, I., Eaves, I. A., Kosoy, R., Morrison, V. A., Heward, J., Gough, S. C., Allahabadia, A., Franklyn, J. A., Tuomilehto, J., Tuomilehto-Wolf, E., Cucca, F., Guja, C., Ionescu-Tirgoviste, C., Stevens, H., Carr, P., Nutland, S., McKinney, P., Shield, J. P., Wang, W., Cordell, H. J., Walker, N., Todd, J. A., and Concannon, P. (2002). Parameters for reliable results in genetic association studies in common disease. *Nat Genet 30*, 149–150.

Daly, M. J., Rioux, J. D., Schaffner, S. F., Hudson, T. J., and Lander, E. S. (2001). High-resolution haplotype structure in the human genome. *Nat Genet 29*, 229–232.

Drysdale, C. M., McGraw, D. W., Stack, C. B., Stephens, J. C., Judson, R. S., Nandabalan, K., Arnold, K., Ruano, G., and Liggett, S. B. (2000). Complex promoter and coding region beta 2-adrenergic receptor haplotypes alter receptor expression and predict in vivo responsiveness. *Proc Natl Acad Sci USA 97*, 10483–10488.

Fearon, E. R. (1997). Human cancer syndromes: Clues to the origin and nature of cancer. *Science 278*, 1043–1050.

FitzGerald, M. G., Bean, J. M., Hegde, S. R., Unsal, H., MacDonald, D. J., Harkin, D. P., Finkelstein, D. M., Isselbacher, K. J., and Haber, D. A. (1997). Heterozygous ATM mutations do not contribute to early onset of breast cancer [see comments]. *Nat Genet 15*, 307–310.

Ford, D., Easton, D. F., Stratton, M., Narod, S., Goldgar, D., Devilee, P., Bishop, D. T., Weber, B., Lenoir, G., Chang-Claude, J., Sobol, H., Teare, M. D., Struewing, J., Arason, A., Scherneck, S., Peto, J., Rebbeck, T. R., Tonin, P., Neuhausen, S., Barkardottir, R., Eyfjord, J., Lynch, H., Ponder, B. A., Gayther, S. A., Zelada-Hedman, M., et al. (1998). Genetic heterogeneity and penetrance analysis of the BRCA1 and BRCA2 genes in breast cancer families. The Breast Cancer Linkage Consortium. *Am J Hum Genet 62*, 676–689.

Fuks, F., Milner, J., and Kouzarides, T. (1998). BRCA2 associates with acetyltransferase activity when bound to P/CAF. *Oncogene 17*, 2531–2534.

Gabriel, S. B., Schaffner, S. F., Nguyen, H., Moore, J. M., Roy, J., Blumenstiel, B., Higgins, J., DeFelice, M., Lochner, A., Faggart, M., Liu-Cordero, S. N., Rotimi, C., Adeyemo, A., Cooper, R., Ward, R., Lander, E. S., Daly, M. J., and Altshuler, D. (2002). The structure of haplotype blocks in the human genome. *Science 296*, 2225–2229.

Gatti, R. A., Tward, A., and Concannon, P. (1999). Cancer risk in ATM heterozygotes: A model of phenotypic and mechanistic differences between missense and truncating mutations. *Mol Genet Metab 68*, 419–423.

Goddard, K. A., Hopkins, P. J., Hall, J. M., and Witte, J. S. (2000). Linkage disequilibrium and allele-frequency distributions for 114 single-nucleotide polymorphisms in five populations. *Am J Hum Genet 66*, 216–234.

Gray, I. C., Campbell, D. A., and Spurr, N. K. (2000). Single nucleotide polymorphisms as tools in human genetics. *Hum Mol Genet 9*, 2403–2408.

Green, M., and Krontiris, T. G. (1993). Allelic variation of reporter gene activation by the HRAS1 minisatellite. *Genomics 17*, 429–434.

Gryfe, R., Di Nicola, N., Gallinger, S., and Redston, M. (1998). Somatic instability of the APC I1307K allele in colorectal neoplasia. *Cancer Res 58*, 4040–4043.

Gryfe, R., Di Nicola, N., Lal, G., Gallinger, S., and Redston, M. (1999). Inherited colorectal polyposis and cancer risk of the APC I1307K polymorphism. *Am J Hum Genet 64*, 378–384.

Halushka, M. K., Fan, J. B., Bentley, K., Hsie, L., Shen, N., Weder, A., Cooper, R., Lipshutz, R., and Chakravarti, A. (1999). Patterns of single-nucleotide polymorphisms in candidate genes for blood-pressure homeostasis. *Nat Genet 22*, 239–247.

Healey, C. S., Dunning, A. M., Teare, M. D., Chase, D., Parker, L., Burn, J., Chang-Claude, J., Mannermaa, A., Kataja, V., Huntsman, D. G., Pharoah, P. D., Luben, R. N., Easton, D. F., and Ponder, B. A. (2000). A common variant in BRCA2 is associated with both breast cancer risk and prenatal viability. *Nat Genet 26*, 362–364.

Jeffreys, A. J., Kauppi, L., and Neumann, R. (2001). Intensely punctate meiotic recombination in the class II region of the major histocompatibility complex. *Nat Genet 29*, 217–222.

Johnson, G. C., Esposito, L., Barratt, B. J., Smith, A. N., Heward, J., Di Genova, G., Ueda, H., Cordell, H. J., Eaves, I. A., Dudbridge, F., Twells, R. C., Payne, F., Hughes, W., Nutland, S., Stevens, H., Carr, P., Tuomilehto-Wolf, E., Tuomilehto, J., Gough, S. C., Clayton, D. G., and Todd, J. A. (2001). Haplotype tagging for the identification of common disease genes. *Nat Genet 29*, 233–237.

Kidd, J. R., Pakstis, A. J., Zhao, H., Lu, R. B., Okonofua, F. E., Odunsi, A., Grigorenko, E., Tamir, B. B., Friedlaender, J., Schulz, L. O., Parnas, J., and Kidd, K. K. (2000). Haplotypes and linkage disequilibrium at the phenylalanine hydroxylase locus, PAH, in a global representation of populations. *Am J Hum Genet 66*, 1882–1899.

Krontiris, T. G., DiMartino, N. A., Colb, M., and Parkinson, D. R. (1985). Unique allelic restriction fragments of the human Ha-ras locus in leukocyte and tumour DNAs of cancer patients. *Nature 313*, 369–374.

Krontiris, T. G., Devlin, B., Karp, D. D., Robert, N. J., and Risch, N. (1993). An association between the risk of cancer and mutations in the HRAS1 minisatellite locus. *N Engl J Med 329*, 517–523.

Kruglyak, L. (1997). The use of a genetic map of biallelic markers in linkage studies. *Nat Genet 17*, 21–24.

Lai, E., Riley, J., Purvis, I., and Roses, A. (1998). A 4-Mb high-density single nucleotide polymorphism-based map around human APOE. *Genomics 54*, 31–38.

Laken, S. J., Petersen, G. M., Gruber, S. B., Oddoux, C., Ostrer, H., Giardiello, F. M., Hamilton, S. R., Hampel, H., Markowitz, A., Klimstra, D., Jhanwar, S., Winawer, S., Offit, K., Luce, M. C., Kinzler, K. W., and Vogelstein, B. (1997). Familial colorectal cancer in Ashkenazim due to a hypermutable tract in APC. *Nat Genet 17*, 79–83.

Lander, E. S. (1996). The new genomics: Global views of biology. *Science 274*, 536–539.

Lee, S. B., Kim, S. H., Bell, D. W., Wahrer, D. C., Schiripo, T. A., Jorczak, M. M., Sgroi, D. C., Garber, J. E., Li, F. P., Nichols, K. E., Varley, J. M., Godwin, A. K., Shannon, K. M., Harlow, E., and Haber, D. A. (2001). Destabilization of CHK2 by a missense mutation associated with Li-Fraumeni syndrome. *Cancer Res 61*, 8062–8067.

Liu, X., and Barker, D. F. (1999). Evidence for effective suppression of recombination in the chromosome 17q21 segment spanning RNU2-BRCA1. *Am J Hum Genet 64*, 1427–1439.

MacDonald, M. E., Novelletto, A., Lin, C., Tagle, D., Barnes, G., Bates, G., Taylor, S., Allitto, B., Altherr, M., Myers, R., Lehrach, H., Collins, F., Wasmuth, J., Frontali, M., and Gusella, J. (1992). The Huntington's disease candidate region exhibits many different haplotypes. *Nat Genet 1*, 99–103.

Meijers-Heijboer, H., van den Ouweland, A., Klijn, J., Wasielewski, M., de Snoo, A., Oldenburg, R., Hollestelle, A., Houben, M., Crepin, E., van Veghel-Plandsoen, M., Elstrodt, F., van Duijn, C., Bartels, C., Meijers, C., Schutte, M., McGuffog, L., Thompson, D., Easton, D., Sodha, N., Seal, S., Barfoot, R., Mangion, J., Chang-Claude, J., Eccles, D., Eeles, R., Evans, D. G., Houlston, R., Murday, V., Narod, S., Peretz, T., Peto, J., Phelan, C., Zhang, H. X., Szabo, C., Devilee, P., Goldgar, D., Futreal, P. A., Nathanson, K. L., Weber, B., Rahman, N., and Stratton, M. R. (2002). Low-penetrance susceptibility to breast cancer due to CHEK2(*)1100delC in noncarriers of BRCA1 or BRCA2 mutations. *Nat Genet 31*, 55–59.

Morrell, D., Chase, C. L., and Swift, M. (1990). Cancers in 44 families with ataxia-telangiectasia. *Cancer Genet Cytogenet 50*, 119–123.

Nickerson, D. A., Taylor, S. L., Weiss, K. M., Clark, A. G., Hutchinson, R. G., Stengard, J., Salomaa, V., Vartiainen, E., Boerwinkle, E., and Sing, C. F. (1998). DNA sequence diversity in a 9.7-kb region of the human lipoprotein lipase gene. *Nat Genet 19*, 233–240.

Olsen, J. H., Hahnemann, J. M., Borresen-Dale, A. L., Brondum-Nielsen, K., Hammarstrom, L., Kleinerman, R., Kaariainen, H., Lonnqvist, T., Sankila, R., Seersholm, N., Tretli, S., Yuen, J., Boice, J. D., Jr., and Tucker, M. (2001). Cancer in patients with ataxia-telangiectasia and in their relatives in the nordic countries. *J Natl Cancer Inst 93*, 121–127.

Patil, N., Berno, A. J., Hinds, D. A., Barrett, W. A., Doshi, J. M., Hacker, C. R., Kautzer, C. R., Lee, D. H., Marjoribanks, C., McDonough, D. P., Nguyen, B. T., Norris, M. C., Sheehan, J. B., Shen, N., Stern, D., Stokowski, R. P., Thomas, D. J., Trulson, M. O., Vyas, K. R., Frazer, K. A., Fodor, S. P., and Cox, D. R. (2001). Blocks of limited haplotype diversity revealed by high-resolution scanning of human chromosome 21. *Science 294*, 1719–1723.

Payne, S. R., Newman, B., and King, M. C. (2000). Complex germline rearrangement of BRCA1 associated with breast and ovarian cancer. *Genes Chromosomes Cancer 29*, 58–62.

Peterson, A. C., Di Rienzo, A., Lehesjoki, A. E., de la Chapelle, A., Slatkin, M., and Freimer, N. B. (1995). The distribution of linkage disequilibrium over anonymous genome regions. *Hum Mol Genet 4*, 887–894.

Peto, J., Collins, N., Barfoot, R., Seal, S., Warren, W., Rahman, N., Easton, D. F., Evans, C., J. Deacon, and Stratton, M. R. (1999). Prevalence of BRCA1 and BRCA2 gene mutations in patients with early-onset breast cancer. *J Natl Cancer Inst 91*, 943–949.

Petrij-Bosch, A., Peelen, T., van Vliet, M., van Eijk, R., Olmer, R., Drusedau, M., Hogervorst, F. B., Hageman, S., Arts, P. J., Ligtenberg, M. J., Meijers-Heijboer, H., Klijn, J. G., Vasen, H. F., Cornelisse, C. J., van't Veer, L. J., Bakker, E., van Ommen, G. J., and Devilee, P. (1997). BRCA1 genomic deletions are major founder mutations in Dutch breast cancer patients. *Nat Genet 17*, 341–345.

Pharoah, P. D., Antoniou, A., Bobrow, M., Zimmern, R. L., Easton, D. F., and Ponder, B. A. (2002). Polygenic susceptibility to breast cancer and implications for prevention. *Nat Genet 31*, 33–36.

Phelan, C. M., Rebbeck, T. R., Weber, B. L., Devilee, P., Ruttledge, M. H., Lynch, H. T., Lenoir, G. M., Stratton, M. R., Easton, D. F., Ponder, B. A., Cannon-Albright, L., Larsson, C., Goldgar, D. E., and Narod, S. A. (1996). Ovarian cancer risk in BRCA1 carriers is modified by the HRAS1 variable number of tandem repeat (VNTR) locus. *Nat Genet 12*, 309–311.

Pritchard, J. K. and Cox, N. J. (2002). The allelic architecture of human disease genes: Common disease-common variant or not? *Hum Mol Genet 11*, 2417–2423.

Pritchard, J. K. and Donnelly, P. (2001). Case-control studies of association in structured or admixed populations. *Theor Popul Biol 60*, 227–237.

Pritchard, J. K., Stephens, M., and Donnelly, P. (2000). Inference of population structure using multilocus genotype data. *Genetics 155*, 945–959.

Rao, D. C., Keats, B. J., Morton, N. E., Yee, S., and Lew, R. (1978). Variability of human linkage data. *Am J Hum Genet 30*, 516–529.

Reich, D. E. and Lander, E. S. (2001). On the allelic spectrum of human disease. *Trends Genet 17*, 502–510.

Reich, D. E., Cargill, M., Bolk, S., Ireland, J., Sabeti, P. C., Richter, D. J., Lavery, T., Kouyoumjian, R., Farhadian, S. F., Ward, R., and Lander, E. S. (2001). Linkage disequilibrium in the human genome. *Nature 411*, 199–204.

Risch, N. (1990). Linkage strategies for genetically complex traits. I. Multilocus models. *Am J Hum Genet 46*, 222–228.

Risch, N. J. (2000). Searching for genetic determinants in the new millennium. *Nature 405*, 847–856.

Risch, N., and Merikangas, K. (1996). The future of genetic studies of complex human diseases. *Science 273*, 1516–1517.

Stankovic, T., Kidd, A. M., Sutcliffe, A., McGuire, G. M., Robinson, P., Weber, P., Bedenham, T., Bradwell, A. R., Easton, D. F., Lennox, G. G., Haites, N., Byrd, P. J., and Taylor, A. M. (1998). ATM mutations and phenotypes in ataxia-telangiectasia families in the British Isles: Expression of mutant ATM and the risk of leukemia, lymphoma, and breast cancer. *Am J Hum Genet 62*, 334–345.

Swift, M., Reitnauer, P. J., Morrell, D., and Chase, C. L. (1987). Breast and other cancers in families with ataxia-telangiectasia. *N Engl J Med 316*, 1289–1294.

Swift, M., Morrell, D., Massey, R. B., and Chase, C. L. (1991). Incidence of cancer in 161 families affected by ataxia-telangiectasia. *N Engl J Med 325*, 1831–1836.

Taillon-Miller, P., Bauer-Sardina, I., Saccone, N. L., Putzel, J., Laitinen, T., Cao, A., Kere, J., Pilia, G., Rice, J. P., and Kwok, P. Y. (2000). Juxtaposed regions of extensive and minimal linkage disequilibrium in human Xq25 and Xq28. *Nat Genet 25*, 324–328.

Thorstenson, Y. R., Shen, P., Tusher, V. G., Wayne, T. L., Davis, R. W., Chu, G., and Oefner, P. J. (2001). Global analysis of ATM polymorphism reveals significant functional constraint. *Am J Hum Genet 69*, 396–412.

Todd, J. A., Mijovic, C., Fletcher, J., Jenkins, D., Bradwell, A. R., and Barnett, A. H. (1989). Identification of susceptibility loci for insulin-dependent diabetes mellitus by trans-racial gene mapping. *Nature 338*, 587–589.

Trepicchio, W. L., and Krontiris, T. G. (1992). Members of the rel/NF-kappa B family of transcriptional regulatory proteins bind the HRAS1 minisatellite DNA sequence. *Nucleic Acids Res 20*, 2427–2434.

Trikka, D., Fang, Z., Renwick, A., Jones, S. H., Chakraborty, R., Kimmel, M., and Nelson, D. L. (2002). Complex SNP-based haplotypes in three human helicases: Implications for cancer association studies. *Genome Res 12*, 627–639.

Unger, M. A., Nathanson, K. L., Calzone, K., Antin-Ozerkis, D., Shih, H. A., Martin, A. M., Lenoir, G. M., Mazoyer, S., and Weber, B. L. (2000). Screening for genomic rearrangements in families with breast and ovarian cancer identifies BRCA1 mutations previously missed by conformation-sensitive gel electrophoresis or sequencing. *Am J Hum Genet 67*, 841–850.

Vahteristo, P., Bartkova, J., Eerola, H., Syrjakoski, K., Ojala, S., Kilpivaara, O., Tamminen, A., Kononen, J., Aittomaki, K., Heikkila, P., Holli, K., Blomqvist, C., Bartek, J., Kallioniemi, O. P., and Nevanlinna, H. (2002). A CHEK2 genetic variant contributing to a substantial fraction of familial breast cancer. *Am J Hum Genet 71*, 432–438.

Vorechovsky, I., Luo, L., Lindblom, A., Negrini, M., Webster, A. D., Croce, C. M., and Hammarstrom, L. (1996). ATM mutations in cancer families. *Cancer Res 56*, 4130–4133.

Weiss, K. M., and Clark, A. G. (2002). Linkage disequilibrium and the mapping of complex human traits. *Trends Genet 18*, 19–24.

Woodage, T., King, S. M., Wacholder, S., Hartge, P., Struewing, J. P., McAdams, M., Laken, S. J., Tucker, M. A., and Brody, L. C. (1998). The APCI1307K allele and cancer risk in a community-based study of Ashkenazi Jews. *Nat Genet 20*, 62–65.

Wu, X., Webster, S. R., and Chen, J. (2001). Characterization of tumor-associated Chk2 mutations. *J Biol Chem 276*, 2971–2974.

Yan, H., Yuan, W., Velculescu, V. E., Vogelstein, B., and Kinzler, K. W. (2002). Allelic variation in human gene expression. *Science 297*, 1143.

Yu, C. E., Oshima, J., Fu, Y. H., Wijsman, E. M., Hisama, F., Alisch, R., Matthews, S., Nakura, J., Miki, T., Ouais, S., Martin, G. M., Mulligan, J., and Schellenberg, G. D. (1996). Positional cloning of the Werner's syndrome gene. *Science 272*, 258–262.

5

EXPRESSION PROFILING OF BREAST CANCER: FROM MOLECULAR PORTRAITS TO CLINICAL UTILITY

Therese Sørlie, Anne-Lise Børresen-Dale, Per E. Lønning, Patrick O. Brown, and David Botstein

INTRODUCTION

Knowledge of the sequence of the human genome has created a nearly unlimited horizon of opportunities to study human genes. Much of the challenge lies in developing new technology for these studies as well as for the statistical and mathematical approaches necessary to interrogate the massive data that are produced. In particular, the use of DNA microarray technology, in which the expression or copy number of genes can be determined genome-wide, offers great potential for improving understanding of the causes and progression of disease, for the discovery of new molecular markers, for therapeutic intervention, and for development of new prevention strategies.

As discussed in Chapter 1, the many diseases that collectively are called cancer arise as a result of the accumulation of mutations, chromosomal instabilities, and epigenetic changes. Together these facilitate an increased rate of cellular evolution and damage that progressively impairs the complex systems of regulation of cell growth and death. Changes in gene activities are further influenced by the microenvironment within and in the vicinity of tumor cells as well as exogenous factors, such as diet. When all of these factors are combined with inborn genetic variations among individuals, there is every reason to expect tumors to display prodigiously diverse phenotypes.

Oncogenomics: Molecular Approaches to Cancer, Edited by Charles Brenner and David Duggan
ISBN 0-471-22592-4 © 2004 John Wiley & Sons, Inc.

Microarray technologies applied to the study of DNA, RNA, and protein profiles, as well as to the genome-wide distribution of epigenetic changes such as DNA methylation, can be used to portray a tumor's detailed phenotype in its unique context. These methods can generate molecular signatures that can be correlated to clinical information. Eventually, advances in tumor portraiture will naturally lead to improved and individualized treatments for cancer patients.

Breast cancer is the most common malignancy and the most common cause of cancer death in women worldwide (Parkin et al., 2001). As for most solid tumors, breast cancers are heterogeneous and consist of several pathologic subtypes with different histological appearances of the malignant cells, different clinical presentations and outcomes, and a diverse range of responses to a given treatment. Furthermore, breast tumor tissue shows heterogeneity with respect to its microenvironment including specifically the types and numbers of infiltrating lymphocytes, adipocytes, stromal and endothelial cells. The cellular composition of tumors is a central determinant of the biological and clinical features of an individual's disease. Though breast cancers are typed according to estrogen and progesterone receptor status, further stratifications will be necessary to understand the biology of the disease and to aid in clinical management and treatment decisions.

This chapter mainly covers published studies of breast tumors with only occasional reference to a similar study of lung tumors. Specifically, we describe advances in breast tumor phenotype determination using DNA microarrays to measure the expression of thousands of genes simultaneously and DNA copy numbers to a gene-length resolution over the entire genome. We also discuss the statistical relationships of such measurements with clinical features of the disease of individual patients.

PRINCIPLE AND PRACTICE OF DNA MICROARRAY TECHNOLOGY

The ability of nucleic acids (DNA and RNA) to hybridize specifically based only on their nucleotide sequence is the principle that underlies all DNA microarray technology. Arraying DNA sequences of many genes (ideally every gene in a genome) allows for the simultaneous measurement and monitoring of the expression levels of all these genes in complex samples, including tumor biopsies. Currently, arrays with ~50,000 features are readily manufactured; thus, the revelation that the human genome consists of fewer than 25,000 genes makes a high-density microarray representing all human genes inevitable in the near future. We can look forward to studies in which an assessment of the transcriptome—i.e., the comprehensive genome-wide pattern of gene expression—is routinely produced.

Most published studies have used spotted cDNA microrrays introduced by Schena et al. (1995). Today these arrays are still produced by individual laboratories using PCR-amplified clone inserts, but alternative oligonucleotide-based arrays are increasingly popular (Pease et al., 1994; Hughes et al., 2001; Kane et al., 2000). Most of these platforms allow use of two different fluorescent labels to distinguish, on the same spots, the abundance of gene-specific nucleic acid from two different samples (Box 5-1).

Two general kinds of experiments have been useful. In one, gene expression levels are measured. Briefly, copies of mRNA extracted from tumors are labeled with one fluorescent dye; copies of mRNA extracted from a standard reference consisting of about a dozen cell lines are labeled with a different dye, and the labeled copies are mixed before hybridization. The rationale behind the standard reference includes the

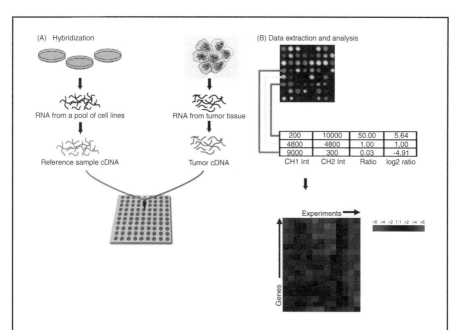

(A) Hybridization

RNA from a pool of cell lines

Reference sample cDNA

RNA from tumor tissue

Tumor cDNA

(B) Data extraction and analysis

CH1 Int	CH2 Int	Ratio	log2 ratio
200	10000	50.00	5.64
4800	4800	1.00	1.00
9000	300	0.03	-4.91

Experiments

Genes

>6 >4 >2 1:1 >2 >4 >6

Box 5-1. Schematic overview of DNA microarray analysis. (A) RNA from a tumor sample and a reference (in this case, a pool of cell lines) are transcribed and differentially labeled with fluorescent nucleotides (by convention Cy 5 for tumor RNA, Cy 3 for reference RNA). The two samples are combined and allowed to hybridize to a DNA microarray in which each gene is represented as a distinct spot. A laser scanner is used to excite the hybridized array at the appropriate wavelengths, and the relative abundance of the two transcripts is visualized in a pseudocolored image by the ratio of the red to green fluorescence intensities at each spot. (B) For further data analysis and interpretation of multiple experiments, the ratios are log transformed and placed in a table in which each row corresponds to a gene and each column corresponds to a single hybridization experiment. The abundance of each transcript is represented by a color: red for relatively increased expression, green for relatively diminished expression. Color saturation reflects the magnitude of the ratio relative to the median for each set of samples (see scale). The procedures summarized in this chapter are standard protocols for labeling and data acquisition for microarray experiments used at Stanford University and can be found in detail at cmgm.stanford.edu/pbrown/protocols.html. See insert for color representation of this figure.

ability to produce a nonzero value in most (in practice, about 86%) of the features on the array and the ability to continually reproduce the same reference.

The other kind of experiment measures, gene by gene, the relative number of copies of the gene sequence itself; this procedure is sometimes called array comparative genomic hybridization, or aCGH (Pollack et al., 1999; see Chapter 3 for more detail). Briefly, the tumor DNA is labeled with one fluorescent dye, normal DNA from leukocytes of a female (for breast cancer) is labeled with a different dye, and the labeled copies are mixed before hybridization. The rationale for using normal DNA as reference is clearly that the tumor's gains and losses will be directly measurable from the ratio of colors observed at each spot on the array.

The great value of microarray experiments when applied to the study of cancer is most clear when a large number of samples is analyzed similarly and combined so that variation in gene expression patterns across a large number of tumors can be investigated. Hierarchical clustering has proved to be a powerful way of organizing the genes and experimental samples into meaningful groups based on similarity in their overall expression patterns in an unsupervised manner (Eisen et al., 1998). Furthermore, by using a reference-based strategy, many diverse experiments can readily be aggregated, analyzed, and compared in a parallel fashion (Eisen and Brown, 1999; Perou et al., 2000; Ross et al., 2000). Using this approach, prominent and recurrent patterns appear that can be related to important characteristics of the tumors. By clustering tumors on the basis of gene expression patterns, biologically coherent subgroups have been observed that are statistically associated with clinical parameters, including survival.

As an alternative to clustering—i.e., searching for patterns in the data with no prior assumptions—we can also apply supervised methods in which predictive models are built based on existing data (Brown et al., 2000; Golub et al., 1999; Hastie et al., 2001; Hedenfalk et al., 2001; Khan et al., 2001; Tibshirani et al., 2002). For example, statistical analysis of microarrays (SAM; Tusher et al., 2001) searches for sets of genes whose expression correlates with a known parameter, e.g., the clinical outcome of patients. In this chapter, we describe how this approach has been used to identify genes that correlate with the *TP53* mutational status in the tumors and with patient outcome.

MOLECULAR PORTRAITS OF BREAST TUMORS: DESCRIPTION OF GENE CLUSTERS

The phenotypic diversity of tumors is accompanied by a corresponding diversity in gene expression patterns that can be gleaned from cDNA microarrays. One of the first such studies of breast tumors reported that clusters of genes with coherent expression patterns could be related to specific features of biological variation among the samples—for example, variation in proliferation rates and activation of the interferon-regulated signal transduction pathway (Perou et al., 1999). Furthermore, clusters of coexpressed genes were identified whose expression patterns derived from different cell types within the grossly dissected breast tumors, including stromal cells and lymphocytes, and this idea was corroborated by immunohistochemistry. These results demonstrated the utility and feasibility of a systematic investigation of the characteristics of a tumor using cDNA microarrays.

This work led to a larger study of 65 surgical specimens of human breast tissue from 42 individuals using cDNA microarrays representing 8102 genes (Perou et al., 2000). Twenty of the forty tumors examined were sampled twice as part of a larger prospective study on locally advanced breast cancer (T3/T4 and/or N2 tumors; see Aas et al., 1996; Geisler et al., 2001). Following an open surgical biopsy to obtain the "before" sample, each of these patients was treated weekly with doxorubicin for an average of 15 weeks (range 12–23), followed by resection of the remaining tumor, in which case the "after" sample was obtained. In addition, primary tumors from two patients were paired with a lymph node metastasis from the same individual. To help provide a framework for interpreting the variation in expression patterns observed in the tumor samples, 17 cultured cell lines were also characterized (one cell line was cultured under three different conditions), and these provided models for many of the cell types encountered in the tissue samples.

A subset of 1753 genes was selected—those whose transcripts varied in abundance by at least fourfold from their median abundance in this sample set in at least three samples—and hierarchical clustering was used to group genes and tissue samples together based on overall similarity in their expression patterns (Fig. 5-1A). The resulting cluster dendrogram showed that there was great molecular heterogeneity among the tumors, with multidimensional variation in the patterns of gene expression. The most striking result was that most of the tumor pairs (15 of the 20 "before" and "after" doxorubicin pairs and both primary tumor/lymph node metastasis pairs) clustered together on terminal branches in the dendrogram (Fig. 5-1B). That is, despite the potential confounding effects of an interval of 16 weeks, cytotoxic chemotherapy, and surgical intervention, independent samples taken from the same tumor were in most cases recognizably more similar to each other than either was to any of the other samples. This implied that every tumor is unique and has a distinctive gene expression signature or portrait. It also implied that the type and number of nonepithelial cells in tumors is a remarkably consistent and enduring feature of each individual tumor. Breast tumors thus appear to be very diverse but are not internally heterogeneous when millions of cells are sampled.

The finding that the two primary tumors and the corresponding metastases were similar in their overall pattern of gene expression suggests that the molecular program of a primary tumor may be retained in its metastases. In a similar study of human lung tumors, six primary tumor/lymph node pairs and one primary tumor/intrapulmonary metastasis pair also clustered together on terminal branches of the dendrogram, indicating that they also shared common expression patterns (Garber et al., 2001). The similarity of the global expression patterns between primary tumors and metastases needs to be further explored in larger studies and other statistical analyses should be applied to reveal important differences between the two. Nevertheless, this suggests that specific expression patterns in primary tumors may help in identifying genes and/or pathways that are important for the metastatic process and for tumor cell biology.

The molecular portraits of the tumors not only uncovered similarities and differences among the tumors but also in many cases pointed to a biological interpretation, based on the clustering of genes according to their expression patterns. Variation in growth rate, the activity of specific signaling pathways, and the cellular composition of the tumors were all reflected in corresponding variation in the expression of specific subsets of genes. The largest distinct cluster of genes within the 1753 gene cluster diagram was the "proliferation cluster," which is a group of genes whose levels of expression correlate with cellular proliferation rates (Perou et al., 1999; Ross et al., 2000; Whitfield et al., 2002). Expression of this cluster of genes varied widely among the tumor samples and was generally well correlated with the mitotic index. Genes encoding two generally used immunohistochemical markers of cell proliferation, Ki-67 and PCNA, were also included in this cluster. More than half of the genes in the proliferation cluster were shown to be cell cycle regulated when the patterns of expression for these genes were analyzed in synchronized HeLa cell cultures (Fig. 5-2; Whitfield et al., 2002). While many of these genes may influence tumorigenesis directly and exhibit transforming activity, such as *PLK* (Smith et al., 1997), *STK15* (Zhou et al.,

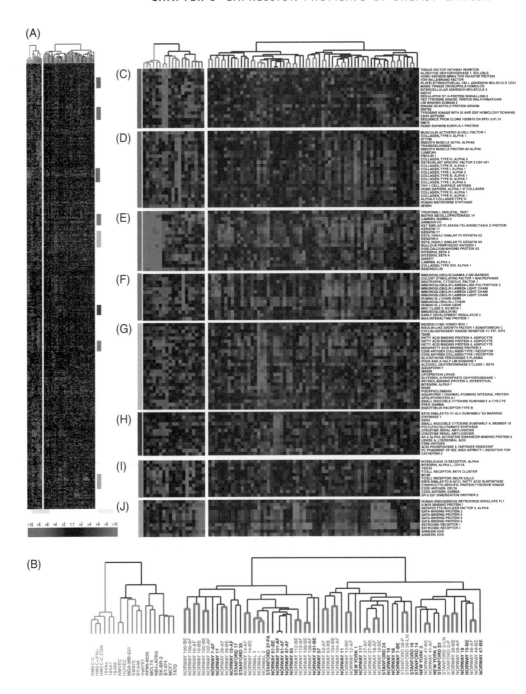

1998), and *CDC25B* (Galaktionov et al., 1995), others may be periodically expressed due to the fact that proliferative tumors contain more cycling cells. The proliferation cluster has been observed in virtually every tumor type examined (Alizadeh et al., 2000; Chen et al., 2002; Perou et al., 2000; Ross et al., 2000; Whitfield et al., 2002).

Another large cluster containing genes regulated by the type I and type II interferon pathways showed substantial variation in expression among the tumors as was previously observed (Perou et al., 1999). These include signal transducer and activator of transcription 1 (*STAT1*), interferon-stimulated gene factor 3 (*ISGF3*), interferon alpha–inducible protein (*G1P3*), and interferon regulatory factor 1 (*IRF1*). When induced in response to a virus infection, interferons, bind to cell surface receptors and induce a tyrosine kinase signaling cascade that leads to activation of STATs which in turn initiate transcription of interferon-stimulated genes that encode proteins with antiviral, antiproliferative, and antitumor effects (Sen, 2001). Only part of the pattern can be accounted for by the contribution of infiltrating lymphocytes in the tumors representing an activated immune response. The carcinoma cells themselves showed high expression of some of the genes (e.g., *STAT1*) by immunohistochemistry in some of the tumors (Perou et al., 1999), suggesting activation of downstream signaling pathways mediated by other factors. This result is strengthened by observations of this gene expression cluster in breast epithelial cells growing in vitro.

As already indicated, the histological complexity of breast tumors with components of various cell types was captured in the expression patterns. The expression patterns observed in the cultured cell lines, as well as the high expression of known cell-type-specific genes within the clusters of genes, were used as guides to infer the lineage of the cells that accounted for the apparently cell-type-specific expression. In this data set, eight independent clusters of genes appeared to reflect variation in specific cell types present within the tumors: endothelial cells, indicated by a cluster of genes containing von Willebrand factor, *CD34* and *CD31* (Fig. 5-1C); stromal fibroblasts, which expressed several isoforms of collagen (Fig. 5-1D); B lymphocytes, indicated by the expression of immunoglobulin genes (Fig. 5-1F); T lymphocytes, known to

←——

Figure 5-1. Cluster analysis of a subset of genes in 84 experimental samples. The ratio of the abundance of each transcript is measured relative to the median abundance of the gene's transcript among all cell lines (left panel) and all tissue samples (right panel). (A) Scaled-down representation of the 1753 gene cluster diagram; the colored bars to the right identify the locations of the inserts displayed in parts C through J. (B) Dendrogram representing similarities in the expression patterns between experimental samples. All tumor pairs that were clustered together on terminal branches are highlighted in red; the two primary tumor/lymph node metastasis pairs are highlighted in light blue; the three clustered normal breast samples are highlighted in light green. The branches representing the four breast luminal epithelial cell lines are displayed in dark blue; breast basal epithelial cell lines are displayed in orange, the endothelial cell lines in dark yellow, the mesynchemal-like cell lines in dark green, and the lymphocyte-derived cell lines in brown. (C) Endothelial cell gene expression cluster. (D) Stromal/fibroblast cluster. (E) Breast basal epithelial cluster. (F) B-cell cluster. (G) Adipose-enriched/normal breast. (H) Macrophage. (I) T cell. (J) Breast luminal epithelial cell. (*Source*: Reprinted by permission from *Nature* 406, 17 August, 747–752, copyright 2000 Macmillan Publishers Ltd.) See insert for color representation of this figure.

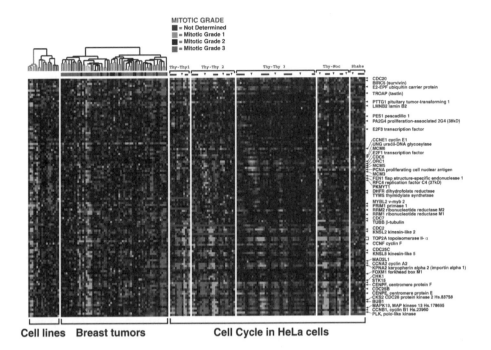

Figure 5-2. Cell cycle regulation of the breast tumor proliferation cluster. The expression patterns of 112 clones in the breast tumor proliferation cluster (Perou et al., 2000) were examined in the HeLa cell cycle data set (Whitfield et al., 2002) and compared with their expression in breast tumors and cell lines. The clones are ordered by their peak expression during the cell cycle such that each row corresponds to a single clone. The purple bars above each column in the HeLa data set represent S phase and the arrows indicate mitoses as estimated by flow cytometry or BrdU labeling. The order of the breast tumor samples based on hierarchical clustering is as in Figure 5-1. The mitotic grade of the tumors is indicated (a higher mitotic grade is indicative of a more proliferative tumor). Of the 112 genes in the proliferation cluster, 69 were identified as cell cycle regulated in this study. (*Source*: Reprinted from *Molecular Biology of the Cell* (2002: 13: 1977–2000), with permission by the American Society for Cell Biology). See insert for color representation of this figure.

express CD3δ and T-cell receptor subunits (Fig. 5-1I); macrophages, expressing the markers CD68, acid phosphatase 5, chitinase, and lysozyme (Fig. 5-1H); adipocyte-enriched normal breast, thought to be the cells of origin for the expression of genes like retinal-binding protein 4 (*RBP4*), lipoprotein lipase (*LPL*), and fatty acid–binding protein 4 (*FABP4*; Fig. 5-1G). Finally, the two distinct types of epithelial cells that are found in the human mammary gland (Ronnov-Jessen et al., 1996) are basal (and/or myoepithelial) cells characterized by the expression of the keratin markers 5, 17, and laminin (Fig. 5-1E), and luminal epithelial cells characterized by keratins 8 and 18 and the estrogen receptor cluster (Fig. 5-1J).

A major theme emerging from DNA microarray studies of tumors is the high degree of similarity among different samples of the same tumor and its metastases, suggesting a higher than generally expected level of histological organization and communication among the cells that comprise the tumors.

MOLECULAR PORTRAITS OF BREAST TUMORS: CLASSIFICATION

To explore the possibilities for refining distinctions among subtypes of breast tumors using microarrays, we took advantage of the paired tumor samples. The specific features of a gene expression pattern that are to be used as the basis for classifying tumors should be similar in any sample taken from the same tumor, and they should vary among different tumors. Therefore, the paired samples provided a unique opportunity for a deliberate and systematic search for genes whose expression levels reflected such intrinsic characteristics of the tumors.

From the genes whose expression was well measured in the 22 paired samples, we selected a subset of 496 genes (termed the intrinsic gene subset) that consisted of genes with significantly greater variation in expression between different tumors than between paired samples from the same tumor. This set of genes was enriched for those genes whose expression patterns were characteristic of each tumor as opposed to those that varied as a function of tissue sampling. When this set of genes was used as the basis for a new clustering analysis, 17 of the 20 "before" and "after" pairs were grouped together as well as both the tumor/lymph node metastasis pairs.

The tissue samples were separated into four discrete subgroups, one of which contained samples characterized by relatively high expression of genes that are known to be expressed by luminal epithelial cells. This was confirmed by an immunohistochemical analysis with antibodies against the luminal epithelial-specific keratins 8/18 (Perou et al., 2000). The expression characteristics of this cluster were anchored by estrogen receptor (*ER*), estrogen-regulated protein *LIV-1*, the transcription factors hepatocyte nuclear factor 3, alpha (*HNF3A*), X-box-binding protein 1 (*XBP1*), and GATA-binding protein 3 (*GATA3*). A second group contained samples that expressed genes characteristic of basal epithelial cells. To corroborate the basal-like (or myoepithelial) characteristics of these tumors, immunohistochemistry was performed using antibodies against the basal cell keratins 5/6 and 17. All six of these tumors showed staining for either keratins 5/6 or 17, or both. Notably, these six tumors also failed to express *ER* and most of the other coexpressed genes.

Overexpression of the *ERBB2* oncogene was associated with high expression of a specific subset of genes, most notably *GRB7* and *MLN64*, which are both located in the same region of chromosome 17. A third group of tumors was identified that was partially characterized by the high level of expression of this subset of genes. These tumors also showed low levels of expression of *ER* and almost all of the other genes associated with *ER* expression—a trait they share with the basal-like tumors. Finally, a few tumor samples and the single fibroadenoma analyzed clustered together with the three normal breast specimens. The accompanying normal breast gene expression pattern was typified by the high expression of genes characteristic of basal epithelial cells and adipose cells, and the low expression of genes characteristic of luminal epithelial cells.

A striking conclusion from these data is the stability, homogeneity, and uniqueness of the molecular portraits provided by the variation in gene expression patterns. We infer that these portraits faithfully represent the *tumor* itself, not merely the particular tumor *sample*, because we could recognize the distinctive expression pattern of a tumor in independent samples. An important implication of this study is that the clinical designation of estrogen receptor–negative breast carcinoma encompasses at least two biologically distinct subtypes of tumors (basal-like and *ERBB2* positive), which may need to be treated as distinct diseases. The implications of this discovery on clinical testing are discussed in Chapter 15.

Encouraged by these results, we extended the analysis to include more samples to further refine the subgroups of tumors and to assess potential clinical implications of these classifications. A set of 78 breast carcinomas, 3 fibroadenomas, and 4 normal breast tissues were analyzed and included the 40 tumors previously described (Sørlie et al., 2001). Using the same intrinsic gene set of 496 cDNA clones, representing 427 unique genes, a total of 85 experiments were analyzed by hierarchical clustering (Fig. 5-3A). The overall expression patterns showed that the main distinction was between tumors that express genes characteristic of luminal epithelial cells and those that are negative for these genes, as previously noted (Perou et al., 2000). The same subgroups of luminal, basal-like, *ERBB2*-overexpressing, and normal breast-like tumors were confirmed, but extending the data set allowed separation of the luminal/ER-positive tumors into two distinct subgroups: luminal A and luminal B (Fig. 5-3B).

The largest group of tumors (termed luminal subtype A, dark blue) demonstrated the highest expression of the estrogen receptor alpha gene (*ER*), GATA-binding protein 3 (*GATA3*), X-box-binding protein 1 (*XBP1*), trefoil factor 3 (*TFF1*), hepatocyte nuclear factor 3 alpha (*HN3A*), and estrogen-regulated LIV-1 protein (*LIV-1*; Fig. 5-3G). The second smaller group of tumors (termed luminal subtype B, light blue) showed low to moderate expression of the luminal-specific genes including the ER cluster but was further distinguished from luminal subtype A by the high expression of a novel set of genes whose coordinated function is unknown (Fig. 5-3D). Expression of this cluster of genes is a feature they share with the basal-like and ERBB2+ subtypes.

The basal-like subtype (red) was characterized by the high expression of keratins 5 and 17, laminin, and fatty acid–binding protein 7 (Fig. 5-3E), while the ERBB2+ subtype (pink) was characterized by the high expression of several genes in the *ERBB2* amplicon at 17q22.24 including *ERBB2, GRB7*, and *MLN64* (Fig. 5-3C). Tumor samples included in the normal breast-like group showed the highest expression of many genes known to be expressed by adipose tissue and other nonepithelial cell types (Fig. 5-3F). These tumors also showed strong expression of basal epithelial genes and low expression of luminal epithelial genes. However, it is unclear whether these tumors represent poorly sampled tumor tissue or a distinct, clinically important group. In summary, based solely on expression patterns of these 427 genes, the breast tissue specimens could be divided into five distinct subtypes.

Correlation to Patient Survival

A major goal in the field of oncogenomics is to try to answer the clinically important questions about which tumors will behave aggressively, which tumors will remain dormant, which patients require systemic therapy, and what type of drugs should be used. To search for genes whose expression correlates to patient survival and hence could prove useful for tumor classification, we performed SAM using overall survival as the supervising variable. This approach resulted in a list of 264 cDNA clones, using a significance threshold expected to produce fewer than 30 false positives. Expression data were retrieved from all 85 experiments using the SAM264 clone set, and hierarchical clustering analysis showed that almost all of the 264 cDNA clones fell into three main gene expression clusters: the luminal/ER+ cluster, the basal epithelial

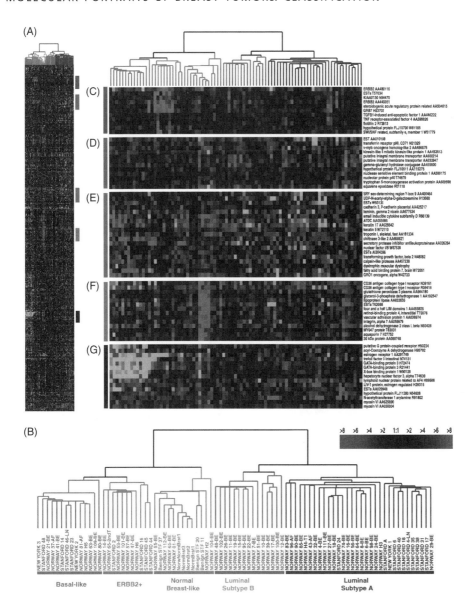

Figure 5-3. Gene expression patterns of 85 experimental samples analyzed by hierarchical clustering using the 496 cDNA intrinsic clone set. A total of 78 carcinomas, 3 benign tumors, and 4 normal tissues are represented in this data set. (A) The full-cluster diagram scaled down. The colored bars on the right represent the inserts presented in parts C through G. The tumor specimens were divided into five subtypes based on differences in gene expression. (B) The cluster dendrogram showing the five subtypes of tumors colored accordingly. Luminal subtype A = dark blue, luminal subtype B = light blue, normal breast-like = green, basal-like = red, and ERBB2+ = pink. (C) *ERBB2* amplicon cluster. (D) Novel unknown cluster highly expressed in luminal subtype B cluster. (E) Basal epithelial cell–enriched cluster. (F) Normal breast-like cluster. (G) Luminal epithelial gene cluster containing *ER*. (*Source:* PNAS, September 11, 2001, vol. 98, no. 19, 10869–10874. Copyright [2001] National Academy of Sciences, U.S.A.) See insert for color representation of this figure.

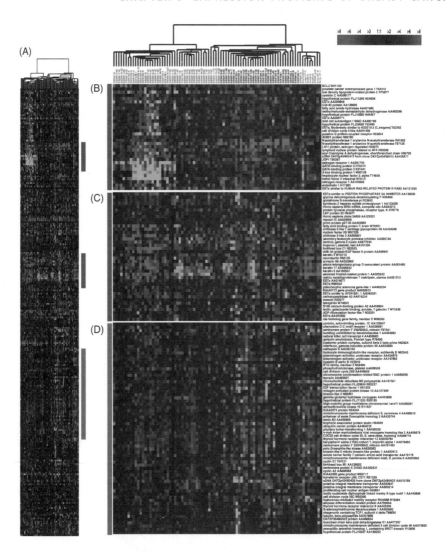

Figure 5-4. Hierarchical clustering using the SAM264 gene set and 78 carcinoma samples. (A) The full-cluster diagram scaled down. (B) The luminal epithelial-specific gene cluster including the estrogen receptor is expressed by the luminal subtype A and B tumors color coded as in Figure 5-3. (C) The basal epithelial gene cluster expressed by the basal-like tumors and the normal breast-like tumors. (D) The proliferation cluster. These genes are mainly expressed by tumors in the basal-like, ERBB2+, and luminal subtype B groups of tumors. (*Source*: PNAS, September 11, 2001, vol. 98, no. 19, 10869–10874. Copyright [2001] National Academy of Sciences, U.S.A.) See insert for color representation of this figure.

cluster that contained keratins 5 and 17, and the previously described proliferation cluster (Fig. 5.4).

The branching patterns in the resulting dendrogram organized the tumors into four main groups. The largest group (dark blue labels) consisted of tumors with the luminal/ER+ characteristics and corresponded almost exactly to the luminal subtype

A from Figure 5-3. The genes comprising the *ERBB2* amplicon from the intrinsic gene list were not included in the SAM clone set, which resulted in a merging of the ERBB2+ subtype with the basal-like tumors into a larger group (red and pink sample names). Notably, all but one of the basal-like tumors clustered together on a distal branch within this larger group. The luminal subtype B and the normal breast-like group were largely grouped as in the original cluster in Figure 5-3. In conclusion, 71 of 78 carcinomas were organized into the same main subtypes when using the list of 264 survival-correlated cDNA clones as compared to using the intrinsic set of 456 clones (with only 81 genes that overlap).

To investigate whether the five different tumor subgroups identified by hierarchical clustering may represent clinically distinct groups of patients, univariate survival analyses comparing the subtypes with respect to overall survival (OS) and relapse-free survival (RFS) were performed. For all survival analyses, only 49 of the patients from a prospective study on locally advanced disease and with no distant metastases were used (Geisler et al., 2001). The Kaplan-Meier curves based on the five subclasses from Figure 5-3 showed a highly significant difference in OS between the patients belonging to the different subclasses (Fig. 5-5A, $p < 0.01$). Specifically, the basal-like and ERBB2+ subtypes were associated with the shortest survival times. Similar results were obtained with respect to RFS (Fig. 5-5B). These two tumor subtypes were characterized by distinct variations in gene expression that were different from the luminal subtype tumors. Overexpression of the ERBB2 oncoprotein is a well-known prognostic factor associated with poor survival in breast cancer.

Perhaps the most intriguing result is the considerable difference in outcome observed between tumors classified as luminal A versus luminal B. While the ER protein value (determined by ligand binding) differed between the two groups (mean 111 and 60, respectively), not all luminal A tumors showed high values (9, > 100 fmol/mg; 5, 30–100 fmol/mg; 4, 10–30 fmol/mg; 1, < 10 fmol/mg). It should also be noted that the ER-positive protein category (>9 fmol/mg) cases based on ligand binding were highly heterogeneous with respect to their gene expression profiles (18/19 luminal A, 15/15 luminal B, 2/7 basal-like, 4/5 ERBB2+, and 4/5 normal breast-like tumors). Indeed, this is reflected in the survival curves when the ER protein expression alone (negative, <9 fmol/mg protein; positive, >9 fmol/mg protein) was used to stratify the cases in a Kaplan-Meier analysis (Fig. 5-5C).

The prognostic value is poorer when compared to a three-group distinction in which expression values of the five main genes in the ER cluster are used to rank the tumors (Fig. 5-5D). The luminal subtype B tumors might represent a clinically distinct group with a more serious disease course, in particular with respect to relapse. Perhaps this subtype reflects a group of patients who will not benefit from adjuvant tamoxifen therapy despite positive receptor values. It should be noted that all patients in this study were given adjuvant tamoxifen provided they had positive receptor values (ER and/or PgR). The potential clinical significance of this molecular subtype is further highlighted by the similarities in expression of some of the genes with the ER-negative tumors in the basal-like and ERBB2+ subtypes, which suggests that the high level of expression of this set of genes is associated with poor disease outcomes.

Corroboration of the Subgroups

Following the identification of these five subtypes, validation in larger data sets and, more importantly, in independent data sets, is essential. For an extended analysis, we

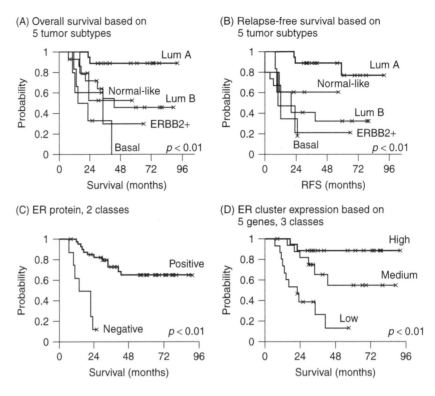

Figure 5-5. Survival analyses of breast cancer patients based on different classification schemes. (A) Overall survival (OS) and (B) relapse-free survival (RFS) for the five expression-based tumor subtypes based on the classification presented in Figure 5-3. (C) Overall survival estimated for a two-group classification based on expression of the estrogen receptor protein. (D) Overall survival based on a three-group classification using the expression values of five genes in the estrogen receptor gene cluster (estrogen receptor, GATA-binding protein 3, hepatocyte nuclear factor 3, X-box-binding protein 1, trefoil factor 3). (*Source*: PNAS, September 11, 2001, vol. 98, no. 19, 10869–10874. Copyright [2001] National Academy of Sciences, U.S.A.)

included 37 additional tumors from a second study on locally advanced breast cancer. These patients were enrolled in a prospective study aimed at evaluating predictive markers for response to chemotherapy (Geisler et al., 2003). This study was designed similarly to the earlier study described (Geisler et al., 2001). Extending the sample size to a total of 115 breast cancer cases corroborated the subgroups and the underlying specific gene expression patterns. Using 45 tumor pairs, a new intrinsic list containing 534 genes was generated using the same criteria as before, by searching for genes whose expression levels varied little between before and after measurements for a subject but showed significant variation between the subjects. A hierarchical clustering analysis using expression data extracted using these 534 genes showed that the tumors were grouped into the same five subtypes characterized by variation in expression of approximately the same specific clusters of genes (Sørlie et al., 2003) (Fig. 5-6).

Moreover, Kaplan-Meier analyses based on four subtypes (excluding the normal-like group) confirmed the significant difference in prognosis for the patients belonging

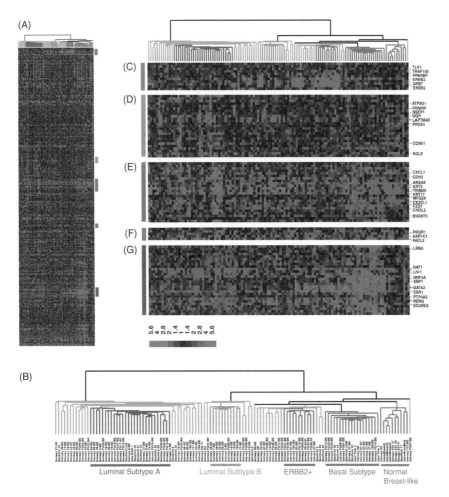

Figure 5-6. Hierarchical clustering of 115 tumor tissues and 7 nonmalignant tissues using the intrinsic gene set. (A) Scaled down representation of the entire cluster of 534 genes and 122 tissue samples based on similarities in gene expression. (B) Experimental dendrogram showing the clustering of the tumors into five subgroups. Branches corresponding to tumors with low correlation to any subtype are shown in gray. (C) Gene cluster showing the *ERBB2* oncogene and other co-expressed genes. (D) Gene cluster associated with luminal subtype B. (E) Gene cluster associated with the basal subtype. (F) Gene cluster relevant for the normal breast-like group. (G) Cluster of genes including the estrogen receptor (*ER*) highly expressed in luminal subtype A tumors. Scale bar represents fold change for any given gene relative to the median level of expression across all samples. (*Source*: PNAS, July 8, 2003, vol. 100, no. 14, 8418–8423. Copyright [2003] National Academy of Sciences, U.S.A.) See insert for color representation of this figure.

to the various subclasses. Again, the relatively poor survival associated with having a tumor with a luminal subtype B profile is particularly interesting. In conclusion, the inherent properties of the tumors seem to be sustained throughout chemotherapy as well as between a primary tumor and its lymph node metastasis, and could be represented by a relatively small number of genes whose variation in expression forms a platform for classification.

The robustness of the tumor subtypes was further tested by conducting an analysis on an independent data set published by van't Veer et al. (2002). The authors investigated tumors from 78 women with lymph node–negative breast cancer, about half of whom had remained disease-free for at least 5 years; the other half developed metastases before 5 years. Expression data were extracted using 461 of the intrinsic genes described previously that were common between the two data sets and analyzed by hierarchical clustering. The same subtypes were identified and characterized by similar variation in gene expression, suggesting that these five subtypes are robust and inherent to breast cancer despite clinical and histopathological differences between the tumors (Sørlie et al., 2003).

THE ROLE OF *TP53*

Differences in biological characteristics of tumors, their aggressiveness and clinical course, are likely to be linked to variation in expression patterns and underlying genetic alterations in regulatory genes. *TP53* plays an important role in directing cellular responses to genotoxic damage and regulates the activation of downstream genes that are involved in apoptosis, cell cycle arrest, and DNA repair (Balint and Vousden, 2001; Guimaraes and Hainaut, 2002; Hussain et al., 2000; Vogelstein et al., 2000). Previous studies have shown that mutations in the *TP53* gene predict poor prognosis and are associated with poor response to systemic therapy (Bergh et al., 1995; Berns et al., 2000; Borresen et al., 1995; Geisler et al., 2001). Even though *TP53* itself is not differentially expressed across this sample set, it is likely that *TP53* has a significant role in shaping the gene expression patterns in the various tumor subtypes. The coding region of the *TP53* gene (exons 2–11) was screened for mutations in all but 8 tumor samples (not including benign tumors; Sørlie et al., 2002). The distribution of the frequency of mutations among the different subclasses was significantly different ($p < 0.001$, two-sided). Luminal subtype A contained only 11% mutated tumors, whereas the luminal B, ERBB2+, and basal-like subclasses had 68%, 72%, and 76% *TP53*-mutated tumors, respectively. The finding of *TP53* mutations in tumors that simultaneously express the *ERBB2* gene at high levels supports previous observations of an interdependent role for *TP53* and *ERBB2* (Nakopoulou et al., 1996; Geisler et al., 2001).

To more directly investigate the effect of *TP53* mutations on the genome-wide expression patterns across the tumors, we searched for genes whose levels of expression were consistently different between *TP53*-mutated and *TP53* wild-type tumors (Wilcoxon rank sum test, $p < 0.1$; Fig. 5-7). As expected, many of the genes that were highly expressed in tumors containing a mutated *TP53* gene are cell cycle–regulated genes such as *BUB1*, *CDC25B*, *S100A8*, and *MCM4* (Whitfield et al., 2002). Oncogenes including *MYBL2* and *YES1*, a number of kinases (*PLK, PTK7, PGK1*), and *ST14*, a protease proposed to play a role in breast cancer invasion and metastasis (Lin et al., 1999), were also included in the list of genes highly correlated with *TP53* mutations.

Interestingly, many of the genes whose high expression and specific pattern distinguished luminal subtype B from subtype A were highly expressed in *TP53*-mutated tumors. Among the genes highly expressed in the tumors with a wild-type *TP53* gene, most of the genes in the luminal/ER+ cluster (*ER, GATA-3*, etc.) were found, and they recapitulate the low *TP53* mutation rate of the luminal subtype A. Further studies

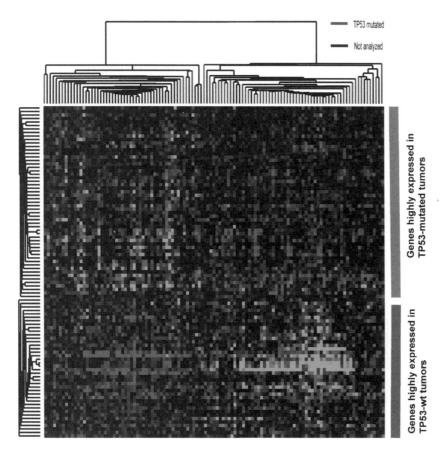

Figure 5-7. Cluster of genes associated with *TP53* mutational status. Hierarchical clustering of 95 genes whose expressions were significantly correlated to the mutation status of the *TP53* gene (Wilcoxon rank sum test, $p < 0.1$). Tumor tissue from 115 patients was included in the analysis of which 51 were *TP53* mutant (red branches) and 56 *TP53* wild type (black branches) (8 not tested). See insert for color representation of this figure.

are needed to determine which of the genes are direct targets of *TP53* and which are only associated with a particular expression phenotype. Finally, the organization of the tumors into two main groups can be used to infer the mutational status of tumors not available for mutational analysis.

COMPARATIVE GENOMIC HYBRIDIZATION ON ARRAYS (aCGH)

The power of microarrays is also illustrated in their broad range of utility; the same cDNA microarrays can be used to investigate both the structural and the expressed genome (see Chapter 3 for more details). Variations in gene expression captured by analyzing the tumor RNA may be caused by underlying genomic DNA copy number alterations, which are key genetic events in the development and progression of human cancers. For example, highly amplified genes that are also highly expressed are a priori the strongest candidate oncogenes within an amplicon. To explore which changes in the genome coincide with changes in expression, genome-wide microarray comparative genomic hybridization (array CGH) analysis was performed on a subset of the breast tumors that were analyzed for variations in gene expression. In total, a profile was generated across 6691 mapped human genes in 45 primary breast tumors and 10 breast cancer cell lines (Pollack et al., 2002). The 6691 cDNAs were ordered according to the "Golden Path" (genome.ucsc.edu/) genome assembly of the draft human genome sequences (Lander et al., 2001). In this way, the arrayed cDNAs not only represent genes of potential interest themselves (e.g., candidate oncogenes within amplicons) but also provide precise genetic landmarks for chromosomal regions of amplification and deletion.

Numerous DNA copy number alterations were detected in the tumors despite the presence of euploid nontumor cell types; the magnitudes of the observed changes were generally lower in the tumor samples than the tumor cell lines. DNA copy number

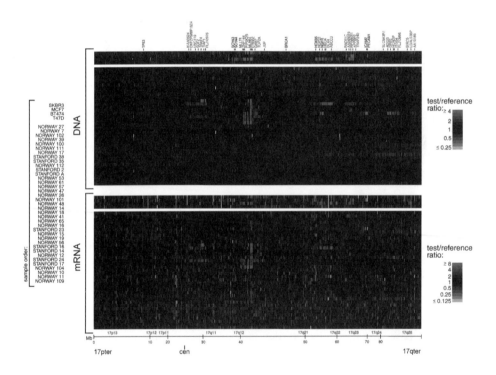

Figure 5-8. Concordance between DNA copy number and gene expression across chromosome 17. DNA copy number alteration (upper panel) and mRNA levels (lower panel) are illustrated for breast cancer cell lines and tumors. Breast cancer cell lines and tumors are separately ordered by hierarchical clustering in the upper panel, and the identical sample order is maintained in the lower panel. The 354 genes present on the microarrays and mapping to chromosome 17, and for which both DNA copy number and mRNA levels were determined, are ordered by position along the chromosome; selected genes are indicated in color-coded text (Pollack et al., 2002). Fluorescence ratios (test/reference) are depicted by separate $\log_2$ pseudocolor scales (indicated). (*Source*: PNAS, October 1, 2002, vol. 99, no. 20, 12963–12968. Copyright [2002] National Academy of Sciences, U.S.A.) See insert for color representation of this figure.

alterations were identified in all cancer cell lines and nearly all (40 of 45) tumors, and on every human chromosome in at least one sample. Recurrent regions of DNA copy number gain and loss were readily identifiable; gains within 1q, 8q, 17q, and 20q were observed in all breast cancer cell lines and a large proportion of tumor samples (75%, 48%, 50%, and 34%, respectively), which are consistent with published cytogenetic studies (Forozan et al., 2000; Kallioniemi et al., 1994; Tirkkonen et al., 1998).

The parallel measurements of mRNA levels and copy number alterations revealed a global impact of widespread DNA copy number alteration on gene expression in tumor cells. The overall patterns of gene amplification and elevated gene expression are quite concordant; i.e., a significant fraction of highly amplified genes appear to be correspondingly highly expressed. Genome-wide, of 117 high-level DNA amplifications (fluorescence ratios > 4, representing 91 different genes), 42% (representing 36 different genes) were associated with comparably highly elevated mRNA levels (mean-centered fluorescence ratios > 4). Furthermore, 62% (representing 54 different genes) were associated with at least moderately elevated mRNA levels (mean-centered fluorescence ratios > 2). The concordance between high-level amplification and increased gene expression is best illustrated for genes on chromosome 17 (Fig. 5-8), where the amplicon containing the oncogene *ERBB2* is located (Coussens et al., 1985). This genome-wide array-based CGH analysis demonstrates the utility of defining amplicon boundaries and shape at high resolution (gene by gene) when attempting to identify candidate oncogenes. Although this method does not show equally good sensitivity in detecting genomic deletions, the global effect of changes in DNA copy number on gene expression can readily be measured.

POTENTIAL CLINICAL IMPLICATIONS AND UTILITY: IDENTIFICATION OF NOVEL MARKERS

The identification of clinically different tumor subtypes based on variation in gene expression patterns of particular subsets of genes and the specific underlying genomic alterations unveil previously unknown genes that may be involved in tumorigenesis. Knowledge about these genes, their products, and how they correlate to different aspects of the disease may improve our understanding of the biology of breast cancer and lead to new prognostic and predictive markers. The distinct expression pattern of the luminal subtype A discussed earlier includes a gene termed *RERG* (ras-related and estrogen-regulated growth inhibitor) that is coexpressed with the estrogen receptor. Its high expression is correlated with a favorable prognosis for patients ($p < 0.01$, univariate analysis; Finlin et al., 2001).

This gene encodes a novel member of the Ras superfamily of small GTPases. *RERG* has biochemical properties characteristic of the Ras proteins, including an intrinsic ability to bind and hydrolyze GTP in a Mg^{2+}-dependent manner, as observed for other GTPases (Bourne et al., 1991). However, contrary to other Ras-related proteins, it lacks any known COOH-terminal prenylation motif (Casey and Seabra, 1996), it demonstrated cytoplastic and nuclear localization, and it showed no interaction with common Ras effectors. The promoter region of *RERG* contains two potential ER-binding sites, suggesting it may be an estrogen-responsive gene. Its expression demonstrates a high degree of correlation with ER in both primary tumors and breast tissue–derived cell lines.

Upon stimulation with β-estradiol, *RERG* was rapidly induced in MCF-7 breast cancer cells, whereas it was completely repressed by tamoxifen, an ER antagonist. By comparing the expression pattern of *RERG* across the breast tumors to the expression of the previously mentioned proliferation cluster, it became evident that the tumors that most highly expressed *RERG* tended to be the least proliferative, and the tumors with low to no *RERG* expression were the most proliferative (Sørlie et al., 2001). The gene is located at 12p12, a chromosomal region that is not amplified in these tumors, which shows that the overexpression of *RERG* is due to other means of regulation. Furthermore, this could indicate that overexpression of *RERG* inhibits growth of tumor cells. Indeed, MCF-7 cells stably overexpressing *RERG* showed reduced rates of cell proliferation, both anchorage dependent and independent. Furthermore, *RERG* tended to slow tumor growth in vivo when overexpressing MCF-7 cells were subcutaneously injected into nude mice. Taken together, these results point to an important role for *RERG* function in the development of breast cancer, particularly in the physiological response to estrogen.

This study sets an example of how genome-wide molecular profiling can be used to search for clinically relevant markers. Similar variation in expression of a set of genes across a set of samples indicates similar means of regulation and function, thus providing a powerful way of identifying novel biologically important genes that could be used as markers and targets for therapy. The strength of this method lies in the ability to identify clusters of genes that in a unique combination will distinguish subgroups of disease and predict outcome or treatment response. Such a multigene approach will undoubtedly be superior to standard clinical markers currently in use.

CONCLUSION

Molecular portraits of tumors identified by specific patterns of gene expression and variation in DNA copy number using microarray technology offer great promise for cancer diagnosis and treatment. This technology represents a new approach to enhance our understanding of the biology of cancer development and progression and the mechanisms behind chemoresistance. By linking genome-wide expression profiles to tumor aggressiveness, patient survival, and response to therapy, better classification schemes may emerge and lead to improved patient care. Importantly, the power of this technology relies on a strong interface between biology and informatics. Bringing together experts from different disciplines is necessary to extract the information embedded in the massive data and to bring the field of molecular medicine forward.

Moreover, development of public informational databases, more uniform platforms, and a common "language" for reporting microarray experiments are required so that researchers can better compare and verify each other's results. Such endeavors are underway with the public repositories Gene Expression Omnibus (GEO; www.ncbi.nlm.nih.gov/geo/) and ArrayExpress (www.ebi.ac.uk/microarray/ArrayExpress/arrayexpress.html), and the two projects MIAME (Minimum Information About a Microarray Experiment) and MAGE-ML (MicroArray Gene Expression Markup Language) developed by the Microarray Gene Expression Data Group (MGED; www.mged.org/). Finally, the public availability of microarray data underlying published studies will be increasingly important because, as we have described, microarray data can be aggregated and analyzed so that the sum is much more than the parts.

REFERENCES

Aas, T., Borresen, A. L., Geisler, S., Smith-Sorensen, B., Johnsen, H., Varhaug, J. E., Akslen, L. A., and Lonning, P. E. (1996). Specific P53 mutations are associated with de novo resistance to doxorubicin in breast cancer patients. *Nat Med 2*, 811–814.

Alizadeh, A. A., Eisen, M. B., Davis, R. E., Ma, C., Lossos, I. S., Rosenwald, A., Boldrick, J. C., Sabet, H., Tran, T., Yu, X., Powell, J. I., Yang, L., Marti, G. E., Moore, T., Hudson, J., Jr., Lu, L., Lewis, D. B., Tibshirani, R., Sherlock, G., Chan, W. C., Greiner, T. C., Weisenburger, D. D., Armitage, J. O., Warnke, R., and Staudt, L. M., et al. (2000). Distinct types of diffuse large B-cell lymphoma identified by gene expression profiling. *Nature 403*, 503–11.

Balint, E. E., and Vousden, K. H. (2001). Activation and activities of the p53 tumour suppressor protein. *Br J Cancer 85*, 1813–1823.

Bergh, J., Norberg, T., Sjogren, S., Lindgren, A., and Holmberg, L. (1995). Complete sequencing of the p53 gene provides prognostic information in breast cancer patients, particularly in relation to adjuvant systemic therapy and radiotherapy. *Nat Med 1*, 1029–1034.

Berns, E. M., Foekens, J. A., Vossen, R., Look, M. P., Devilee, P., Henzen-Logmans, S. C., van Staveren, I. L., van Putten, W. L., Inganas, M., Meijer-van Gelder, M. E., Cornelisse, C., Claassen, C. J., Portengen, H., Bakker, B., and Klijn, J. G. (2000). Complete sequencing of TP53 predicts poor response to systemic therapy of advanced breast cancer. *Cancer Res 60*, 2155–2162.

Borresen, A. L., Andersen, T. I., Eyfjord, J. E., Cornelis, R. S., Thorlacius, S., Borg, A., Johansson, U., Theillet, C., Scherneck, S., and Hartman, S. (1995). TP53 mutations and breast cancer prognosis: Particularly poor survival rates for cases with mutations in the zinc-binding domains. *Genes Chromosomes Cancer 14*, 71–75.

Bourne, H. R., Sanders, D. A., and McCormick, F. (1991). The GTPase superfamily: Conserved structure and molecular mechanism. *Nature 349*, 117–127.

Brown, M. P., Grundy, W. N., Lin, D., Cristianini, N., Sugnet, C. W., Furey, T. S., Ares, M., Jr., and Haussler, D. (2000). Knowledge-based analysis of microarray gene expression data by using support vector machines. *Proc Natl Acad Sci USA 97*, 262–267.

Casey, P. J., and Seabra, M. C. (1996). Protein prenyltransferases. *J Biol Chem 271*, 5289–5292.

Chen, X., Cheung, S. T., So, S., Fan, S. T., Barry, C., Higgins, J., Lai, K. M., Ji, J., Dudoit, S., Ng, I. O., van de, R. M., Botstein, D., and Brown, P. O. (2002). Gene expression patterns in human liver cancers. *Mol Biol Cell 13*, 1929–1939.

Coussens, L., Yang-Feng, T. L., Liao, Y. C., Chen, E., Gray, A., McGrath, J., Seeburg, P. H., Libermann, T. A., Schlessinger, J., Francke, U., et al. (1985). Tyrosine kinase receptor with extensive homology to EGF receptor shares chromosomal location with neu oncogene. *Science 230*, 1132–1139.

Eisen, M. B., and Brown, P. O. (1999). DNA arrays for analysis of gene expression. *Methods Enzymol 303*, 179–205.

Eisen, M. B., Spellman, P. T., Brown, P. O., and Botstein, D. (1998). Cluster analysis and display of genome-wide expression patterns. *Proc Natl Acad Sci USA 95*, 14863–14868.

Finlin, B. S., Gau, C. L., Murphy, G. A., Shao, H., Kimel, T., Seitz, R. S., Chiu, Y. F., Botstein, D., Brown, P. O., Der, C. J., Tamanoi, F., Andres, D. A., and Perou, C. M. (2001). RERG is a novel ras-related, estrogen-regulated and growth-inhibitory gene in breast cancer. *J Biol Chem 276*, 42259–42267.

Forozan, F., Mahlamaki, E. H., Monni, O., Chen, Y., Veldman, R., Jiang, Y., Gooden, G. C., Ethier, S. P., Kallioniemi, A., and Kallioniemi, O. P. (2000). Comparative genomic hybridization analysis of 38 breast cancer cell lines: A basis for interpreting complementary DNA microarray data. *Cancer Res 60*, 4519–4525.

Galaktionov, K., Lee, A. K., Eckstein, J., Draetta, G., Meckler, J., Loda, M., and Beach, D. (1995). CDC25 phosphatases as potential human oncogenes. *Science 269*, 1575–1577.

Garber, M. E., Troyanskaya, O. G., Schluens, K., Petersen, S., Thaesler, Z., Pacyna-Gengelbach, M., van de, R. M., Rosen, G. D., Perou, C. M., Whyte, R. I., Altman, R. B., Brown, P. O., Botstein, D., and Petersen, I. (2001). Diversity of gene expression in adenocarcinoma of the lung. *Proc Natl Acad Sci USA 98*, 13784–13789.

Geisler, S., Lønning, P. E., Aas, T., Johnsen, H., Fluge, Ø., et al. (2001). Influence of TP53 gene alterations and c-erbB2 expression on the response to treatment with doxorubicin in locally advanced breast cancer. *Cancer Res 61*, 2505–2512.

Geisler, S., Børresen-Dale, A.-L., Johnsen, H., Aas, T., Geisler, J., Akslen, L. A., Anker, G., and Lønning, P. E. (2003). *TP53* gene mutations predict the response to neoadjuvant treatment with 5-fluorouracil and mitomycin in locally advanced breast cancer. *Clin Cancer Res 9*, 5582–5588.

Golub, T. R., Slonim, D. K., Tamayo, P., Huard, C., Gaasenbeek, M., Mesirov, J. P., Coller, H., Loh, M. L., Downing, J. R., Caligiuri, M. A., Bloomfield, C. D., and Lander, E. S. (1999). Molecular classification of cancer: Class discovery and class prediction by gene expression monitoring. *Science 286*, 531–537.

Guimaraes, D. P., and Hainaut, P. (2002). TP53: A key gene in human cancer. *Biochimie 84*, 83–93.

Hastie, T., Tibshirani, R., Botstein, D., and Brown, P. (2001). Supervised harvesting of expression trees. *Genome Biol 2*, RESEARCH0003. 1–0003.12.

Hedenfalk, I., Duggan, D., Chen, Y., Radmacher, M., Bittner, M., Simon, R., Meltzer, P., Gusterson, B., Esteller, M., Kallioniemi, O. P., Wilfond, B., Borg, A., and Trent, J. (2001). Gene-expression profiles in hereditary breast cancer. *N Engl J Med 344*, 539–548.

Hughes, T. R., Mao, M., Jones, A. R., Burchard, J., Marton, M. J., Shannon, K. W., Lefkowitz, S. M., Ziman, M., Schelter, J. M., Meyer, M. R., Kobayashi, S., Davis, C., Dai, H., He, Y. D., Stephaniants, S. B., Cavet, G., Walker, W. L., West, A., Coffey, E., Shoemaker, D. D., Stoughton, R., Blanchard, A. P., Friend, S. H., and Linsley, P. S. (2001). Expression profiling using microarrays fabricated by an ink-jet oligonucleotide synthesizer. *Nat Biotechnol 19*, 342–347.

Hussain, S. P., Hollstein, M. H., and Harris, C. C. (2000). p53 tumor suppressor gene: At the crossroads of molecular carcinogenesis, molecular epidemiology, and human risk assessment. *Ann NY Acad Sci 919*, 79–85.

Kallioniemi, A., Kallioniemi, O. P., Piper, J., Tanner, M., Stokke, T., Chen, L., Smith, H. S., Pinkel, D., Gray, J. W., and Waldman, F. M. (1994). Detection and mapping of amplified DNA sequences in breast cancer by comparative genomic hybridization. *Proc Natl Acad Sci USA 91*, 2156–2160.

Kane, M. D., Jatkoe, T. A., Stumpf, C. R., Lu, J., Thomas, J. D., and Madore, S. J. (2000). Assessment of the sensitivity and specificity of oligonucleotide (50mer) microarrays. *Nucleic Acids Res 28*, 4552–4557.

Khan, J., Wei, J. S., Ringner, M., Saal, L. H., Ladanyi, M., Westermann, F., Berthold, F., Schwab, M., Antonescu, C. R., Peterson, C., and Meltzer, P. S. (2001). Classification and diagnostic prediction of cancers using gene expression profiling and artificial neural networks. *Nat Med 7*, 673–679.

Lander, E. S., et al. (2001). Initial sequencing and analysis of the human genome. *Nature 409*, 860–921.

Lin, C. Y., Anders, J., Johnson, M., Sang, Q. A., and Dickson, R. B. (1999). Molecular cloning of cDNA for matriptase, a matrix-degrading serine protease with trypsin-like activity. *J Biol Chem 274*, 18231–18236.

Nakopoulou, L. L., Alexiadou, A., Theodoropoulos, G. E., Lazaris, A. C., Tzonou, A., and Keramopoulos, A. (1996). Prognostic significance of the co-expression of p53 and c-erbB-2 proteins in breast cancer. *J Pathol 179*, 31–38.

Parkin, D. M., Bray, F., Ferlay, J., and Pisani, P. (2001). Estimating the world cancer burden: Globocan 2000. *Int J Cancer 94*, 153–156.

Pease, A. C., Solas, D., Sullivan, E. J., Cronin, M. T., Holmes, C. P., Folor, S. P. (1994). Light-generated oligonucleotide arrays for rapid DNA sequence analysis. *Proc Natl. Acad. Sci. USA 91*, 5022–5026.

Perou, C. M., Jeffrey, S. S., van de Rijn, M., Rees, C. A., Eisen, M. B., Ross, D. T., Pergamenschikov, A., Williams, C. F., Zhu, S. X., Lee, J. C., Lashkari, D., Shalon, D., Brown, P. O., and Botstein, D. (1999). Distinctive gene expression patterns in human mammary epithelial cells and breast cancers. *Proc Natl Acad Sci USA 96*, 9212–9217.

Perou, C. M., Sorlie, T., Eisen, M. B., van de, R. M., Jeffrey, S. S., Rees, C. A., Pollack, J. R., Ross, D. T., Johnsen, H., Akslen, L. A., Fluge, O., Pergamenschikov, A., Williams, C., Zhu, S. X., Lonning, P. E., A. L., Brown,P. O., and Botstein,D. (2000). Molecular portraits of human breast tumours. *Nature 406*, 747–752.

Pollack, J. R., Perou, C. M., Alizadeh, A. A., Eisen, M. B., Pergamenschikov, A., Williams, C. F., Jeffrey, S. S., Botstein, D., and Brown, P. O. (1999). Genome-wide analysis of DNA copy-number changes using cDNA microarrays. *Nat Genet 23*, 41–46.

Pollack, J. R., Sørlie, T., Perou, C. M., Rees, C., Lønning, P. E., Tibhirani, R., Botstein, D., Børresen-Dale, A. L., and Brown, P. O. (2002). Microarray analysis reveals a major direct role of DNA copy number alteration in the transcriptional program of human breast tumors. *Proc Natl Acad Sci USA 99*, 12963–12968.

Ronnov-Jessen, L., Petersen, O. W., and Bissell, M. J. (1996). Cellular changes involved in conversion of normal to malignant breast: Importance of the stromal reaction. *Physiol Rev 76*, 69–125.

Ross, D. T., Scherf, U., Eisen, M. B., Perou, C. M., Rees, C., Spellman, P., Iyer, V., Jeffrey, S. S., van de Rijn, M., Waltham, M., Pergamenschikov, A., Lee, J. C., Lashkari, D., Shalon, D., Myers, T. G., Weinstein, J. N., Botstein, D., and Brown, P. O. (2000). Systematic variation in gene expression patterns in human cancer cell lines. *Nat Genet 24*, 227–235.

Schena, M., Shalon, D., Davis, R. W., and Brown, P. O. (1995). Quantitative monitoring of gene expression patterns with a complementary DNA microarray. *Science 270*, 467–470.

Sen, G. C. (2001). Viruses and interferons. *Annu Rev Microbiol 55*, 255–281.

Smith, M. R., Wilson, M. L., Hamanaka, R., Chase, D., Kung, H., Longo, D. L., and Ferris, D. K. (1997). Malignant transformation of mammalian cells initiated by constitutive expression of the polo-like kinase. *Biochem Biophys Res Commun 234*, 397–405.

Sørlie, T., Perou, C. M., Tibshirani, R., Aas, T., Geisler, S., Johnsen, H., Hastie, T., Eisen, M. B., van de, R. M., Jeffrey, S. S., Thorsen, T., Quist, H., Matese, J. C., Brown, P. O., Botstein, D., Eystein, L. P., and Børresen-Dale, A. L. (2001). Gene expression patterns of breast carcinomas distinguish tumor subclasses with clinical implications. *Proc Natl Acad Sci USA 98*, 10869–10874.

Sørlie, T., Johnsen, H., Vu, P., Lind, G. E., Lothe, R., and Børresen-Dale, A.-L. (2004). Protocol for mutation screening of the *TP53* gene by temporal temperature gel electrophoresis (TTGE). In P. Keohavong, and S. G. Grant (eds.). *Molecular Toxicology Protocols*, Humana Press, Totowa, New Jersey.

Sørlie, T., Tibshirani, T., Parker, J., Hastie, T., Marron, J. S., Nobel, A., Deng, S., Johnsen, H., Pesich, R., Geisler, S., Perou, C. M., Lønning, P. E., Brown, P. O., Børresen-Dale, A.-L., and Botstein, D. (2003). Repeated observation of breast tumor subtypes in independent gene expression data sets. *Proc Natl Acad Sci USA 100*, 8418–8423.

Tibshirani, R., Hastie, T., Narasimhan, B., and Chu, G. (2002). Diagnosis of multiple cancer types by shrunken centroids of gene expression. *Proc Natl Acad Sci USA 99*, 6567–6572.

Tirkkonen, M., Tanner, M., Karhu, R., Kallioniemi, A., Isola, J., and Kallioniemi, O. P. (1998). Molecular cytogenetics of primary breast cancer by CGH. *Genes Chromosomes Cancer 21*, 177–184.

Tusher, V. G., Tibshirani, R., and Chu, G. (2001). Significance analysis of microarrays applied to the ionizing radiation response. *Proc Natl Acad Sci USA 98*, 5116–5121.

van't Veer, L. J., Dai, H., van de Vijver, M. J., He, Y. D., Hart, A. A., Mao, M., Peterse, H. L., van der, K. K., Marton, M. J., Witteveen, A. T., Schreiber, G. J., Kerkhoven, R. M., Roberts, C., Linsley, P. S., Bernards, R., and Friend, S. H. (2002). Gene expression profiling predicts clinical outcome of breast cancer. *Nature 415*, 530–536.

Vogelstein, B., Lane, D., and Levine, A. J. (2000). Surfing the p53 network. *Nature 408*, 307–310.

Whitfield, M. L., Sherlock, G., Saldanha, A. J., Murray, J. I., Ball, C. A., Alexander, K. E., Matese, J. C., Perou, C. M., Hurt, M. M., Brown, P. O., and Botstein, D. (2002). Identification of genes periodically expressed in the human cell cycle and their expression in tumors. *Mol Biol Cell 13*, 1977–2000.

Zhou, H., Kuang, J., Zhong, L., Kuo, W. L., Gray, J. W., Sahin, A., Brinkley, B. R., and Sen, S. (1998). Tumour amplified kinase STK15/BTAK induces centrosome amplification, aneuploidy and transformation. *Nat Genet 20*, 189–193.

WEB RESOURCES

Stanford Microarray Database (SMD): www.genome-www5.stanford.edu/MicroArray/SMD/

Stanford breast cancer portal: http://genome-www.stanford.edu/breast_cancer/

Stanford Functional Genomics Facility (SFGF): http://genome-www4.stanford.edu/cgi-bin/sfgf/home.pl

SOURCE: http://genome-www5.stanford.edu/cgi-bin/SMD/source/sourceSearch

Brown lab page: http://cmgm.stanford.edu/pbrown/

Stanford Genomic Resources: http://genome-www.stanford.edu/

6

CLASSIFYING HEREDITARY CANCERS AND PHENOCOPIES OF HEREDITARY CANCERS USING EXPRESSION ARRAYS

Mary B. Daly, Alicia Parlanti, and David Duggan

INTRODUCTION

The Human Genome Project has provided new opportunities to define cancer in genetic terms that will alter the practice of medicine in several ways. The growing understanding of the molecular basis of carcinogenesis will have clinical applications in understanding cancer etiology and assigning more precise estimates of risk both for those rare heritable forms of cancer associated with a high penetrance germ-line mutation and for sporadic cancers in which multigenic polymorphisms are likely to play a role. Using hereditary breast cancer as an example, we first review the status quo of the genetics of familial breast cancer. Since their discovery in the early 1990s, *BRCA1* and *BRCA2* have been shown conclusively to be involved in hereditary breast cancer. It is just as clear that despite intensive effort, additional genes predisposing to hereditary breast cancer have yet to be identified. Next, we look at how the separation of the heterogeneous group of hereditary breast cancers into homogeneous subgroups based on gene expression profiling may facilitate the search for breast cancer predisposing

Oncogenomics: Molecular Approaches to Cancer, Edited by Charles Brenner and David Duggan
ISBN 0-471-22592-4 © 2004 John Wiley & Sons, Inc.

genes. These findings suggest a diagnostic model in which loss of *BRCA1* activity either through mutation or by downregulation of gene expression can be diagnosed with the use of gene expression profiling. Last, the application of such promising technologies must be accompanied by attention to the social and ethical issues they raise.

The role of genetics in understanding and treating cancer was initially limited to observation of cytogenetic abnormalities in certain tumor types. Examples include Burkitt's lymphoma in which the t(8;14)(q24;q32) rearrangement results in transloca-tion of the *MYC* gene from chromosome 8 into the immunoglobin heavy-chain gene on chromosome 14. This results in the overexpression of the normal *MYC* product, which initiates altered cell growth and tumor development.

The commencement of the Human Genome Project in the early 1990s acceler-ated the identification of molecular abnormalities. The Morbid Map of the Human Genome (Amberger et al., 2001), a catalog of genetic diseases with known clinical associations and their cytogenetics map locations, provides a view of the genome to which more than 2200 disease phenotypes have been mapped. Today, the molecular basis for nearly 1400 of these phenotypes have been identified.

Before the draft human genome sequence was released (Lander et al., 2001) sophis-ticated high-throughput technologies were being developed to gain an understanding of the genes and the cells that express them. High-throughput molecular tools such as microarray technology have the potential to create a taxonomy of tumors that will reflect their molecular diversity. This approach, for example, has been used to identify subsets of ER-negative breast tumors derived from different cells in the ductal epithe-lium having unique molecular profiles (Perou et al., 2000; see also Chapter 5). As argued in Chapters 5 and 15, improvements in genomic classification and integration with traditional genetic approaches hold promise for understanding the biology of var-ious tumors and for optimizing the clinical management of individual patients (Mohr et al., 2002; Bertucci et al., 2001).

This growing understanding of the molecular basis of carcinogenesis will have clinical applications in understanding cancer etiology and assigning more precise esti-mates of risk; in tailoring screening and prevention approaches to populations at defined levels of risk; in improving accuracy of diagnosis and prognosis based on molecular profiles; and in the rational design of therapeutic modalities based on molecular tar-gets. This chapter will further explore the application of genetics and genomics to the clinical diagnosis of hereditary *BRCA1*- and *BRCA2*-mutation-positive and *BRCAx* (non-*BRCA1/2*) breast cancers. First, we look at the introduction and application of *BRCA1* and *BRCA2* genetics to the clinic, which in many respects has only just begun. Second, we describe the identification of genome-wide gene expression profiles spe-cific to each of these tumor types and consider the future potential of genomics to the clinic. Finally, we look at the ethical, legal, and social implications associated with the application of genetics and genomics in the clinic.

INHERITED BREAST CANCER SYNDROMES

Although site-specific cancer clusters in some families have been appreciated for decades, it was not until identification of genes like *BRCA1* and *BRCA2* that the hereditary patterns of cancer could be definitively linked to discrete germ-line muta-tions. Although high-penetrance hereditary cancer syndromes account for less than

10% of all cancer, identification of these genes and the attention devoted to these discoveries have heightened awareness of the genetic contribution to cancer in general among both the medical profession and the lay community, and have provided a means to begin to recognize individuals and families with an increased risk of cancer.

Because deleterious mutations in genes associated with hereditary cancer syndromes diagnose a *risk* for cancer, not the disease itself, knowledge of germ-line cancer susceptibility genes has stimulated intense interest in preventive strategies that may be employed to alter an individual's risk and that of his or her family members. Studies are underway to understand the functions of cancer susceptibility genes and how their alteration contributes to carcinogenesis. A full understanding of the genes and pathways of carcinogenesis will have profound implications for the development of targeted prevention, detection, and treatment. This work is likely to elucidate the causal mechanisms of the traditional epidemiologic factors associated with cancer, which will have implications for the more common sporadic forms.

In 1990, a susceptibility gene for breast cancer was mapped by genetic linkage to the long arm of chromosome 17 in the interval 17q12-21. The linkage between breast cancer and genetic markers on chromosome 17q was soon confirmed by others, and evidence for the coincident transmission of both breast and ovarian cancer susceptibility in linked families was observed (Narod et al., 1991). The *BRCA1* gene was subsequently identified by positional cloning methods and has been found to encode a protein of 1863 amino acids. This susceptibility gene appears to be responsible for disease in 45% of families with multiple cases of breast cancer only and up to 90% of families with both breast and ovarian cancer.

A second breast cancer susceptibility gene, *BRCA2*, was localized through linkage studies of 15 families with multiple cases of breast cancer to the long arm of chromosome 13. Germ-line mutations in *BRCA2* are thought to account for approximately 35% of multiple-case breast cancer families and are also associated with male breast cancer, ovarian cancer, prostate cancer, and pancreatic cancer (Wooster et al., 1994; Gayther et al., 1997). The risk for breast cancer in female *BRCA2* mutation carriers appears similar to that for *BRCA1* carriers, but the age of onset is shifted to an older distribution.

Of the several hundred mutations described in these genes, most lead to a frameshift resulting in missing or nonfunctional proteins. In addition, tumors from individuals born heterozygous for *BRCA1/2* mutations show loss of the wild-type allele, consistent with a role in tumor suppression. Both *BRCA1* and *BRCA2* are also involved in the control of meiotic and mitotic recombination and in the maintenance of genomic stability, suggesting a role in DNA repair (Tutt and Ashworth, 2002; Venkitaraman, 2002).

The frequency of *BRCA1* mutation carriers in the general population has been estimated to be 1 in 800. *BRCA1* and *BRCA2* also share differential prevalence rates in certain ethnic groups. Most notably, three specific mutations—the 185delAG mutation and the 5382insC mutation on *BRCA1*, and the 6174delT mutation on *BRCA2*—have been found to be common in Ashkenazi Jews. The frequency of these three mutations approaches 1 in 40 in this population and accounts for up to 25% of early-onset breast cancer and up to 90% of families with both breast and ovarian cancer (Streuwing et al., 1997). Additional founder effects have been described in the Netherlands and in Iceland (Thorlacius et al., 1996).

The actual expression of disease in gene mutation carriers, known as penetrance, is estimated to range from 36% to 85% for breast cancer and from 16% to 60% for ovarian cancer. Among female *BRCA1* carriers who have already developed a primary breast cancer, estimates for a second contralateral breast cancer are as high as 64% by age 70, and for ovarian cancer as high as 44% by age 70 (Greene, 1997). Clearly, different alleles confer different degrees of penetrance. Ongoing studies are addressing the role of reproductive factors, endogenous and exogenous hormone exposure, diet, and lifestyle factors in the modulation of risk among mutation carriers.

OTHER BREAST CANCER SYNDROMES

Breast cancer is part of the disease spectra in several multicancer syndromes of known genetic origin. These rare syndromes can explain only a small proportion of hereditary breast cancer. Breast cancer is a component of the rare Li-Fraumeni syndrome in which germ-line mutations of the p53 gene on chromosome 17p have been documented (Garber et al., 1991). A germ-line mutation in the p53 gene has been identified in over 50% of families exhibiting this syndrome, and inheritance is autosomal dominant with a penetrance of at least 50% by age 50. Although highly penetrant, the Li-Fraumeni gene is thought to account for less than 1% of breast cancer cases.

One of the over 50 cancer-related genodermatoses, Cowden's syndrome is also characterized by an excess of breast cancer. Germ-line mutations in *PTEN*, a protein tyrosine phosphatase with homology to tensin, located on chromosome 10q23, are responsible for this syndrome. Loss of heterozygosity observed in a high proportion of related cancers suggests that *PTEN* functions as a tumor suppressor gene. Disruption of *PTEN* appears to occur late in tumorigenesis and may act as a regulatory molecule of cytoskeletal function. Although it accounts for a small fraction of hereditary breast cancer, the characterization of *PTEN* function will provide valuable insights into signal pathways and the maintenance of normal cell physiology (Eng, 1998; Myers and Tonks, 1997).

Ataxia telangiectasia is an autosomal-recessive disorder characterized by neurologic deterioration, telangiectasias, immunodeficiency, and hypersensitivity to ionizing radiation. Several epidemiologic studies have suggested a statistically increased risk of breast cancer among female heterozygote carriers, with an estimated relative risk of 3.9 (Easton, 1994), and more recent studies have described specific candidate AT mutations associated with increased breast cancer risk (Concannon, 2002). AT cells are sensitive to ionizing radiation and radiomimetic drugs and lack cell cycle regulatory properties after exposure to radiation. It is estimated that approximately 1% of the general population may be heterozygotic for ATM mutations. Given the high carrier rate in the population, this association could account for a significant proportion of hereditary breast cancer and poses a potential risk related to diagnostic radiation exposure in these individuals.

Women who appear to meet criteria for one of the hereditary breast/ovarian cancer syndromes should be offered the opportunity to participate in clinical genetic counseling delivered by a team of trained health care professionals. The goals of counseling include a better understanding of the genetic, biological, and environmental factors related to an individual's risk of disease; assistance in decisions regarding genetic testing; formulation of appropriate management options based on level of risk; and the provision of psychosocial support to adjust to risk perception and adhere to recommended actions. Management strategies for mutation carriers are beginning to emerge, with limited clinical evidence of efficacy. Because of the early age of onset of many of these tumors, screening often begins at a younger age. Primary prevention in the forms of prophylactic surgery and chemoprevention may be appropriate options.

BIOLOGY OF *BRCA1* AND *BRCA2* BREAST CANCERS: MICROARRAY-BASED DIAGNOSTICS

We used complementary DNA (cDNA) microarrays to explore the patterns of gene expression in samples of primary breast tumors that had mutations in *BRCA1*, *BRCA2*, or neither gene (sporadic cases) (Duggan et al., 1999; Hedenfalk et al., 2001). Studies of the pathological features (Breast Cancer Linkage Consortium, 1997; Lakhani et al., 1998), genomic alterations (Tirkkonen et al., 1997; Kainu et al., 2000), and steroid receptor levels (Johannsson et al., 1997; Loman et al., 1998) support the idea that cancers with underlying germ-line mutations in *BRCA1* and *BRCA2* differ molecularly from each other and from cancers that do not carry these mutations. Thus, it would be useful to classify hereditary breast tumors with a single method that is not limited by the underlying tissue heterogeneity, gene defect, or receptor status and that will provide information about the full range of phenotypic alterations (Box 6-1).

Statistical analyses of the gene expression profiles were used to determine which of the genes expressed by the tumors correlated with the *BRCA1*-mutation-positive tumors,

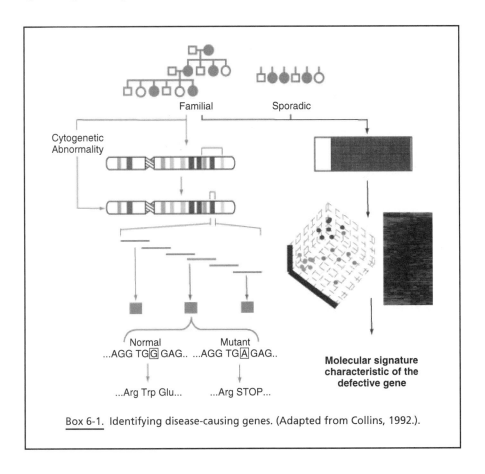

Box 6-1. Identifying disease-causing genes. (Adapted from Collins, 1992.).

the *BRCA2*-mutation-positive tumors, and the sporadic tumors. Results yielded a list of genes whose variation in expression among all experiments best differentiated among these types of cancers. These data were visualized using a multidimensional scaling plot demonstrating that the patterns of gene expression among the *BRCA1*-mutation-positive tumors, the *BRCA2*-mutation-positive tumors, and the sporadic tumors were largely distinctive (Fig. 6-1). In this three-dimensional rendering of the data, samples with similar expression profiles lie closer to each other that those with dissimilar profiles.

A class prediction method was used to determine whether the gene expression patterns in tumors with *BRCA1* mutations and tumors with *BRCA2* mutations could be used to identify the status of each sample in the data set according to the presence or absence of *BRCA1* and *BRCA2* mutations. The misclassification rate was estimated using a leave-one-out cross-validation method whereby one of the samples was left out and the results from the remaining samples were used to predict the status of the withheld sample. This process was repeated for each of the samples. Finally, random permutations of the class membership indicators (*BRCA1*, *BRCA2*, sporadic) were used to determine the significance of the result.

With the use of this approach, most of the samples were correctly classified. Gene expression patterns of the breast tumor samples accurately identified them as positive or negative for *BRCA1* mutations or as positive or negative for *BRCA2* mutations.

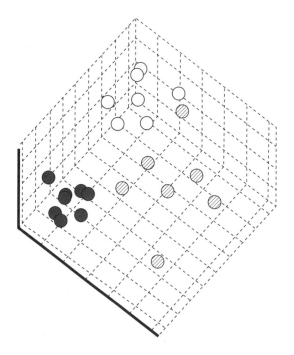

Figure 6-1. Classification of hereditary *BRCA1* and *BRCA2* and sporadic breast cancer tumors. A multidimensional scaling plot of the primary tumor samples is shown as determined by the individual tumor gene expression patterns. The physical separation of the clusters suggests that the gene list used to generate this MDS plot is capable of differentiating the three types of tumors. *BRCA1*-mutation-positive tumor samples (open circles); *BRCA2*-mutation-positive tumor samples (filled circles); sporadic breast cancer tumor samples (hashed circles).

With respect to identifying *BRCA1* mutations, all tumors with *BRCA1* mutations and 14 of 15 tumors without *BRCA1* mutations were correctly identified in the *BRCA1* classification. Only 0.3 percent of data sets in which *BRCA1* classifications were randomly permuted resulted in the misclassification of one or fewer samples; thus, the accuracy of these classifications was significant as compared with randomized data. From a diagnostic point of view, the result was significant because *BRCA1* and *BRCA2* mutations can often be missed in traditional DNA-based diagnostics (Ford et al. 1998).

This study illustrates the potential of genome-wide views to influence the diagnosis of cancer. These results indicate that a heritable mutation influences the gene expression profile of a tumor. Samples from patients with germ-line mutations in *BRCA1* and those from patients with such mutations in *BRCA2* differ significantly in their global patterns of gene expression (Fig. 6-2), even though both mutant genes lead to breast and ovarian cancer. These complex patterns of gene expression can serve as proxies for abnormalities in entire molecular pathways with or without the need to identify the genetic changes that cause the disturbance. Notwithstanding the tremendous power of mutation detection technologies described in Chapter 2, it is likely that in the future the integrity of functionally important pathways in tumors will be

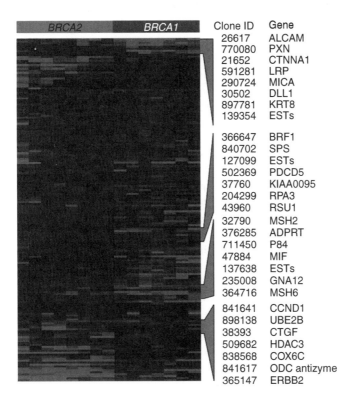

Figure 6-2. Statistical analysis of genes differentiating the *BRCA1*-mutation-positive breast tumor samples from the *BRCA2*-mutation-positive breast tumor samples. Red = increased gene expression relative to the reference sample; green = decreased gene expression. See insert for color representation of this figure.

evaluated by transcriptional profiling. As demonstrated in Chapter 3 and 5, genomics and transcriptomics are complementary technologies that can sometimes share the same high throughput platform.

DIAGNOSING PHENOCOPIES OF HEREDITARY DISEASE

In our analysis of hereditary *BRCA1*- and *BRCA2*-mutation-positive and sporadic breast cancer tumor samples, one sporadic tumor was misclassified as positive for a *BRCA1* mutation. Compared to the other specimens from patients with sporadic breast cancer, this specimen had a markedly reduced level of expression of *BRCA1*, perhaps because of an unrecognized mutation of *BRCA1* in this patient. On further investigation, the tumor was found to have phenotypic characteristics (e.g., negativity for estrogen receptors, a high grade, and a ductal location) that were consistent with the common clinical and pathological profiles of a *BRCA1*-mutation-positive breast cancer.

This unexpected finding prompted consideration of whether to contact the patient to request that she undergo testing for *BRCA1* mutations. The investigators and the institutional review boards evaluated this unanticipated finding, noting that patients with breast cancer who have a *BRCA1* mutation are at greater risk for ovarian cancer and breast cancer in the contralateral breast than patients with breast cancer who do not have *BRCA1* mutations (Burke et al., 1997) and that preventive surgery (oophorectomy and mastectomy) might increase the life expectancy of such patients (Schrag et al., 2000). Upon approval by the institutional review board, the patient was contacted through her family physician and agreed to be tested for a germ-line mutation in *BRCA1*.

Using sequence-based mutation analysis and a chip-based system of mutation detection, we found no mutation in the *BRCA1* gene. We then analyzed the *BRCA1* promoter region for aberrant methylation, which is known to silence *BRCA1* in sporadic cancers with no mutations in the gene (Esteller et al., 2000; Lakhani et al., 2000). Testing (in a blinded fashion) of all specimens of sporadic tumors from our study indicated that the misclassified tumor was the only one with hypermethylation of the *BRCA1* promoter region, which is indicative of epigenetic inactivation of *BRCA1*.

These findings suggest a diagnostic model in which loss of *BRCA1* activity, whether through germ-line mutations or by downregulation of gene expression, can be diagnosed with the use of gene expression profiling. While decreased expression of the *BRCA1* gene has been shown in sporadic tumors (Thompson et al., 1995), the frequency of these reduced levels has not been extensively studied. Given all that is likely to be learned about treatment of *BRCA1* mutation positive breast cancer cohorts, identification of sporadic patients who present as *BRCA1*-phenocopies will embrace additional individuals into appropriately targeted treatment.

BRCAx

Despite the considerable variation in the contribution to breast cancer from *BRCA1*, *BRCA2*, *TP53*, *PTEN*, and *ATM*, it remains evident that additional breast cancer susceptibility genes are still to be identified. The genes known to be involved in familial breast cancer account for fewer than 25% of the observed familial clustering (Fig. 6-3). In principle, the remaining 75% of familial risks might have a genetic or environmental

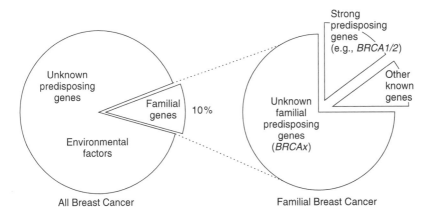

Figure 6-3. Frequency of known (and unknown) genes in breast cancer.

origin, but evidence from studies of breast cancer in twins (Peto, 2001; Lichtenstein et al., 2000), tumor incidence in the contralateral breast of affected individuals (Peto, 2001; Lichtenstein et al., 2000), and the pattern of inheritance in families (Cui et al., 2001; Antoniou et al., 2002) suggests that genetic factors predominate. A large number of these hereditary breast cancer cases are believed to be due to unidentified breast cancer predisposition genes (*BRCAx*).

Several genomic regions have been suggested as candidate loci for these additional breast cancer susceptibility genes. Genetic linkage analysis of *BRCAx* families has been performed and identified 8p12-p22 and 13q21 as chromosomal regions potentially harboring a breast cancer susceptibility gene (Seitz et al., 1997; Kainu et al., 2000). However, these loci have either subsequently been excluded as major predisposing loci on a global perspective (Rahman et al., 2000; Thompson et al., 2002), or remain to be confirmed. The identification of additional breast cancer predisposition genes is likely due to genetic heterogeneity, low penetrance, polygenic mechanisms, or population-specific effects within *BRCAx* kindreds (Nathanson and Weber, 2001).

These *BRCAx* breast cancer families comprise a histopathologically heterogeneous group, indicating the presence of multiple underlying genetic events. A study of the histological features of cancers in families not attributable to mutations in *BRCA1* or *BRCA2* indicated that these breast cancers differed histologically from both *BRCA1* and *BRCA2* breast cancers (Lakhani et al., 2000). The study also suggested that non-*BRCA1/2* breast cancers differ from nonfamilial (sporadic) breast cancers. Thus, it is likely that the different tumor phenotypes reflect the multiple genetic origins of breast cancers.

In a follow-up study to the *BRCA1*, *BRCA2*, and sporadic breast cancer study, Hedenfalk et al. (2003) successfully subdivided *BRCAx* families into recognizable groups using a combination of gene expression profiling, array-based comparative genomic hybridization (array CGH; see also Chapters 3 and 5), and information from genetic linkage analysis. Here they showed that gene expression profiling can discover novel classes among *BRCAx* tumors and differentiate them from *BRCA1* and *BRCA2* tumors. Moreover, array-based CGH to cDNA arrays revealed specific somatic genetic alterations within the *BRCAx* subgroups.

Based on the gene expression profiles, their class discovery method identified two distinct groups of *BRCAx* tumors. This classification was supported by 60 statistically significant genes ($p < 0.001$), whereas only 5 were expected by chance. To exclude the possibility that the discriminatory genes were related to unidentified *BRCA1* and *BRCA2* mutations, a number of tumors from known *BRCA1* and *BRCA2* mutation carriers were included in the analysis. Multidimensional scaling analysis and hierarchical clustering with the 60 genes that best separated the *BRCAx* tumors into two groups were performed. It was found that neither *BRCA1* nor *BRCA2* tumors clustered with the *BRCAx* samples, supporting their underlying difference. Furthermore, in families where multiple individuals were expression-profiled, individual samples tended to cluster together from within a family.

Given the heterogeneity of *BRCAx* tumors and the previous difficulty in distinguishing this group, these findings illustrate that homogeneous subsets of *BRCAx* families can be identified using gene expression profiling. Results such as these when used in combination with array-based CGH, linkage analysis, or positional cloning information could potentially increase the power of genetic analysis. Unfortunately, due to small sample sizes, further studies are needed to pinpoint whether the partitioning reflects a hereditary predisposition or is a manifestation of similarities in tumor progression within each group. Nevertheless, the family clustering supports an underlying hereditary cause for the partitioning.

COMBINED LINKAGE AND MICROARRAY ANALYSIS

Three recent studies have combined the use of DNA microarrays with genetic linkage analysis, leading to identification of the disease genes under study. In the first report, microarrays were used to identify genes that were differentially expressed between a rat strain with insulin resistance and a normal, insulin-sensitive control strain (Aitman et al., 1999). One of the genes identified in this microarray study, Cd36 or fatty acid translocase, mapped to a chromosomal location previously shown to contain an insulin resistance gene (Aitman et al., 1997). Defects in the gene were then shown to result in glucose intolerance and defective fatty acid metabolism in this rat strain (Aitman et al., 1999; Pravenec et al., 2001) and in humans (Miyaoka et al., 2001). In the second report, a combination of gene expression microarrays, genetic mapping, and biochemical studies was used to identify the *ABC1* transporter as the defect in Tangier disease (Lawn et al., 1999). In the third report, gene expression profiling and single-nucleotide polymorphism-based genotyping, combined with quantitative trait locus analysis, were used to identify the gene encoding complement factor 5 as a susceptibility locus for asthma (Karp et al., 2000).

As yet, it is too soon to know if the combined microarray and linkage/genetic abnormality approach will be more generally applicable to identification of monogenic or complex trait genes, but adoption of the approach in a growing number of gene mapping laboratories will answer this question in the near future. We are also enthusiastic about disease classification studies reported in Chapter 5 for their potential power to segregate patients into treatment groups. As discussed in Chapter 15, however, the potential clinical benefits brought by microarrays will have to be evaluated prospectively and weighed against their costs before their introduction into routine clinical use.

ETHICAL, LEGAL, AND SOCIAL ISSUES

The exciting potential of the work emanating from the Human Genome Project has created enthusiasm about our ability to improve public health through population screening for cancer predisposition, through a more sophisticated understanding of the molecular profiles of cancer phenotypes, and through new gene-targeted drug development. The new technologies have also spawned ethical issues concerning patients and their families, the health care profession, and society at large.

Most of the ethical debate for the public has centered around the ability to genetically characterize individuals for inherited cancer susceptibility syndromes. Limitations of test accuracy and the relative uncertainties about effective preventive strategies for those who test positive have led many to advise caution about the widespread adoption of genetic testing in the clinical setting. The public has also expressed concern that the explosion of genetic information may result in an environment in which people will be labeled and disadvantaged in the workplace and in their ability to obtain insurance. In fact, the most common reason cited for not considering genetic testing for mutations in the *BRCA1/2* genes is fear of insurance discrimination.

Responsibility to other family members is another concern voiced by individuals who undergo genetic testing. Privacy and confidentiality issues place the burden of communicating genetic test results with the first individual diagnosed, who may not have a sophisticated medical background and who may face difficult family dynamics in the communication process. The application of novel genetic technologies to the diagnosis, characterization, and treatment of cancer has not generated as much concern and attention among cancer patients, who are often overwhelmed by their situation and feel incapable of fully understanding the details of the treatments proposed to them.

Among members of the health care profession, knowledge regarding the criteria for hereditary cancer syndromes, the indications for associated genetic testing, and the role that molecular genetics plays in the prevention, diagnosis, and treatment of cancer is limited. Health care providers are often at a loss about how to understand and communicate genetic test results to individuals, what is their responsibility to inform other at-risk relatives of their potential genetic risk, and how to assure confidentiality and privacy of genetic information in the medical record system.

Primary care providers will assume a more pivotal role in the provision of clinical genetic services at the bedside, including providing education to patients and their families about genetic information in general, genetic testing in particular, and the use of genetic technologies in cancer risk-reduction surveillance, diagnosis, and treatment. The involvement of the entire health care team will be critical to assess the outcomes of family decisions regarding genetic information and to guide individuals and their families through the complex world of cancer genetics.

Limited physician knowledge of genetics may pose a barrier to the referral of appropriate candidates for genetic testing and the standardized utilization of genetic predictive testing in clinical practice for increased cancer surveillance, screening, and prevention options. Based on the potential for identification, classification, prevention, and treatment for a wide variety of cancer types, physicians and other health care providers and their patients would greatly benefit from training in interpretation and use of the results of genetic technologies as part of their clinical practice.

The promise of genomic technologies is emerging at a time when health costs are expanding and access to care is not shared by all members of society. Although advances in technology may reduce costs of existing diagnostics, new diagnostic and treatment options are likely to increase costs overall. Thus, disparities in cancer care may grow as more advanced technologies are introduced. The role of insurance companies in providing coverage for these new costs is unclear. The magnitude of insurance and/or employment risks from discrimination on the basis of genetic risk information is also a major concern for state and federal governmental agencies and the insurance industry. Legislation for protection against discrimination based on genetic test results is incomplete and has not been thoroughly challenged in the court system. Finally, the ability to characterize individuals genetically facilitates the application of this technology more generally. Thus, it is likely that databases potentially designed to provide predictive data on individual cancer risks could also reveal associations with ancestry, ethnicity, and aspects of human behavior with potential for misuse. These issues call for public education about the genomic revolution and a general discourse on the use of genomics and genetics in the oncology setting.

REFERENCES

Aitman, T. J., Gotoda, T., Evans, A. L., Imrie, H., Heath, K. E., Trembling, P. M., Truman, H., Wallace, C. A., Rahman, A., Dore, C., Flint, J., Kren, V., Zidek, V., Kurtz, T. W., Pravenec, M., and Scott, J. (1997). Quantitative trait loci for cellular defects in glucose and fatty acid metabolism in hypertensive rats. *Nat Genet 16*, 197–201.

Aitman, T. J., Glazier, A. M., Wallace, C. A., Cooper, L. D., Norsworthy, P. J., Wahid, F. N., Al-Majali, K. M., Trembling, P. M., Mann, C. J., Shoulders, C. C., Graf, D., St. Lezin, E., Kurtz, T. W., Kren, V., Pravenec, M., Ibrahimi, A., Abumrad, N. A., Stanton, L. W., and Scott, J. (1999). Identification of Cd36 (Fat) as an insulin-resistance gene causing defective fatty acid and glucose metabolism in hypertensive rats. *Nat Genet 21*, 76–83.

Amberger, J. S., Hamosh, A., and McKusick, V. A. (2001). Morbid anatomy of the human genome. In *The Metabolic and Molecular Bases of Inherited Disease*, 8th ed. C. R. Scriver, A. L. Beaudet, W. S. Sly, and D. Valle, (eds.). New York: McGraw-Hill, pp. 47–111.

Antoniou, A. C., Pharoah, P. D., McMullan, G., Day, N. E., Stratton, M. R., Peto, J., Ponder, B. J., and Easton, D. F. (2002). A comprehensive model for familial breast cancer incorporating BRCA1, BRCA2 and other genes. *Br J Cancer 86*, 76–83.

Bertucci, F., Houlgatte, R., Nguyen, C., Viens, P., Jordan, B. R., and Birnbaum, D. (2001). Gene expression profiling of cancer by use of DNA arrays: How far from the clinic? *Lancet Oncol 2*, 674–682.

Breast Cancer Linkage Consortium (1997). Pathology of familial breast cancer: Differences between breast cancers in carriers of BRCA1 and BRCA2 mutations and sporadic cases. *Lancet 349*, 1505–1510.

Burke, W., Petersen, G., Lynch, P., Botkin, J., Daly, M., Garber, J., Kahn, M. J., McTiernan, A., Offit, K., Thomson, E., and Varricchio, C. (1997). Recommendations for follow-up care of individuals with an inherited predisposition to cancer. I. Hereditary nonpolyposis colon cancer. Cancer Genetics Studies Consortium. *JAMA 277*, 915–919.

Collins, F. S. (1992). Positional cloning: Let's not call it reverse anymore. *Nat Genet 1*, 3–6.

Concannon, P. (2002), ATM heterozygosity and cancer risk. *Nat Genet 32*, 89–90.

Cui, J., Antoniou, A. C., Dite, G. S., Southey, M. C., Venter, D. J., Easton, D. F., Giles, G. G., McCredie, M. R., and Hopper, J. L. (2001). After BRCA1 and BRCA2—what next? Multifactorial segregation analyses of three-generation, population-based Australian families affected by female breast cancer. *Am J Hum Genet 68*, 420–431.

Duggan, D. J., Bittner, M., Chen, Y., Meltzer, P., and Trent, J. M. (1999). Expression profiling using cDNA microarrays. *Nat Genet 21*, 10–14.

Easton, D. F. (1994). Cancer risks in A-T heterozygotes. *Int J Radiat Biol 66*, S177–182.

Eng, C. (1998). Genetics of Cowden syndrome: through the looking glass of oncology. *Int J Oncol 12*, 701–710.

Esteller, M., Silva, J. M., Dominguez, G., Bonilla, F., Matias-Guiu, X., Lerma, E., Bussaglia, E., Prat, J., Harkes, I. C., Repasky, E. A., Gabrielson, E., Schutte, M., Baylin, S. B., and Herman, J. G. (2000). Promoter hypermethylation and BRCA1 inactivation in sporadic breast and ovarian tumors. *J Natl Cancer Inst 92*, 564–569.

Esteller, M., Corn, P. G., Baylin, S. B., and Herman, J. G. (2001). A gene hypermethylation profile of human cancer. *Cancer Res 61*, 3225–3229.

Ford, D., Easton, D. F., Stratton, M., Narod, S., Goldgar, D., Devilee, P., Bishop, D. T., Weber, B., Lenoir, G., Chang-Claude, J., Sobol, H., Teare, M. D., Struewing, J., Arason, A., Scherneck, S., Peto, J., Rebbeck, T. R., Tonin, P., Neuhausen, S., Barkardottir, R., Eyfjord, J., Lynch, H., Ponder, B. A., Gayther, S. A., Zelada-Hedman, M., et al. (1998). Genetic heterogeneity and penetrance analysis of the BRCA1 and BRCA2 genes in breast cancer families. The Breast Cancer Linkage Consortium. *Am J Hum Genet 62*, 676–689.

Garber, J. E., Goldstein, A. M., Kantor, A. F., Dreyfus, M. G., Fraumeni, J. F. Jr., Li, F. P. (1991). Follow-up study of twenty-four families with Li-Fraumeni Syndrome. *Cancer Res. 51*, 6094–6097.

Gayther, S. A., Mangion, J., Russell, P., Seal, S., Barfoot, R., and Ponder, B. A. (1997). Variation of risks of breast and ovarian cancer associated with different germline mutations of the BRCA2 gene. *Nat Genet 15*, 103–105.

Greene, M. H. (1997). Genetics of breast cancer. *Mayo Clin Proc 72*, 54–65.

Hedenfalk, I., Duggan, D., Chen, Y., Radmacher, M., Bittner, M., Simon, R., Meltzer, P., Gusterson, B., Esteller, M., Kallioniemi, O. P., Wilfond, B., Borg, A., and Trent, J. (2001). Gene-expression profiles in hereditary breast cancer. *N Engl J Med 344*, 539–548.

Hedenfalk, I., Ringner, M., Ben-Dor, A., Yakhini, Z., Chen, Y., Chebil, G., Ach, R., Loman, N., Olsson, H., Meltzer, P., Borg, A., and Trent, J. (2003). Molecular classification of familial non-BRCA1/BRCA2 breast cancer. *Proc Natl Acad Sci USA 100*, 2532–2537.

Huntington's Disease Collaborative Research Group (1993). A novel gene containing a trinucleotide repeat that is expanded and unstable on Huntington's disease chromosomes. *Cell 72*, 971–983.

Johannsson, O. T., Idvall, I., Anderson, C., Borg, A., Barkardottir, R. B., Egilsson, V., and Olsson, H. (1997). Tumour biological features of BRCA1-induced breast and ovarian cancer. *Eur J Cancer 33*, 362–371.

Johannsson, O. T., Ranstam, J., Borg, A., and Olsson, H. (1998). Survival of BRCA1 breast and ovarian cancer patients: A population-based study from southern Sweden. *J Clin Oncol 16*, 397–404.

Kainu, T., Juo, S. H., Desper, R., Schaffer, A. A., Gillanders, E., Rozenblum, E., Freas-Lutz, D., Weaver, D., Stephan, D., Bailey-Wilson, J., Kallioniemi, O. P., Tirkkonen, M., Syrjakoski, K., Kuukasjarvi, T., Koivisto, P., Karhu, R., Holli, K., Arason, A., Johannesdottir, G., Bergthorsson, J. T., Johannsdottir, H., Egilsson, V., Barkardottir, R. B., Johannsson, O., Haraldsson, K., Sandberg, T., Holmberg, E., Gronberg, H., Olsson, H., Borg, A., Vehmanen, P., Eerola, H., Heikkila, P., Pyrhonen, S., and Nevanlinna, H. (2000). Somatic deletions in hereditary breast cancers implicate 13q21 as a putative novel breast cancer susceptibility locus. *Proc Natl Acad Sci USA 97*, 9603–9608.

Karp, C. L., Grupe, A., Schadt, E., Ewart, S. L., Keane-Moore, M., Cuomo, P. J., Kohl, J., Wahl, L., Kuperman, D., Germer, S., Aud, D., Peltz, G., and Wills-Karp, M. (2000).

Identification of complement factor 5 as a susceptibility locus for experimental allergic asthma. *Nat Immunol 1*, 221–226.

Lakhani, S. R., Jacquemier, J., Sloane, J. P., Gusterson, B. A., Anderson, T. J., van de Vijver, M. J., Farid, L. M., Venter, D., Antoniou, A., Storfer-Isser, A., Smyth, E., Steel, C. M., Haites, N., Scott, R. J., Goldgar, D., Neuhausen, S., Daly, P. A., Ormiston, W., McManus, R., Scherneck, S., Ponder, B. A., Ford, D., Peto, J., Stoppa-Lyonnet, D., Easton, D. F., et al. (1998). Multifactorial analysis of differences between sporadic breast cancers and cancers involving BRCA1 and BRCA2 mutations. *J Natl Cancer Inst 90*, 1138–1145.

Lakhani, S. R., Gusterson, B. A., Jacquemier, J., Sloane, J. P., Anderson, T. J., van de Vijver, M. J., Venter, D., Freeman, A., Antoniou, A., McGuffog, L., Smyth, E., Steel, C. M., Haites, N., Scott, R. J., Goldgar, D., Neuhausen, S., Daly, P. A., Ormiston, W., McManus, R., Scherneck, S., Ponder, B. A., Futreal, P. A., Peto, J., Stoppa-Lyonnet, D., Bignon, Y. J., and Stratton, M. R. (2000). The pathology of familial breast cancer: Histological features of cancers in families not attributable to mutations in BRCA1 or BRCA2. *Clin Cancer Res 6*, 782–789.

Lander, E. S., Linton, L. M., Birren, B., et al. (2001). Initial sequencing and analysis of the human genome. *Nature 409*, 860–921.

Lawn, R. M., Wade, D. P., Garvin, M. R., Wang, X., Schwartz, K., Porter, J. G., Seilhamer, J. J., Vaughan, A. M., and Oram, J. F. (1999). The Tangier disease gene product ABC1 controls the cellular apolipoprotein-mediated lipid removal pathway. *J Clin Invest 104*, R25–R31.

Lichtenstein, P., Holm, N. V., Verkasalo, P. K., Iliadou, A., Kaprio, J., Koskenvuo, M., Pukkala, E., Skytthe, A., and Hemminki, K. (2000). Environmental and heritable factors in the causation of cancer—analyses of cohorts of twins from Sweden, Denmark, and Finland. *N Engl J Med 343*, 78–85.

Loman, N., Johannsson, O., Bendahl, P. O., Borg, A., Ferno, M., and Olsson, H. (1998). Steroid receptors in hereditary breast carcinomas associated with BRCA1 or BRCA2 mutations or unknown susceptibility genes. *Cancer 83*, 310–319.

Miyaoka, K., Kuwasako, T., Hirano, K., Nozaki, S., Yamashita, S., and Matsuzawa, Y. (2001). CD36 deficiency associated with insulin resistance. *Lancet 357*, 686–687.

Mohr, S., Leikauf, G. D., Keith, G., and Rihn, B. H. (2002). Microarrays as cancer keys: An array of possibilities *J Clin Oncol 20*, 3165–3175.

Myers, M. P., and Tonks, N. K. (1997). PTEN: Sometimes taking it off can be better than putting it on. *Am J Hum Genet 61*, 1234–1238.

Narod, S. A., Feunteun, J., Lynch, H. T., Watson, P., Conway, T., Lynch, J., and Lenoir, G. M. (1991). Familial breast-ovarian locus on chromosome 17q12–23. *Lancet 338*, 82.

Nathanson, K. L., and Weber, B. L. (2001). "Other" breast cancer susceptibility genes: Searching for more holy grail. *Hum Mol Genet 10*, 715–720.

Perou, C. M., Sorlie, T., Eisen, M. B., van de Rijn, M., Jeffrey, S. S., Rees, C. A., Pollack, J. R., Ross, D. T., Johnsen, H., Akslen, L. A., Fluge, O., Pergamenschikov, A., Williams, C., Zhu, S. X., Lonning, P. E., Borresen-Dale, A. L., Brown, P. O., and Botstein, D. (2000). Molecular portraits of human breast tumours. *Nature 406*, 747–752.

Peto, J. (2001). Cancer epidemiology in the last century and the next decade. *Nature 411*, 390–395.

Pravenec, M., Landa, V., Zidek, V., Musilova, A., Kren, V., Kazdova, L., Aitman, T. J., Glazier A. M., Ibrahimi, A., Abumrad, N. A., Qi, N., Wang, J. M., St Lezin, E. M., and Kurtz, T. W. (2001). Transgenic rescue of defective Cd36 ameliorates insulin resistance in spontaneously hypertensive rats. *Nat Genet 27*, 156–158.

Rahman, N., Teare, M. D., Seal, S., Renard, H., Mangion, J., Cour, C., Thompson, D., Shugart, Y., Eccles, D., Devilee, P., Meijers, H., Nathanson, K. L., Neuhausen, S. L., Weber, B., Chang-Claude, J., Easton, D. F., Goldgar, D., and Stratton, M. R. (2000). Absence of evidence for a familial breast cancer susceptibility gene at chromosome 8p12-p22. *Oncogene 19*, 4170–4173.

Riordan, J. R., Rommens, J. M., Kerem, B., Alon, N., Rozmahel, R., Grzelczak, Z., Zielenski, J., Lok, S., Plavsic, N., Chou, J. L., et al. (1989). Identification of the cystic fibrosis gene: Cloning and characterization of complementary DNA. *Science 245*, 1066–1073.

Rommens, J. M., Iannuzzi, M. C., Kerem, B., Drumm, M. L., Melmer, G., Dean, M., Rozmahel, R., Cole, J. L., Kennedy, D., Hidaka, N., et al. (1989). Identification of the cystic fibrosis gene: Chromosome walking and jumping. *Science 245*, 1059–1065.

Schrag, D., Kuntz, K. M., Garber, J. E., and Weeks, J. C. (2000). Life expectancy gains from cancer prevention strategies for women with breast cancer and BRCA1 or BRCA2 mutations. *JAMA 283*, 617–624.

Seitz, S., Rohde, K., Bender, E., Nothnagel, A., Kolble, K., Schlag, P. M., and Scherneck, S. (1997). Strong indication for a breast cancer susceptibility gene on chromosome 8p12-p22: Linkage analysis in German breast cancer families. *Oncogene 14*, 741–743.

Streuwing, J. P., Hartge, P., Wacholder, S., Baker, S. M., Berlin, M., McAdams, M., Timmerman, M. M., Brody, L. C., and Tucker, M. A. (1997). The risk of cancer associated with specific mutations of BRCA1 and BRCA2 among Ashkenazi Jews. *N Engl J Med 336*, 1401–1408.

Thompson, D., Szabo, C. I., Mangion, J., Oldenburg, R. A., Odefrey, F., Seal, S., Barfoot, R., Kroeze-Jansema, K., Teare, D., Rahman, N., Renard, H., Mann, G., Hopper, J. L., Buys, S. S., Andrulis, I. L., Senie, R., Daly, M. B., West, D., Ostrander, E. A., Offit, K., Peretz, T., Osorio, A., Benitez, J., Nathanson, K. L., Sinilnikova, O. M., Olah, E., Bignon, Y. J., Ruiz, P., Badzioch, M. D., Vasen, H. F., Futreal, A. P., Phelan, C. M., Narod, S. A., Lynch, H. T., Ponder, B. A., Eeles, R. A., Meijers-Heijboer, H., Stoppa-Lyonnet, D., Couch, F. J., Eccles, D. M., Evans, D. G., Chang-Claude, J., Lenoir, G., Weber, B. L., Devilee, P., Easton, D. F., Goldgar, D. E., and Stratton, M. R. (2002). Evaluation of linkage of breast cancer to the putative BRCA3 locus on chromosome 13q21 in 128 multiple case families from the Breast Cancer Linkage Consortium. *Proc Natl Acad Sci USA 99*, 827–831.

Thompson, M. E., Jensen, R. A., Obermiller, P. S., Page, D. L., and Holt, J. T. (1995). Decreased expression of BRCA1 accelerates growth and is often present during sporadic breast cancer progression. *Nat Genet 9*, 444–450.

Thorlacius, S., Olafsdottir, G., Kryggvadottir, L., Neuhausen, S., Jonasson, J. G., Tavtigian, S. V., Tulinius, H., Ogmundsdottir, H. M., and Eyfjord, J. E. (1996). A single BRCA2 mutation in male and female breast cancer families from Iceland with varied cancer phenotypes. *Nat Genet 13*, 117–119.

Tirkkonen, M., Johannsson, O., Agnarsson, B. A., Olsson, H., Ingvarsson, S., Karhu, R., Tanner, M., Isola, J., Barkardottir, R. B., Borg, A., and Kallioniemi, O. P. (1997). Distinct somatic genetic changes associated with tumor progression in carriers of BRCA1 and BRCA2 germ-line mutations. *Cancer Res 57*, 1222–1227.

Tutt, A., and Ashworth, A. (2002). The relationship between the roles of BRCA genes in DNA repair and cancer predisposition. *Trends Mol Med 8*, 571–576.

Venkitaraman, A. R. (2002). Cancer susceptibility and the functions of BRCA1 and BRCA2. *Cell 108*, 171–182.

Wooster, R., Neuhausen, S. L., Mangion, J., Quirk, Y., Ford, D., Colllins, N., Nguyen, K., Seal, S., Tran, T., Averill, D., Fields, P., Marshall, G., Narod, S., Lenoir, G. M., Lynch, H., Feunteun, J., Devilee, P., Cornelisse, C. J., Menko, F. H., Daly, P. A., Ormiston, W., McManus, R., Pye, C., Lewis, C. M., Cannon-Albright, L. A., Peto, J., Ponder, B. A. J., Skolnick, M. H., Easton, D. F., Goldgar, D. E., and Stratton, M. R. (1994). Localization of a breast cancer susceptibility gene, BRCA2, to chromosome 13q12–13. *Science 265*, 2088–2090.

7

LINKING DRUGS AND GENES: PHARMACOGENOMICS, PHARMACOPROTEOMICS, BIOINFORMATICS, AND THE NCI-60

John N. Weinstein

INTRODUCTION

Each new paradigm in drug discovery and development is claimed to be more rational, or at least more reasonable, than what came before. In the case of the pharmacogenomic and pharmacoproteomic approaches, however, the claim has considerable substance. We are beginning to see the hoped-for individualization of therapy and molecular subsetting of patients. The 60-cell line panel (the NCI-60) used by the National Cancer Institute to screen compounds for anticancer activity constitutes a "60-square chess board" for working out both experimental and bioinformatic links between molecular characteristics of cancer cells and the drug discovery process.

The vision is clear: Use information on the molecular profiles of tumor cells to individualize therapy for cancer—or at least to select more appropriate therapy for particular subgroups of patients. For the most part, that vision is being pursued through the study of clinical tumors. But that pursuit has proved more difficult than might have been expected. There are several reasons: (1) Clinical tumors are heterogeneous—a mixture

Oncogenomics: Molecular Approaches to Cancer, Edited by Charles Brenner and David Duggan
ISBN 0-471-22592-4 © 2004 John Wiley & Sons, Inc.

of cancer cells, stromal components, endothelial cells, and infiltrating leukocytes. Any molecular profile obtained for bulk tumor is a compromise among the characteristics of those components. The alternative approach is to obtain relatively homogeneous microscopic portions of the tumor by a technique such as laser capture microdissection (Emmert-Buck et al., 1996; see also Chapter 8). Such techniques can be used to isolate the cancer cells—for example, in pseudoglandular epithelial structures within the tumors. The technique is precise enough to isolate even single cells. But then an amplification method must generally be used to generate enough DNA or mRNA for study. Methods of amplification are available (e.g., T7-viral amplification, rolling circle amplification, two-primer PCR, and single-primer PCR), but their fidelity is still a significant question. For proteins, there is no equivalent method, but given sufficient patience and dedication, it has been possible to obtain enough material from a large number of laser shots for analysis by a technique such as two-dimensional polyacrylamide gel electrophoresis or hybridization to a protein array. (2) Clinical tumors are difficult to study, given anesthesia effects, surgical trauma, and the many logistical and ethical constraints discussed in Chapter 15 on the design of clinical trials. (3) Clinical materials often have fragmentary, complex histories. Demographic and clinical information may be difficult or impossible to obtain because of ethical and/or legal issues. (4) Clinical studies are expensive.

In contrast, cell lines have the advantages that they are relatively homogeneous, at least in cell lineage (though not in cell cycle state); they are reproducible from experiment to experiment and year to year; they can be obtained in quantity; they can be manipulated by transfection, knockout, selection for resistant forms, or treatment with siRNA, antisense RNA, drugs, or radiation to address particular experimental questions. The problem, of course, is that they are not fully representative of cancer cells in vivo. Even primary cultures of tumor cells have been removed from their natural society of other cell types, cytokines, and three-dimensional architecture. They have been selected for growth on plastic in standard medium with a relatively quick rate of cell cycling. Therefore, predictions from cultured cells toward the clinic are uncertain; we can, at best, obtain clues to formulate hypotheses to be validated in real tumors, either clinically or through pathological studies. A valuable tool for the latter is the tissue array (see Chapter 8). When one extrapolates backwards from cell line studies to the basic biology or pharmacology, however, one is on reasonably sound ground. Most of our knowledge of the biology and pharmacology, after all, has been obtained from cultured cells or from molecular studies, not from clinical materials.

As researchers consider the various ways of screening for anticancer agents (Shoemaker et al., 2002), the currently dominant approach involves biochemical (i.e., molecular) targets rather than cells or clinical tumors. As illustrated in Section III, biochemical screens are powerful because they can identify compounds with selectivity for particular functioning molecules or pathways. As our understanding of potential target molecules and the interactions among them increases, we should be able to translate that knowledge into new therapies. A limitation of the biochemical approach, however, is that activity against a target does not imply *selective* activity; the compound must, in principle, be tested against an indefinitely large number of additional targets to reduce the likelihood of "off-target" effects. Even then, as illustrated in Chapter 14's discussion of farnesyl transferase inhibitors, there are surprises when the compounds are tested in cells, in animals, or in the clinic.

The problem is worse for cancer than for most other diseases because researchers are usually targeting molecules in highly redundant pathways and networks with relatively small differences between the cancer cells and rapidly proliferating normal cell types—for example, in the bone marrow and gastrointestinal lining. Furthermore, as discussed in Chapter 1, tumors undergo evolution through a process of natural (or unnatural, drug-induced) selection. They tend to develop resistance to the compounds used against them. Increasingly, the aim is to find drugs with targets that are fundamental to selective proliferation of the tumor cells. Conceptually attractive current examples are Herceptin for HER2-positive metastatic breast cancer, Gleevec for adult Philadelphia chromosome-positive chronic myeloid leukemia, and adenoviruses such as ONYX-015 engineered to multiply selectively in cells with defects in pathways related to the tumor suppressor p53. But clinical experience to date indicates that it is rarely sufficient to attack just one target. Most current nonsurgical cancer treatments are based on combinations of drugs, with or without radiation. Potential targets must be considered not in isolation but in their cellular milieu (Monga and Sausville, 2002). For that reason, cells and then animal models must be invoked early in the drug discovery process, even if the starting point is a molecular screen or molecular drug design.

THE NCI'S CELL-BASED SCREEN

As noted in the introduction, an additional disadvantage of clinical materials from a pharmacological perspective is that their treatment histories are generally fragmentary and difficult to interpret. For many pharmacological purposes, we would like to study cancer cell types that have been tested with a large number of potential drugs. The most obvious such cells are the 60 human cancer lines (the NCI-60) used by the Developmental Therapeutics Program (DTP) of the National Cancer Institute (NCI) to test for potential anticancer agents. They have been characterized pharmacologically by exposure to more than 100,000 defined chemical compounds (plus a large number of natural product extracts), one at a time and independently.

Prior to 1985, NCI's DTP was using P388 leukemias of mice to screen compounds for anticancer activity. That strategy identified agents active against leukemias but was not deemed effective in identifying agents active against the common solid tumors of humans. Hence, the decision was made to seek a different strategy for screening. Between 1985 and 1989, under the leadership of Michael Boyd and Bruce Chabner, with the advice of committees of international experts in drug discovery, a variety of cell-based screening methods were tried and analyzed. After competing factors were taken into account, the result was the NCI-60 screening protocol.

After a period of pilot testing, the screen went into production mode in April 1990. Since that time, >100,000 chemically defined compounds plus natural product extracts have been tested. Since 1991, the 60 cell lines have included leukemias, melanomas, and cancer cells of ovarian, renal, breast, prostate, colon, lung, and central nervous system origin. That is by no means a complete list of tumor categories, but it includes the most common ones. The aim was to include at least 6 lines of each type (except prostate, for which 6 suitable lines were not available) to provide sufficient statistical power to identify organ selectivity of the tested compounds. The guiding hypothesis was that selective activity against cancers from a particular organ would predict activity against the same type of tumor in the clinic. That type of predictiveness has not been demonstrated, but the screen quickly took on a new role and a new character: It became a system for profiling, or "fingerprinting," the tested compounds and, later, the cell lines themselves. The NCI-60 system is called a screen, but increasingly it has been used for secondary testing of compounds that have been found in screens by the DTP or others to attack a defined molecule or pathway. Increasingly, DTP is establishing molecular target screens to identify candidate compounds.

The top part of Box 7-1 shows the screening strategy in highly schematic form. The bottom part shows how it produces a database (A) of activities, which can be mapped into a database (S) of structural characteristics of the tested compounds and a database (T) of molecular targets and other characteristics of the cells used for testing. This set of databases provides the conceptual structure for the pharmacogenomic and pharmacoproteomic studies described in this chapter. Not shown is a 3 cell line pre-screen that was recently introduced to filter out compounds with little or no activity. The first topic discussed is the screen itself. After that, in order, are the A, S, and T databases. Finally, we consider how they can be integrated with each other to serve pharmacogenomic and pharmacoproteomic aims.

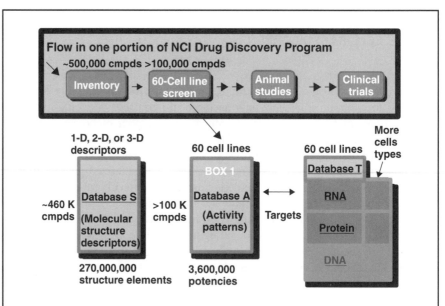

Box 7-1. Simplified schematic overview of an information-intensive approach to cancer pharmacogenomics and pharmacoproteomics based on the NCI-60 cancer cell lines. Each row of the activity (A) database represents the pattern of activity of a particular compound across the 60 cell lines. The A database can be mapped into a structure (S) database containing 2-D or 3-D chemical structure descriptors of the compounds and a target (T) database containing molecular profile information on the cells. The T database consists of data on individual molecules and omic data at the DNA, mRNA, protein, and functional levels. The bioinformatic challenge is to analyze and understand each of these databases separately, then to integrate them with each other and with public information resources for pharmacogenomic purposes. (*Source*: Modified from Weinstein et al., 1997.)

The NCI-60 Screen: Methodology

The methodology of the NCI-60 screen has been described in detail elsewhere (see www.dtp.nci.nih.gov). Briefly, on day zero the human tumor cell lines are plated in 96-well microtiter format in RPMI 1640 medium with 5% fetal calf serum and 2 mM L-glutamine. Twenty-four hours later, the drug (dissolved in DMSO) is added to achieve five concentrations at 10-fold intervals (plus a negative control). Usually, the concentration range is from 10^{-4} down to 10^{-8} M. After 48 hours of drug exposure at $37^{o}C$ (in 5% CO_2, 95% air, 100% relative humidity), the cells are fixed in situ with trichloroacetic acid. The supernatant is discarded (along with floating cells and cell fragments), and the plates are washed five times, then air-dried. Colorimetric measurement of sulforhodamine B (SRB) dye is used to quantitate the amount of cell material left attached to the well at the end of the incubation period.

Three indices are calculated by straight-line interpolation (with appropriate quality-control checks) from the 5-point dose-response curves: The 50% growth inhibition (GI_{50}) is the concentration of drug required to inhibit cell growth by a factor of 2 (as judged from the SRB signal). The total growth inhibition (TGI) is the concentration required to maintain the SRB signal at its predrug level. The 50% lethal concentration (LC_{50}) is the concentration required to decrease the SRB signal by 50%. In terms of the concentrations required, $GI_{50} < TGI < LC_{50}$.

The Activity (A) Database

Since more compounds reach GI_{50} than reach the other indices, we consider only calculations based on GI_{50} in this chapter. For relatively inactive compounds, all that can be said is that the GI_{50} is greater than the highest concentration tested. In statistical terms, the data point is censored. As with dose-response curves in general, the data are best treated by log-transforming them. The fundamental parameter used as a measure of potency is $-\log_{10} GI_{50}$. During pilot studies for the screen in the late 1980s, Kenneth Paull realized that the absolute potency of a compound did not give much information on its mechanisms of action and resistance; rather, the *pattern* of relative activities across the cell lines contained the important information. He therefore subtracted out the log mean over the 60 cell lines (including censored, but not missing, values) to obtain the very useful "mean graph" representation of activity data. The lack of information inherent in absolute potency was later corroborated more formally by principal components analysis (Koutsoukos et al., 1994; Keskin et al., 2000; Shi et al., 2000).

The mean graph representation of patterns led to the COMPARE algorithm (Paull et al., 1989; Boyd, 1992). Given one compound as a "seed," COMPARE searches the database of screened agents for those most similar to the seed in their patterns of activity against the NCI-60. Similarity in pattern often indicates similarity in mechanism of action, mode of resistance, and/or molecular structure. The similarity metric was initially taken as the Euclidean distance and later as the Pearson correlation coefficient. COMPARE has been applied productively to topoisomerase inhibitors (Solary, 1993; Leteurtre et al., 1994, 1995; Gupta et al., 1995; Koo et al., 1996), pyrimidine biosynthesis inhibitors (Cleveland et al., 1995), antimitotics (Bai et al., 1991; Paull et al., 1992; Kuo et al., 1993; Hamel et al., 1996), compounds with preferential effects against Nm23-expressing cells (Freije et al., 1997), and agents active against epidermal growth factor-expressing cells (Wosikowski et al., 1997), among many other classes of agents.

In 1992, to discriminate among various possible mechanisms of drug action on the basis of activity patterns, we introduced feed-forward, back-propagation neural networks, with statistical validation by cross-validation and sensitivity analysis (Weinstein et al., 1992). Since then, a variety of additional statistical and artificial intelligence methods have yielded detailed information on the relationship between pattern and mechanism. Included have been principal components analysis (Koutsoukos et al., 1994) and Kohonen self-organizing maps (van Osdol et al., 1994, 2000; Keskin et al., 2000). Self-organizing maps in this context are used to represent the structural or functional similarities of compounds in the form of two-dimensional maps.

In 1994, we introduced clustering and clustered image maps (CIMs) for analysis and visualization of the pharmacological and molecular data (Weinstein et al., 1994, 1997). Figure 7-1 shows a CIM correlating the activity patterns with molecular characteristics (targets) of the cells, including gene and protein expression data. CIMs have since become the most popular way to represent expression data sets globally, although they by no means capture all of the information available in those data.

The Structure (S) Database

The chemical structures in S can be coded in terms of any set of one-, two-, or three-dimensional descriptors. Useful codings can be found at the DTP's web site (dtp.nci.nih.gov). Analyses that relate the S and A databases can be thought of as quite general formulations of Q-SARs (quantitative structure-activity relationships). A number of studies have highlighted various aspects of these relationships for the NCI-60 (Shi et al., 1996, 1997, 1998a, 1998b, 1998c, 2000; Fan et al., 1998, 2001; Rabow et al., 2002). Genetic function approximation (an amalgam of genetic algorithm for variable selection and regression splines for data fitting; Rogers and Hopfinger, 1994) proved a useful approach (Shi et al., 1996, 1998b, 2000; Fan et al., 2001). Since structural descriptors are available for >500,000 compounds (Milne et al., 1994), it has been possible to map interesting patterns of activity into the S database and develop abstract pharmacophore templates with which to search the >400,000 compounds not yet screened, bringing candidate compounds into the testing process.

The Target (T) Database

The first molecular target analyzed experimentally and analytically was the drug resistance transporter P-glycoprotein (Pgp) encoded by the multidrug resistance gene Mdr-1 (Wu et al., 1992; Lee et al., 1994; Alvarez et al., 1995; Izquierdo et al., 1996). Figure 7-1, a clustered image map obtained by combining information from the T and A databases, shows the importance of Pgp/Mdr-1 to the pattern of drug sensitivities of the cell lines. The dark blue patch for compounds 513–667 indicates that those compounds are highly negative in correlation with targets 81 to 88, which are the indices of Pgp/Mdr-1 expression and function.

The statistics were striking. We analyzed cell screen data for a set of 35 compounds of diverse structure and mechanism that had been reported previously on the basis of transport assays to be Mdr-1 substrates (Chin et al., 1993; Gottesman and Pastan, 1993; Lee et al., 1994; Alvarez et al., 1995). Of those, 18 (51%) fell within the blue patch,

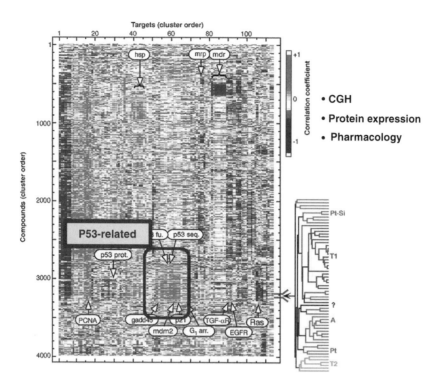

Figure 7-1. Clustered image map of the relationship between tested compounds and molecular targets in the NCI-60 cells. This normalized $A \cdot T^T$ product matrix (where the superscript T indicates the matrix transpose) correlates target patterns with patterns of growth inhibition for a set of 3989 important compounds. A red or orange point (high positive Pearson correlation coefficient) indicates that the agent tends to be selectively active in the SRB assay against cell lines that express the target in large amounts (or in functional form). A dark blue point (high negative correlation) indicates the opposite. The 113 columns correspond to 76 distinct target molecules or functions, some represented multiple times in different mathematical transformations. Compounds and targets have been cluster-ordered by an average linkage algorithm to bring like together with like. To the right is shown one 61-leaf "twig" of the overall 3989-leaf cluster tree of compounds. Symbols for mechanisms of action are as follows: T1, topoisomerase 1 inhibitors; T2, topoisomerase 2 inhibitors; A, alkylating agents; Pt, platinum compounds; Pt-Si, platinum agents containing a silane moiety;?, mechanism unknown. The most prominent features are a red patch that indicates compounds (2802–3309) that tend to be active in the assay in cell lines with intact p53 function and a blue patch that indicates compounds (513–667) selectively inactive in Mdr-1/Pgp-expressing cells. (*Source*: Modified from Weinstein et al., 1997.) See insert for color representation of this figure.

whereas only 4% would have been expected to do so by chance. That represented a 13-fold enrichment with respect to random assignment. The probability (exact binomial) of such an extreme enrichment being found by chance is <0.0001. Although 18 of the 35 reported substrates fell within the blue patch, 0 of 12 compounds were reported not to be substrates (Chin et al., 1993; Gottesman and Pastan, 1993; Lee et al., 1994; Alvarez et al., 1995) did so ($P = 0.001$ by Fisher's exact test).

Mdr-1 substrates tend to be natural products of high molecular weight and are often cationic. We found (by linear discriminant analysis) that those three factors could predict with a specificity of 84% and sensitivity of 78% which compounds would be found in the blue patch ($P < 0.0001$). Columns 76 and 77 in Figure 7-1 are indices of mRNA expression for Mrp-1, another transporter molecule associated with multidrug resistance (Izquierdo et al., 1996). As expected, there was little overlap in the families of compounds sensitive to Mrp-1 and Pgp/Mdr-1. These calculations provide a sort of proof of principle for the pattern recognition process (Weinstein et al., 1997). Various other molecular targets have been assessed in the NCI-60, prominently including a set of molecular characteristics associated with p53 function (O'Connor et al., 1997).

Omic Profiling

For the remainder of this chapter, we are concerned with a different approach, which can be termed "omic" characterization of the cells (Weinstein, 1998, 2002)—that is, characterization of the molecules in aggregate at the DNA, RNA, or protein level. Omics began with genomics and proteomics. Then there emerged, not entirely in jest, such designations as transcriptomics, kinomics, immunomics, metabolomics, CHOmics (i.e., glycomics) clinomics, and integromics. This book is titled *Oncogenomics*. Other compound forms include chemical, structural, and functional genomics, as well as specialized areas such as oncopharmacomethylomics (referring to cytosine methylation in the promoter regions of cancer genes; Weinstein, 2000).

We hardly need more jargon, but it did seem that there ought to be a generic way of distinguishing between classical hypothesis-driven research and exploratory research that generates and/or applies large databases of biological information. In the latter case, a specifically biological hypothesis may motivate generation of the data, but the enterprise often takes on a life of its own; it is not known in advance what aspect or use of the data will prove most important. The paradigmatic example is, of course, the genome project. The draft human sequence was reported in *Science* and *Nature* in the year 2001 (Lander et al., 2001; Venter et al., 2001) in the form of several manuscripts that made particular uses of the information or organized the sequences in particular ways. But no one would seriously claim that the chief long-term value of the information, or of its publication, resided in that immediate set of contributions. The still-developing sequence database is a resource of much more general utility, a time capsule (Weinstein, 2002).

In light of the preceding discussion, what is the difference between pharmacogenetics and pharmacogenomics? It may not be possible to distinguish the two precisely, but, broadly speaking, pharmacogenomics is the study of large numbers of genes at a time for their interactions with drug responses, whereas pharmacogenetics focuses on one or a few genes at a time. A pharmacogenomic study may, of course, lead to a pharmacogenetic one if it identifies particular genes of interest. As an alternative definition of pharmacogenetics, it could be considered as the generic term, with pharmacogenomics as the omic subcategory.

Many laboratories, including ours, have characterized the NCI-60 one or a few molecules or functions at a time. For the most part, however, we have taken an "omic" approach, characterizing them more broadly in terms of molecular types in aggregate at the DNA, RNA, and protein levels. The result is the richest, most varied profiling of any set of cells. Figure 7-2 presents the overall array of databases generated. Because most pharmacological targets are proteins rather than mRNA, we began our expression profiling studies in the mid-1990s with 2D-PAGE, in collaboration with Leigh Anderson at Large Scale Biology, Inc. That project led to a database of 1014 spots indexed across the 60 cell lines. We then spent a year refining a method (Li et al., 1997) for identification of the spots by in-gel digestion using combinations of proteases, followed by MALDI-TOF (matrix-assisted laser desorption ionization–time-of-flight) peptide mapping. However, by that time it was clear that identification of hundreds or thousands of proteins was not a job for a small academic laboratory. We decided to wait for the proteomic technologies to improve and dropped back to the transcript level, where the task appeared easier. The wait has been a long one.

In part, the challenge at the mRNA level appeared easier because there are "only" about 25,000 independent transcripts and perhaps 200,000 splice variants of those transcripts, rather than millions of functional protein states. We were able to generate transcript profiles for the NCI-60 using four different platforms: a 7907-clone cDNA array with the Brown/Botstein laboratory (Ross et al., 2000; Scherf et al., 2000), a 6800-gene Affymetrix oligonucleotide chip (Hu6800) with the Golub/Lander group (Staunton et al., 2001), and the 60,000-gene U95 and 30,000-gene U133 Affymetrix oligonucleotide chips with Uwe Scherf at Gene Logic, Inc. Versions of the first two used for our calculations are available at discover.nci.nih.gov.

In parallel with those studies, we have undertaken collaborations with a number of laboratories for profiling at the DNA level, as indicated in Figure 7-2: with the laboratory of Kenneth Buetow (NCI) using Affymetrix SNP chips for single-nucleotide polymorphisms (Alexander et al., in preparation); with that of Ilan Kirsch and Anna Roschke (NCI) for spectral karyotyping (SKY) and comparative genomic hybridization (CGH; Reinhold et al., 2003; Roschke et al., submitted); with that of Joe Gray at the University of California, San Francisco Cancer Center for CGH based on BAC arrays

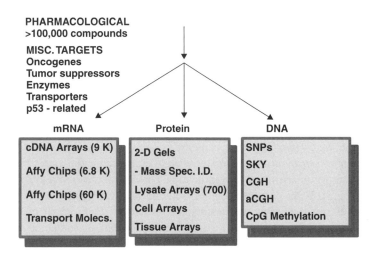

Figure 7-2. Molecular profiling of the NCI-60 cancer cell lines. Methods noted in the DNA, RNA, and protein boxes are those used by the Genomics & Bioinformatics Group and collaborating laboratories to profile the cells. The pharmacological database was generated by the NCI-60 screen in DTP, and the miscellaneous targets are from various laboratories. Tissue arrays of clinical tumors are used for validation of hypotheses developed on the basis of data from the NCI-60.

(Chin et al. and Bussey et al., in preparation); with the laboratories of David Munroe (NCI) and Andrew Feinberg (Johns Hopkins University) for detailed sequence analysis of cytosine methylation in the CpG islands of promoter regions of cancer-interesting genes (Reinhold et al. and Maunakea et al., in preparation). Most recently, at the protein level, with Lance Liotta (NCI) and Emanuel Petricoin (Food and Drug Administration), we have developed a high-density reverse-phase protein lysate microarray for proteomic profiling of the 60 lines without the need for spot identification (Nishizuka et al., 2003a, and Nishizuka et al., 2003b).

For validation of hypotheses directed toward the clinic, we have used tissue arrays produced by the TARP (Tissue Array Program) Consortium at NCI (Nishizuka et al., 2003a). The arrays consist of cores from 503 human tumors of disparate types and 62 normal human tissues.

Transcript Expression Profiling by cDNA Array. The methods used in this study are described in detail elsewhere (Ross et al., 2000; Scherf et al., 2000). Very briefly, cells were harvested carefully (with less than 1 minute from incubator to stabilization of the preparation) at approximately 80% confluence. Total RNA was stored, then further purified to obtain poly-A mRNA shortly prior to hybridization with microarrays (Synteni, Inc.; now Incyte, Inc.) consisting of robotically spotted, PCR-amplified cDNAs on coated glass slides (Shalon et al., 1996).

The 9703 DNA elements on the array were cDNAs from the Washington University/Merck IMAGE set, obtained from Research Genetics, Inc. The array included 3700 named genes, 1900 human genes homologous to those of other organisms, and 4104 ESTs of unknown function but defined chromosome map location. For each hybridization, cDNA synthesized from the test cell's mRNA was labeled by incorporation of Cy5-dNTP during reverse transcription. cDNA synthesized from pooled mRNA of 12 highly diverse cell lines out of the 60 (Scherf et al., 2000) was analogously labeled by incorporation of Cy3-dNTP. Cells for the pool were selected to satisfy three criteria (Scherf et al., 2000): (1) at least one cell line from each organ of origin; (2) diversity of growth rates; (3) diversity in terms of protein expression pattern based on prior two-dimensional gel studies (Myers et al., 1997). After appropriate filtering, we settled on a data set of approximately 1400 genes for detailed analysis.

Figure 7-3A shows a cluster tree that represents the patterns of gene expression across the cell lines. As indicated by the accompanying annotations, there is considerable regularity by organ of origin of the cells. Figure 3B shows the remarkably different cluster tree obtained when the same cells are clustered on the basis of drug activity. The correlation of correlations (Scherf et al., 2000) between the two trees was only +0.21 (0 indicating no similarity; 1 indicating perfect identity). Figure 7-4 shows a CIM that summarizes all pairwise relationships between the gene database and a set of 118 drugs of putatively known mechanism of action. Each patch of color represents a story. It may be causally interesting, epiphenomenal, or statistical coincidence. There is clearly not sufficient statistical power to eliminate most of the false positive associations without losing too many of the true positives. Hence, we must generally consult the literature for clues to determine which relationships are worth pursuing. An interesting vignette is presented at the end of this chapter.

Gene Expression Profiling by Affymetrix Oligonucleotide Chip. The methods used have been described previously (Staunton et al., 2001). Very briefly, mRNA

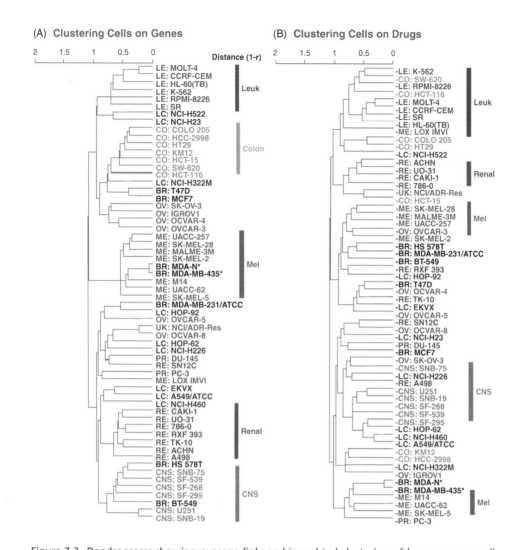

Figure 7-3. Dendrograms showing average linkage hierarchical clustering of human cancer cell lines. (A) Cluster tree of the 60 cell lines based on their gene expression profiles for 1376 genes and 40 individual targets. One hundred percent of the colon cancer lines (CO; 7/7), the central nervous system lines (CNS; 6/6), and the leukemias (LE; 6/6) clustered together. Seven out of eight melanoma lines (ME) clustered together, the exception being the one reported to lack melanin production (LOX-IMVI). Seven out of eight renal carcinoma lines (RE) clustered together, as did four out of six ovarian lines (OV). Non-small-cell lung cancer cells (LC) clustered on two different branches, and those of breast origin (BR) appeared most heterogeneous. The estrogen receptor–positive breast lines, T-47D and MCF7, appeared together and grouped with the colon lines, whereas the estrogen receptor–negative HS578T and BT-549 clustered with CNS malignancies. NCI/ADR-Res is of unknown origin (UK). (B) Cluster tree for the cells based on their patterns of sensitivity to 1400 tested compounds. The distance metric used was (1 − Pearson correlation coefficient). *Indicates two cell lines (MDA MB435 and MDA-N) with the gene expression and drug sensitivity signatures of melanotic melanoma but putatively derived from the pleural effusion of a breast cancer patient. (Source: Modified from Scherf et al., 2000.)

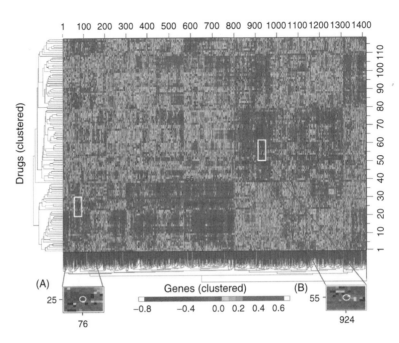

Figure 7-4. Clustered image map (CIM) relating activity patterns of 118 tested compounds to the expression patterns of 1376 genes in the 60 cell lines. Included in addition to the gene expression levels are data for 40 molecular targets assessed one at a time in the cells. A red point (high positive Pearson correlation coefficient) indicates that the agent tends to be more active (in the 2-day assay) against cell lines that express more of the gene; a blue point (high negative correlation) indicates the opposite tendency. Genes were cluster-ordered on the basis of their correlations with drugs (mean-subtracted, average linkage clustered with correlation metric); drugs were clustered on the basis of their correlations with genes (mean-subtracted, average linkage clustered with correlation metric). Sharp edges of the colored patches reflect deep forks in the corresponding cluster tree. Insert (A) shows a magnified view of the region around the point (white circle) representing the correlation between the dihydropyrimidine dehydrogenase gene and 5-fluorouracil. Insert (B) is an analogous magnified view for the asparagine synthetase gene and the drug L-asparaginase. (*Source*: Modified from Scherf, et al., 2000.) See insert for color representation of this figure.

was obtained from the cells (Scherf et al., 2000) and used to prepare biotinylated cDNA, which was hybridized to Hu6800 arrays (Affymetrix, Santa Clara, CA). The results generally reflected what we had found with the cDNA arrays. We then cross-compared the oligonucleotide and cDNA array data to establish a robust database of >1600 transcripts for which results from the two very different technologies are reasonably concordant across the 60 cell types (Lee et al., 2003). That database has since proved useful as a firm statistical basis for further analyses.

THE BIOINFORMATICS OF PHARMACOGENOMIC PROFILING

Anyone who does gene expression profiling (or similar omic experiments) for molecular targets finds that most of the time and energy are spent *after* the experiment in statistical analysis of the data and in biological interpretation. The problems are particularly acute for us because we are trying to integrate so many types of information—at the DNA, RNA, protein, functional, and pharmacological levels. Motivated by the needs of our experimental program, we developed a number of algorithms and computer program packages to assist in the analysis and interpretation steps. These programs, publicly available at discover.nci.nih.gov, are proving useful to others as well.

CIM-Miner

This program generates color-coded clustered image maps (CIMs; also called clustered heat maps) to represent "high-dimensional" data sets such as gene expression profiles. We introduced CIMs in the mid-1990s for data on drug activities, target expression levels, gene expression values, and proteomic profiles (Weinstein et al., 1994, 1997; Myers et al., 1997). The clustering of both axes (or sometimes only one if there is another organizing principle for the second axis) puts like together with like to create patterns of color. A program for producing CIMs can be found at discover.nci.nih.gov, and Figure 7-4 shows a CIM for drug-target relationships. Each patch of color in the CIM represents a possible story. But how can we determine whether a patch represents a causally interesting story, an epiphenomenal correlation (which still may identify a useful molecular marker), or statistical coincidence? Most often, the answer is that we must consult the biomedical literature and public databases.

To streamline the process of searching and organizing the biomedical literature, we developed the program packages MedMiner (Tanabe et al., 1999) and EDGAR (Rindflesch et al., 2000). Similarly, to facilitate use of the public gene and protein databases, we developed MatchMiner (Bussey et al., 2003) and GoMiner (Zeeberg et al., 2003). To link genomics firmly to drug discovery, we and our collaborators developed LeadScope/LeadMiner (Blower et al., 2002). These programs are proving useful to both clinical and preclinical researchers.

MedMiner

MedMiner (publicly available at discover.nci.nih.gov; Tanabe et al., 1999) can be used for gene, gene-gene, gene-drug, or more general literature queries. It uses a combination of GeneCards from the Weizmann Institute, PubMed from the National Library of Medicine, syntactic analysis, truncated keyword filtering of relationals, and user-controlled sculpting of Boolean queries to generate key sentences from pertinent abstracts. Those sentences are then organized so that the user can access the most pertinent ones directly by clicking on a relevance term. Whole abstracts of interest can then be accessed fluently and dropped into a "shopping basket" for display or for automated entry into a library under EndNote (ISI ResearchSoft, Berkeley, CA) or other bibliographic software. Experienced users have estimated that MedMiner speeds up 5- to 10-fold the process of capturing and organizing the literature from PubMed searches on lists of gene-gene and gene-drug relationships. MedMiner is fast enough and transparent enough for real-world use on the web, but it does not capture all of the information that is theoretically available in the free text of an abstract.

EDGAR

Natural language processing (NLP) is one of the great intellectual challenges, and a number of attempts are being made to harness NLP principles for omic studies. Our own effort in this direction is EDGAR, (Extraction of Data on Genes and Relationships), a software tool for semantic analysis and organization of the literature relevant to our studies in the pharmacogenomics of cancer (Rindflesch et al., 2000). EDGAR is based on an underspecified parser and the Unified Medical Language System.

MatchMiner

MatchMiner (publicly available at discover.nci.nih.gov; Bussey et al., 2003) provides a solution to the major problem of translating among various gene identifier types for lists of hundreds or thousands of genes. Currently included are GenBank accession numbers, IMAGE clone ids, common gene names, gene symbols, UniGene clusters, FISH-mapped BAC clones, Affymetrix identifiers, and chromosome locations. The LookUp function in MatchMiner makes such translations, providing the user with diagnostics that indicate how the translation was done. The Merge function finds the

(A)

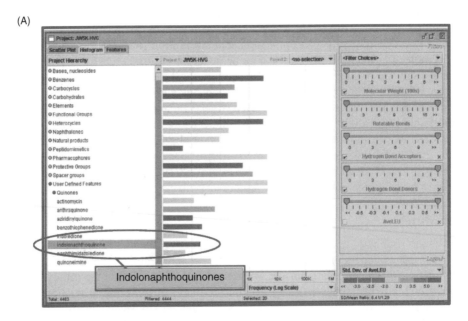

Figure 7-5. The LeadScope/LeadMiner program package. This program package performs the central task of pharmacogenomics: In terms of Figure 7-1, it relates molecular substructures of the screened compounds to molecular profiles of the cells used for screening—that is, it projects the substructures through the drugs and through the cells, all the way to molecular characteristics of the cells. (A) Screen shot of one of the visualizations. For example, the fact that the bar is colored red by Leadscope for indolonaphthoquinones indicates that an indolonaphthoquinone moiety tends to be found in compounds that are active in cells that express large amounts of a particular transcript. The length of the bar indicates the number of compounds in the pertinent sublibrary. At the left is a clickable hierarchical listing of the approximately 27,000 substructures included. At the right are sliders for restricting the compounds to be analyzed (e.g., restricting in terms of molecular weight). (B) A color-coded sublibrary identified by the program for one particular query (for compounds active in cell lines that highly express a particular transcript). (*Source*: Based on algorithms in Blower et al., 2002. Courtesy of P. Blower, LeadScope, Inc.)

(B)

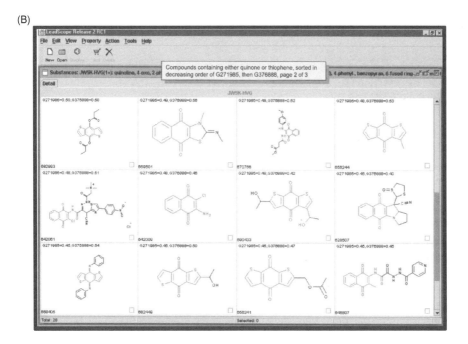

Figure 7-5. (*continued*)

intersection of two lists of genes, which may be designated by either the same or different identifiers. This functionality is particularly important to our "integromic" efforts to meld information from the variety of different data types on the NCI-60.

GoMiner

GoMiner (publicly available at discover.nci.nih.gov; Zeeberg et al., 2003) provides an answer to the question, "Now that I've done the gene expression experiment and identified a set of "interesting" genes, what do those genes mean biologically?" To address the question, GoMiner batch-processes and organizes lists of thousands or tens of thousands of genes and provides two fluent, robust visualizations of the genes embedded within the framework of the Gene Ontology hierarchy. It calculates summary statistics that indicate for each GO category whether it is enriched with, or depleted of, interesting genes and gives *p*-values with which to assess the statistical robustness of the enrichment or depletion.

LeadScope/LeadMiner™

LeadScope/LeadMiner (Blower et al., 2002) provides a firm link between molecular markers and the drug discovery process. More precisely, it links gene expression profiles for the NCI-60 (or other cell panels used for screening) to a set of 27,000 chemical substructure descriptors of the compounds that have been tested against the cells. One can use it, for example, to identify substructure classes that are found in compounds active in the screen against cell types that express large amounts of a particular gene.

Figure 7-5A and B shows screenshots of two aspects of the performance. The potential utility for identification and validation of therapeutic targets should be clear.

CLINICAL PHARMACOGENOMIC MARKERS: THE CASE OF ASPARAGINASE

The two white rectangles on the gene expression vs. drug sensitivity CIM in Figure 7-4 indicate stories with likely causal significance on the basis of literature information. The case of asparagine synthetase and L-asparaginase is particularly instructive.

Many acute lymphoblastic leukemias (ALL) lack asparagine synthetase and therefore must scavenge exogenous L-asparagine to survive. This dependence is exploited by treating ALL with bacterial L-asparaginase, which depletes extracellular L-asparagine and selectively starves the cancer cells. Figure 7-6 shows the relationship between L-asparaginase activity and asparagine synthetase expression across the NCI-60. As might have been predicted on the basis of the above mechanism, there was a statistically robust negative correlation (-0.44; bootstrap 95% confidence interval -0.59 to -0.25) between expression of the asparagine synthetase gene and L-asparaginase sensitivity in the 60 cell lines (Scherf et al., 2000). The correlation was moderately, but not very, strong. We knew, however, to focus specifically on the leukemic subpanel, and in that case the correlation was a striking -0.98 (bootstrap 95% confidence interval -1.00 to -0.93). This value survived even a Bonferroni correction for statistical multiple comparisons. Furthermore, the two ALL-derived lines expressed the lowest levels of

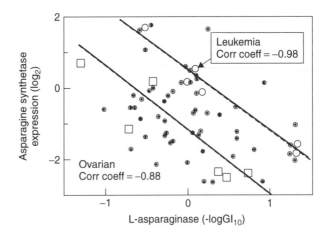

Figure 7-6. Relationship between asparagine synthetase expression levels and chemosensitivity of the NCI cell lines to L-asparaginase. Main effects have been removed for both cells and drugs. Hence, a negative $\log(GI_{50})$ value of 1 for sensitivity indicates a 10-fold higher-than-average sensitivity of the cell line to the agent. The asparagine synthetase expression level is plotted as the abundance of the asparagine synthetase transcript relative to its abundance in the reference pool of 12 cell lines. A value of +2 indicates 4-fold higher expression than in the reference pool. The large, open circles and squares indicate leukemia and ovarian cell lines, respectively. The linear regression lines were fitted to the leukemia and ovarian cancer data. (*Source*: Modified from Scherf et al., 2000.)

asparagine synthetase mRNA and were the most sensitive to L-asparaginase, as might have been expected. These results supported the possible use of asparagine synthetase as a marker for clinical decisions about L-asparaginase therapy (Scherf et al., 2000).

We then asked whether any other cell line panel showed similar correlation. The answer was yes, though not as strongly. The correlation coefficient for the ovarian lines was -0.88 (confidence interval -0.23 to -0.99; Scherf et al., 2000). Early clinical trials done with an assortment of solid tumors showed occasional responses to L-asparaginase in melanoma, chronic granulocytic leukemia, lymphosarcoma, and reticulum cell sarcoma but not in other tumor types (see Scherf et al., 2000, for references). The microarray findings, however, support a closer look at L-asparaginase therapy for solid tumors, particularly for a subset of ovarian cancers low in asparagine synthetase. The preferred material for a clinical trial would be the polyethylene glycol-modified forms of L-asparaginase, which show much better pharmacokinetic and immunological properties than does the native bacterial form of the enzyme. Further studies of this correlation are underway in collaboration with Von Hoff at the Arizona Cancer Center.

CONCLUDING REMARKS

When it comes to finding or designing the next generation of anticancer drugs, there is no sure bet. But it does appear likely that pharmacogenomic and pharmacoproteomic approaches to individualization of therapy and subsetting of patients will play significant roles. The bench-to-bedside and bedside-to-bench possibilities of those approaches are just too powerful to fail. The discovery process can begin in silico, in molecular screens, in screens based on engineered, isogenic cell sets, on wild-type cell panels, or in animals. Regardless of the starting point, however, exposure to a variety of cell types at an early stage in the process makes sense. The NCI-60 cells are not necessarily those that would be chosen to form a panel if we were starting now, but their legacy of pharmacological and molecular biological characterization makes them an invaluable resource—for discovery and also as a "60-square chess board" on which to design the foundations of next-generation pharmacomic inquiry. In the near term, as more patient samples are expression-profiled, we anticipate that researchers will be able to ask which reference cell sample is most similar to the tumor in order to try drugs with demonstrated efficacy against a particular molecular profile.

REFERENCES

Alvarez, M., Paull, K. D., Hose, C., Lee, J. S., Weinstein, J. N., Grever, M., Bates, S., and Fojo, T. (1995). Generation of a drug resistance profile by quantitation of MDR-1/P-glycoprotein expression in the cell lines of the NCI anticancer drug screen. *J Clin Invest* 95, 2205–2214.

Bai, R., Paull, K. D., Herald, C. L., Malspeis, L., Pettit, G. R., and Hamel, E. (1991). Halichondrin B and homohalichondrin B, marine natural products binding in the vinca domain of tubulin. Discovery of tubulin-based mechanism of action by analysis of differential cytotoxicity data. *J Biol Chem* 266, 15882–15889.

Blower, P. E., Jr., Yang, C., Fligner, M. A., Verducci, J. S., Yu, L., Richman, S., and Weinstein, J. N. (2002). Pharmacogenomic analysis: Correlating molecular substructure classes with microarray gene expression data. *Pharmacogenomics J* 2, 259–271.

Boyd, M. R. (1992). The future of new drug development. In *Current Therapy in Oncology*, J. E. Neiderhuber (ed.). Philadelphia: Decker, pp. 11–22.

Bussey, K. J., Kane, D., Sunshine, M., Narasimhan, S., Nishizuka, S., Reinhold, W. C., Zeeberg, B., Ajay, W., and Weinstein, J. N. (2003). MatchMiner: A tool for batch navigation among gene and gene product identifiers. *Genome Biol 4*, R27.

Chin, K. V., Pastan, I., and Gottesman, M. M. (1993). Function and regulation of the human multidrug resistance gene. *Adv Cancer Res 60*, 157–180.

Cleveland, E. S., Monks, A., Vaigro-Wolff, A., Zaharevitz, D. W., Paull, K., Ardalan, K., Cooney, D. A., and Ford, H., Jr. (1995). Site of action of two novel pyrimidine biosynthesis inhibitors accurately predicted by the compare program. et al. *Biochem Pharmacol 49*, 947–954.

Emmert-Buck, M. R., Bonner, R. F., Smith, P. D., Chuaqui, R. F., Zhuang, Z., Goldstein, S. R., Weiss, R. A., and Liotta, L. A. (1996). Laser capture microdissection. *Science 274* (5289), 998–1001.

Fan, Y., Weinstein, J. N., Kohn, K. W., Shi, L. M., and Pommier, Y. (1998). Molecular modeling studies of the DNA–topoisomerase 1 ternary cleavable complex with camptothecin. *J Med Chem 38*, 2216–2226.

Fan, Y., Shi, L. M., Myers, T. G., Kohn, K. W., Pommier, Y., and Weinstein, J. N. (2001). Quantitative structure-antitumor activity relationships of camptothecins: Cluster analysis and genetic algorithm-based studies. *J Med Chem 44*, 3254–3263.

Freije, J. M., Lawrence, J. A., Hollingshead, M. G., De la Rosa, A., Narayanan, V., Grever, M., Sausville, E. A., Paull, K., and Steeg, P. S. (1997). Identification of compounds with preferential inhibitory activity against low-Nm23-expressing human breast carcinoma and melanoma cell lines. *Nat Med 3*, 395–401.

Gottesman, M. M., and Pastan, I. (1993). Biochemistry of multidrug resistance mediated by the multidrug transporter. *Annu Rev Biochem 62*, 385–427.

Gupta, M., Fujimori, A., and Pommier, Y. (1995). DNA topoisomerase I. *Biochim Biophys Acta 1262*, 1–14.

Hamel, E., Lin, C. M., Plowman, J., Wang, H. K., Lee, K. H., and Paull, K. D. (1996). Antitumor 2,3-dihydro-2-(aryl)-4(1H)-quinzolinone derivatives. Interactions with tubulin. *Biochem Pharmacol 51*, 53–59.

Izquierdo, M. A., Shoemaker, R. H., Flens, M. J., Scheffer, G. L., Wu, L., and Prather, T. R. (1996). Overlapping phenotypes of multidrug resistance among panels of human cancer-cell lines. *Int J Cancer 65*, 230–237.

Keskin, O., Bahar, I., Jernigan, R. L., Beutler, J. A., Shoemaker, R. H., Sausville, E. A., and Covell, D. G. (2000). Characterization of anticancer agents by their growth inhibitory activity and relationships to mechanism of action and structure. *Anticancer Drug Des 15*, 79–98.

Koo, H. M., Monks, A., Mikheev, A., Rubinstein, L. V., Gray-Goodrich, M., McWilliams, M. J., Alvord, W. G., Oie, H. K., Gazdar, A. F., Paull, K. D., et al. (1996). Enhanced sensitivity to 1-beta-D-arabinofuranosylcytosine and topoisomerase II inhibitors in tumor cell lines harboring activated ras oncogenes. *J Natl Cancer Inst 56*, 5211–5216.

Koutsoukos, A., Rubinstein, L., Faraggi, D., Kalyandrug, S., Weinstein, J. N., Paull, K. D., Kohn, K. W., and Simon, R. M. (1994). Discrimination techniques applied to the NCI in vivo antitumor drug screen: Predicting biochemical mechanism of action. *Stat Med 13*, 719–730.

Kuo, S. C., Lee, H. Z., Juang, J. P., Lin, Y. T., Wu, T. S., Chang, J. J., Lednicer, D., Paull, K. D., Lin, C. M., Hamel, E., et al. (1993). Synthesis and cytotoxicity of 1,6,7,8-substituted 2-(4′-substituted phenyl)-4-quinolones and related compounds: identification as antimitotic agents interacting with tubulin. *J Med Chem 36*, 1146–1156.

Lander, E. S., Linton, L. M., Birren, B., Nusbaum, C., Zody, M. C., Baldwin, J., Devon, K., Dewar, K., Doyle, M., and FitzHugh, W. (2001). Initial sequencing and analysis of the human genome. *Nature 409*, 860–921.

Lee, J. K., Scherf, U., Bussey, K. J., Gwadry, F. G., Reinhold, W. C., Riddick, G., and Weinstein, J. N. (2003). Comparing cDNA and oligonucleotide array data: Concordance of gene expression across platforms for the NCI-60 cancer cell lines. *Genome Biol 4*, R82.

Lee, J. S., Paull, K. D., Alvarez, M., Hose, C., Monks, A., Grever, M., Fojo, A. T., and Bates, S. E. (1994). Rhodamine efflux patterns predict P-glycoprotein substrates in the National Cancer Institute drug screen. *Mol Pharmacol 46*, 627–638.

Leteurtre, F., Kohlhagen, G., Paull, K. D., and Pommier, Y. (1994). *J Natl Cancer Inst 86*, 1239–1290.

Leteurtre, F., Sacrett, D. L., Madalengoitia, J., Kohlhagen, G., MacDonald, T., Hamel, E., Paull, K. D., and Pommier Y. (1995). Azatoxin derivatives with potent and selective action on topoisomerase II. *Biochem Pharmacol 49*, 1283–1290.

Li, G., Waltham, M., Unsworth, E., Treston, A., Mushine, J., Anderson, N. L., Kohn, K. W., and Weinstein, J. N. (1997). Rapid protein identification from two-dimensional polyacrylamide gels by MALDI mass spectrometry. *Electrophoresis 18*, 647–653.

Milne, G. W. A., Nicklaus, M. C., Driscoll, J. S., Wang, S., and Zaharevitz, D. (1994). National Cancer Institute drug information system 3D database. *J Chem Inf Comput Sci 34* (5), 1219–1224.

Monga, M., and Sausville, E. A. (2002). Overview: The art of cancer drug screening: Molecular target versus milieu-based screens. *Curr Opin Invest Drugs 3*, 478–481.

Myers, T. G., Waltham, M., Li, G., Buolamwini, J. K., Scudiero, D. A., Rubinstein, L. V., Paull, K. D., Sausville, E. A., Anderson, N. L., and Weinstein, J. N. (1997). A protein expression database for the molecular pharmacology of cancer. *Electrophoresis 18*, 647–653.

Nishizuka, S., Chen, S. T., Gwadry, F. G., Alexander, J., Scherf, U., Reinhold, W. C., Waltham, M., Charboneau, L., Young, L., Bussey, K. J., et al. (2003a). Diagnostic markers that distinguish colon and ovarian adenocarcinomas: Identification by genomic, proteomic, and tissue array profiling. *Cancer Res. 65*, 5243–5250.

Nishizuka, S., Charboneau, L., Young, L., Major, S., Reinhold, W. C., Waltham, M., Kouros-Mehr, H., Bussey, K. J., Munson, P. J., Petricoin, E., III, et al. (2003b). Proteomic profiling of the NCI-60 cancer cell lines using new high-density "reverse-phase" proteomic arrays. *Proc Natl Acad Sci USA 100*, 14229–14234.

O'Connor, P. M., Jackman, J., Bae, I., Myers, T. G., Fan, S., Mutoh, M., Scudiero, D. A., Monks, A., Sausville, E. A., Weinstein, J. N., et al. (1997). Characterization of the p53-tumor suppressor pathway in cells of the National Cancer Institute anticancer drug screen and correlations with the growth-inhibitory potency of 123 anticancer agents. *Cancer Res 57*, 4285–4300.

Paull, K. D., Shoemaker, R. H., Hodes, L., Monks, A., Scudiero, D. A., Rubinstein, L., Plowman, J., and Boyd, M. R. (1989). Display and analysis of patterns of differential activity of drugs against human tumor cell lines: Development of mean graph and COMPARE algorithm. *J Natl Cancer Inst 81*, 1088–1092.

Paull, K. D., Lin, C. M., Malspeis, L., and Hamel, E. (1992). Identification of novel antimitotic agents acting at the tubulin level by computer-assisted evaluation of differential cytotoxicity data. *Cancer Res 52*, 3892–3900.

Rabow, A. A., Shoemaker, R. H., Sausville, E. A., and Covell, D. G. (2002). Mining the National Cancer Institute's tumor-screening database: Identification of compounds with similar cellular activities. *J Med Chem 45*, 818–840.

Reinhold, W. C., Kouros-Mehr, H., Kohn, K. W., Maunakea, A. K., Lababidi, S., Roschke, A., Stover, K., Alexander, J., Pantazis, P., Miller, L., et al. (2003). Apoptotic susceptibility of cancer cells selected for camptothecin resistance: Gene expression profiling, functional analysis, and molecular interaction mapping. *Cancer Res 63*, 1000–1011.

Rindflesch, T. C., Tanabe, L., Weinstein, J. N., and Hunter, L. (2000). EDGAR: Drugs, genes and relations from the biomedical literature. *Pac Symp Biocomput* 517–528.

Rogers, D., and Hopfinger, A. J. (1994). Application of genetic function approximation to quantitative structure-activity relationships and quantitative structure-property relationships. *J Chem Inf Comput Sci 34* (4), 854–866.

Ross, D. T., Scherf, U., Eisen, M. B., Perou, C. M., Rees, C., Spellman, P., Iyer, V., Jeffrey, S. S., Van de Rijn, M., Waltham, M., et al. (2000). Systematic variation in gene expression patterns in human cancer cell lines. *Nat Genet 24*, 227–235.

Scherf, U., Ross, D. T., Waltham, M., Smith, L. H., Lee, J. K., Tanabe, L., Kohn, K. W., Reinhold, W. C., Myers, T. G., Andrews, D. T., et al. (2000). A gene expression database for the molecular pharmacology of cancer. *Nat Genet 24*, 236–244.

Shalon, D., Smith, S. J., and Brown, P. O. (1996). A DNA microarray system for analyzing complex DNA samples using two-color fluorescent probe hybridization. *Genome Res 6* (7), 639–645.

Shi, L. M., Myers, T. G., Fan, Y., and Weinstein, J. N. (1996). Application of Genetic Function Approximation to the QSAR Study of Anticancer Ellipticine Analogs. Jackson, MS, pp. 1–5.

Shi, L. M., Fan, Y., Myers, T. G., and Weinstein, J. N. (1997). Genetic function approximation in the molecular pharmacology of cancer. *Proceedings of the International Conference on Neural Networks 4*, 2490–2493.

Shi, L. M., Fan, Y., Myers, T. G., O'Connor, P. M., Paull, K. D., Friend, S. H., and Weinstein, J. N. (1998a). Mining the NCI anticancer drug discovery databases: Genetic function approximation for the QSAR study of anticancer ellipticine analogues. *J Chem Inf Comput Sci 38*, 189–199.

Shi, L. M., Fan, Y., Myers, T. G., Waltham, M., Paull, K. D., and Weinstein, J. N. (1998b). Mining the anticancer activity database generated by the U.S. National Cancer Institute's drug discovery program using statistical and artificial intelligence techniques. *J Chem Inf Comput Sci*.

Shi, L. M., Myers, T. G., Fan, Y., O'Connor, P. M., Paull, K. D., Friend, S. H., and Weinstein, J. N. (1998c). Mining the National Cancer Institute Anticancer Drug Discovery Database: Cluster analysis of ellipticine analogs with p53-inverse and central nervous system–selective patterns of activity. *Mol Pharmacol 53*, 241–251.

Shi, L. M., Lee, J. K., Fan, Y., Waltham, M., Andrews, D. T., Scherf, U., Paull, K. D., and Weinstein, J. N. (2000). Mining and visualizing large anticancer drug discovery databases. *J Chem Inf Comput Sci 40*, 367–379.

Shoemaker, R. H., Scudiero, D. A., Melillo, G., Currens, M. J., Monks, A. P., Rabow, A. A., Covell, D. G., and Sausville, E. A. (2002). Application of high-throughput, molecular-target screening to anticancer drug discovery. *Curr Top Med Chem 2*, 229–246.

Solary, E., Leteurtre, F., Paull, K. D., Scudiero, D., Hamel, E., and Pommier, Y. (1993). Dual inhibition of topoisomerase II and tubulin polymerization by azatoxin, a novel cytotoxic agent. *Biochem Pharmacol 45*, 2449–2454.

Staunton, J. E., Slonim, D. K., Coller, H. A., Tamayo, P., Angelo, M. J., Park, J., Scherf, U., Lee, J. K., Weinstein, J. N., Mesirov, J. P., et al. (2001). Chemosensitivity prediction by transcriptional profiling. *Proc Natl Acad Sci USA 98*, 10787–10792.

Tanabe, L., Smith, L. H., Lee, J. K., Scherf, U., Hunter, L., and Weinstein, J. N. (1999). MedMiner: An internet tool for mining information, with application to gene expression profiling. *BioTechniques 27*, 1210–1217.

van Osdol, W. W., Myers, T. G., Paull, K. D., Kohn, K. W., and Weinstein, J. N. (1994). Use of the Kohonen self-organizing map to study the mechanisms of action of chemotherapeutic agents. *J Natl Cancer Inst 86*, 1853–1859.

van Osdol, W. W., Myers, T. G., and Weinstein, J. N. (2000). Neural network techniques for the informatics of cancer drug discovery. *Methods Enzymol 321*, 369–395.

Venter, J. C., Adams, M. D., Myers, E. W., Li, P. W., Mural, R. J., Sutton, G. G., Smith, H. O., Yandell, M., Evans, C. A., and Holt, R. A. (2001). The sequence of the human genome. *Science 291*, 1304–1351.

Wada, H., Imamura, I., Sako, M., Katagiri, S., Tarui, S., Nishimura, H., and Inada, Y. (1990). Antitumor enzyme: Polyethylene glycol–modified asparaginase. *Ann NY Acad Sci 613*, 95–108.

Weinstein, J. N. (1998). Fishing expeditions. *Science 282*, 627–628.

Weinstein, J. N. (2000). Pharmacogenomics: Teaching old drugs new tricks. *N Engl J Med 343*, 1408–1409.

Weinstein, J. N. (2002). "Omic" and hypothesis-driven research in the molecular pharmacology of cancer. *Curr Opin Pharmacol 2*, 361–365.

Weinstein, J. N., Kohn, K. W., Grever, M. R., Viswanadhan, V. N., Rubinstein, L. V., Monks, A. P., Scudiero, D. A., Welch, L., Koutsoukos, A. D., Chiausa, A. J., et al. (1992). Neural computing in cancer drug development: Predicting mechanism of action. *Science 258* (5081), 447–451.

Weinstein, J. N., Myers, T. G., Buolamwini, J. K., Raghavan, K., van Osdol, W., Licht, J., Viswanadhan, V. N., Kohn, K. W., Rubinstein, L. V., Koutsoukos, A. D., et al. (1994). Predictive statistics and artificial intelligence in the U.S. National Cancer Institute's drug discovery program for cancer and AIDS. *Stem Cells 12*, 13–22.

Weinstein, J. N., Myers, T. G., O'Connor, P. M., Friend, S. H., Fornace, A. J., Kohn, K. W., Fojo, T., Bates, S. E., Rubinstein, L. V., Anderson, N. L., et al. (1997). An information-intensive approach to the molecular pharmacology of cancer. *Science 275*, 343–349.

Wosikowski, K., Schuurhuis, D., Johnson, K., Paull, K. D., Myers, T. G., Weinstein, J., and Bates, S. E. (1997). Identification of epidermal growth factor receptor and c-erbB2 pathway inhibitors by correlation with gene expression patterns. *J Natl Cancer Inst 89*, 1505–1513.

Wu, L., Smythe, A. M., Stinson, S. F., Mullendore, L. A., Monks, A., Scudiero, D. A., Paull, K. D., Koutsoukos, A. D., Rubinstein, L. V., Boyd, M. R., et al. (1992). Multidrug-resistant phenotype of disease-oriented panels of human tumor cell lines used for anticancer drug screening. *Cancer Res 52*, 3029–3034.

Zeeberg, B., Feng, W., Wang, G., Wang, M. D., Fojo, A. T., Kane, D. W., Reinhold, W. C., and Weinstein, J. N. (2003). GoMiner: A resource for biological interpretation of genomic and proteomic data. *Genome Biol 4*, R28.

8

TISSUE MICROANALYSIS: PROFILING CANCER STAGES

Michael A. Tangrea and Michael R. Emmert-Buck

INTRODUCTION

The genetic events underlying cancer development and progression are not fully known. There are many uncertainties regarding how malignancies will progress in patients, the toxicity of imprecise therapeutic agents, and the significant potential for treatment failure. As our understanding of the molecular nature of cancer increases, it becomes clear that we must move toward more tailored approaches to treatment for each patient. Tissue microanalysis enables investigators to examine normal, premalignant, and tumor cell populations from preserved patient specimens. The use of tissue microdissection (e.g., laser capture microdissection), in addition to molecular profiling techniques, has broadened the current understanding of cancer. The identification of the specific molecular events responsible for tumor progression will allow for the design of optimal treatments, ultimately resulting in a significant improvement in patient survival and quality of life. This chapter focuses on the molecular analysis and characterization of human tumors, using prostate cancer as an example.

At present, few cancer patients have tumors whose underlying genetic defects are known. As a result, the diagnosis and treatment of cancer remains a significant

Oncogenomics: Molecular Approaches to Cancer, Edited by Charles Brenner and David Duggan
ISBN 0-471-22592-4 © 2004 John Wiley & Sons, Inc.

challenge. Often, a cell undergoes a gradual transformation from normal to malignant that can go undetected for years. Therefore, the identification of the genetic differences between normal, premalignant, and cancerous cells will contribute to a greater understanding of the disease process. These discoveries will then provide a way to identify precancerous cells and improve methods of early detection. Because of the multigenic and diverse nature of malignancies, there is no single molecular marker that can be used to detect cancer development. Instead, the evolution of the tumor genotype and gene expression patterns through the use of high-throughput techniques such as cDNA microarrays and proteomics, provide genetic and epigenetic signatures of cancer progression.

It has been shown that phenotypically similar tumors in patients can have very different outcomes despite receiving the same treatment. Thus, the determination of the genetic events responsible for tumorigenesis is a primary objective of the scientific community, with the hope that the identification of these specific molecular events will allow for the design of optimal treatments, resulting in significant improvements in patient survival. In fact, as articulated in chapter 16, NCI Director Andrew C. von Eschenbach has challenged the cancer research community to transform cancer into manageable diseases that patients live with rather than die from.

The global study of the molecular composition of a cell, termed *molecular profiling*, is a relatively new concept that has developed due to an influx of innovative techniques that enable a "shotgun" approach to the study of gene expression and protein content in cells. Tissue microanalysis enables investigators to examine normal, premalignant, and tumor cell populations from preserved patient specimens, providing a more accurate molecular profile of specific cell types. In any type of cell, only limited sets of the genes are switched on at any given time. Therefore, from one cell type to another, the limited set of expressed genes will vary. Thus, each cellular phenotype can be identified by its unique pattern of gene expression.

Comparing the molecular signatures of normal versus tumor cells highlights genes that by their suspicious absence, presence, or change in level deserve further scrutiny to determine whether such suspects play a role in cancer or can be exploited in a test for early detection. The use of tissue microdissection (e.g., laser capture microdissection), in addition to molecular profiling techniques, has broadened the current understanding of cancer progression. Molecular profiling and tissue microanalysis may lead to the discovery of novel genes and the identification of molecular and cellular interactions important for drug development (Box 8-1).

This chapter focuses on the microanalysis and characterization of human prostate cancer. Prostate cancer is the second leading cause of cancer deaths in men within the United States, and the incidence of this disease is highly correlated with age and race. For example, African-American men are at higher risk than Asian men, and men older than 65 are also at a much higher risk (Vogelstein and Kinzler, 1998). Although the molecular profile of prostate cancer is still unclear, the development of new techniques discussed in this chapter has aided in our current understanding of the molecular progression of prostate malignancies. Despite these new discoveries, current markers and methodologies are still unable to differentiate between an aggressive tumor and an indolent tumor in a consistent manner (Gopalkrishnan et al., 2001).

This chapter begins with a discussion on the processing and preservation of tissue, with methods amenable to molecular profiling, followed by an introduction to laser capture microdissection. An overview of high-throughput techniques essential

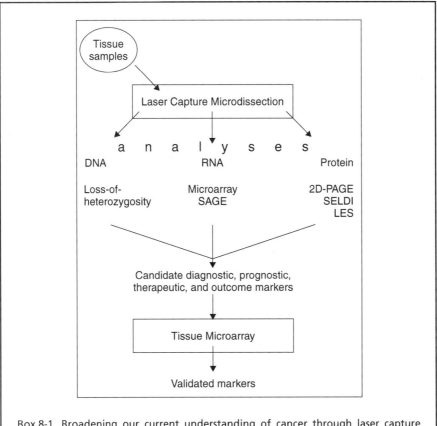

Box 8-1. Broadening our current understanding of cancer through laser capture microdissection.

for microanalysis is presented, including DNA microarrays, serial analysis of gene expression, the NCI's Cancer Genome Anatomy Project, surface-enhanced laser desorption and ionization, and tissue microarrays. An example of the latest in technological developments (i.e., layered expression scanning) is discussed prior to a few remarks on ethical considerations associated with global genetic analysis. These high-throughput approaches allow for the simultaneous analysis of hundreds of genes or proteins that may lead to the improvement of cancer diagnosis and treatment.

TISSUE FIXATION

There are many valuable and complimentary techniques that can be utilized to study molecular profiles in tissues, such as the use of cell lines and animal models, in addition to the direct study of human tissue specimens. In most cases, tissue specimens provide the most accurate sampling of genetic changes that exist in vivo. Despite this advantage, tissue specimens are typically difficult to handle and it is usually a challenge to obtain a large amount of material, especially in the case of a needle biopsy.

The manner in which tissues are handled from patient to bench top is directly related to the success or failure of subsequent molecular analyses (Gillespie et al., 2001). It is important to keep in mind that tissue must be preserved for histological diagnosis, as well as for molecular analysis. Historically, tissue specimens have been preserved using an aldehyde-based fixation process (e.g., formalin). This fixative is ideal for maintaining tissue histology but has been found to harm the quality of biomolecules used for molecular profiling studies. In addition, the tissue is typically embedded in paraffin, which requires a series of dehydration steps, allowing the paraffin to penetrate the tissue.

At the time that these protocols were developed, investigators did not have molecular-based studies in mind (Cole et al., 1999). Formalin fixation results in extensive protein and nucleic acid cross-linking and thus makes the recovery of high-quality biomolecules difficult (Ben-Ezra et al., 1991; Foss et al., 1994). Although the diagnostic integrity of the tissue is preserved, molecular information is difficult to obtain and is compromised by the presence of the aldehyde-based fixative. If a tissue is preserved through an alternative method such as freezing, it becomes easier to recover biomolecules, but the histology of the sample is often compromised (Cole et al., 1999). Any tissue microanalysis downstream of fixation is directly dependent on the initial condition of the biomolecules in the sample. In the future, new tissue processing methods must be developed that produce high-quality histological detail and also allow for the recovery of optimal levels and quality of DNA, mRNA, and protein for molecular profiling studies.

In a recent prostate cancer study, 70% ethanol fixation and paraffin embedding of clinical tissue specimens was shown to result in better biomolecular preservation for tissue microanalysis when compared to formalin fixation, while also preserving the morphology of the tissue (Gillespie et al., 2002). Prostate tissue specimens preserved in 70% ethanol were found to produce good-quality histology and also permit the recovery of nucleic acids and proteins sufficient for many downstream molecular analyses. An earlier study further supported these results, where the effect of fixation on RNA extraction and amplification from microdissected mouse liver tissue was evaluated (Goldsworthy et al., 1999). Goldsworthy et al. showed that ethanol fixation consistently provided more RT-PCR product than other forms of fixation, such as formalin. Thus, the use of ethanol preservation has been shown to be adequate for the use of high-throughput molecular analysis of clinical tissue specimens, while also preserving the histology of the tissue for patient diagnosis. In the future, as argued in Chapter 15, it will be important to apply these new tissue preservation techniques in standard hospital pathology laboratories, with the hope of preserving as much molecular information from processed tissue specimens as possible for future tissue microanalysis.

LASER CAPTURE MICRODISSECTION

Tissue processing and preservation are the first steps in accurately profiling clinical tissue specimens. The next point to consider is the technology required for specific isolation of cell populations from the tissue specimen. Historically, cancer classification has been based on the interpretation of tumor morphology, histochemistry, immunophenotyping, and cytogenetic analysis by an experienced pathologist (Golub et al., 1999). In the case of the prostate gland, the tissue is highly complex in nature and contains many diverse cell and tissue types. The normal epithelial component of the prostate gland only represents a small percentage (5–10%) of the entire prostate (Rubin, 2001). Epithelium adjacent to the tumor may not be "normal" in the molecular sense, even though the cells may appear "normal" phenotypically at the light microscopic level (Cole et al., 1999). In addition, multiple tumor regions in various stages of cancer progression can be found within the complex tissue.

Several cases have been shown to express differing patterns of allelic loss, despite tumor foci occurring in the same patient (Emmert-Buck et al., 1995). It is now widely accepted that prostate cancer is a multifocal disease. Tumor development in the prostate gland is a complicated phenomenon that is thought to progress through several distinct pathological stages, from early premalignant lesions to neoplasms of increasing invasiveness, and finally to metastatic cancer (McWilliams et al., 2002). Since the histology of normal and cancerous epithelium is complex and cells can display a wide spectrum of phenotypic features, it is difficult to isolate specific cells from a region of interest within a tissue specimen and determine discrete molecular changes within those cells using manual dissection techniques. The development of a method for isolating specific cells from a tissue specimen with as much accuracy and precision as possible becomes very important.

In response to the challenge of more precisely isolating cell populations, laser capture microdissection (LCM) was developed at the National Cancer Institute in 1996 (Emmert-Buck et al., 1996; Bonner et al., 1997). LCM is a technology for rapid and easy acquisition of a microscopic and pure cellular subpopulation away from its complex tissue milieu, under direct microscopic visualization (Fig. 8-1). A thin polymer film is placed in direct contact with a frozen or fixed tissue section and a laser beam activates the polymer, transferring the selected cell(s) out of the tissue and onto the polymer film. This positive selection method is done repeatedly until all of the desired tissue is embedded onto the polymer.

An extraction buffer is applied to the polymer film so that DNA, RNA, or proteins can be solubilized from the captured cells. LCM fully preserves the state of biological molecules for quantitative analysis. These molecules can be used as the starting material for genomic DNA analysis including loss of heterozygosity; messenger RNA analysis including cDNA libraries, microarrays, and serial analysis of gene expression; and protein analysis including surface-enhanced laser desorption and ionization (SELDI), layered expression scanning (LES), and two-dimensional polyacrylamide gel electrophoresis (2D-PAGE) (Box 8-1).

One caveat of analyzing microdissected tissue is the need for amplification of nucleic acids via the polymerase chain reaction (PCR) or reverse transcriptase PCR following microdissection. A typical yield of total RNA from 10,000 microdissected cells is approximately 10–20 nanograms, of which only 1–5% is mRNA; the majority consists of ribosomal RNA. An amplification step is often necessary to generate enough DNA or RNA from a small cell population for downstream molecular profiling studies.

When compared with nonlaser-based methods of microdissection, LCM is faster, more precise, and requires less dexterity. LCM technology also provides an excellent opportunity for documentation, as dissection occurs in real time and can be photographed. Both single cells and cell populations can be selected based not only on morphology but also on their immunohistochemical phenotype and genotype (Fend et al., 1999; Simone et al., 2000). LCM provides an opportunity to study the molecular profile of cells within a tissue. The combination of laser capture microdissection and

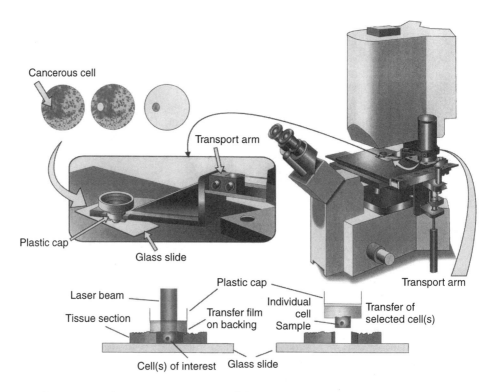

Figure 8-1. A schematic representation of the laser capture microdissection technology.

molecular profiling techniques is enhancing the field of tissue microanalysis and may provide a better understanding for the molecular events characterizing each histological stage of cancer progression.

Ornstein et al. (2000) showed for the first time that LCM can be used to study differences in expressed proteins in benign and malignant prostate cells. Specific populations of normal and malignant epithelium from radical prostatectomy tissue specimens were obtained by LCM and analyzed by 2D-PAGE. Several proteins were found to be differentially expressed between the malignant cells and benign epithelium. Furthermore, one of the proteins found to be overexpressed in microdissected tumor cells was determined to be prostate-specific antigen (PSA). This type of direct comparison of protein fingerprints between different lineages of tissue cells enables the prioritization of candidate proteins for further analysis (see tissue microarray later).

Since the early 1990s, several new techniques/technologies have been developed to advance tissue microanalysis of cancer. Some of these methods include cDNA microarrays (Schena et al., 1995, 1998; DeRisi et al., 1996; Ramsay, 1998), serial analysis of gene expression (SAGE; Zhang et al., 1997; Velculescu et al., 1995), SELDI (Hutchens and Yip, 1993), tissue microarrays (Kononen et al., 1998), and layered expression scanning (Englert et al., 2000). Along with these new methods, older methods, such as 2D-PAGE, have been applied in new ways to analyze protein expression patterns within different cell populations.

cDNA/OLIGONUCLEOTIDE MICROARRAYS

In combination with tissue arrays and laser capture microdissection, microarrays (reviewed in Chapters 5 and 6) provides a powerful tool for globally analyzing gene expression levels within distinct cell populations. However, an amplification step must follow microdissection through the use of a PCR or a linear mRNA amplification step ("aRNA"). Microarrays are often used to compare and contrast gene expression levels in two different cell populations, for example, normal versus tumor (Duggan et al., 1999).

Despite these advantages of microarrays over lower throughput methods such as Northern analysis, there are pitfalls. For example, inconsistent results may be detected due to problems with sample preparation—e.g. tissue quality, condition of cells grown in culture, etc. In addition, significant differences in gene expression may be masked by either weak or saturated signal intensities.

Microarrays have been used in experiments to elucidate the gene expression levels in prostate cancer and other tissues. Ernst et al. analyzed the gene expression profiles of total and microdissected prostate tissue sections (Ernst et al., 2002). The expression level of 63 genes was found to be significantly increased in a total prostate tissue study and was further confirmed to be upregulated in microdissected cancerous epithelium (Ernst et al., 2002). This study validated the use of microdissection and the examination of gene expression levels.

SERIAL ANALYSIS OF GENE EXPRESSION

Serial analysis of gene expression (SAGE) is a sequencing-based method for the analysis of global gene expression (Zhang et al., 1997; Velculescu et al., 1995). This method is especially useful for the discovery of novel genes. The SAGE technique utilizes 10-base cDNA tags obtained from each gene transcript, which are then concatenated and sequenced (Velculescu et al., 1995). These 10-base tags are produced from the total RNA of a cell population. An average of approximately 50 transcripts can be determined per procedure (Waghray et al., 2001). SAGE can allow for the quantification of every gene expressed in the cells of study, provided that enough tags are analyzed (Waghray et al., 2001) A major disadvantage of this technique is the requirement of a large amount (2.5–5 µg) of high-quality mRNA starting material. To address this problem, Datson et al. developed a modified SAGE procedure termed microSAGE (Datson et al., 1999). MicroSAGE requires 500- to 5000-fold less RNA starting material compared to the standard SAGE technique and therefore allows for the use of microdissected tissue.

In prostate cancer, SAGE has been successfully used to identify 156 differentially expressed genes between normal and tumor tissue (Waghray et al., 2001). Xu et al. (2001) also studied prostate cancer with the use of the SAGE technique. Xu et al. performed their own SAGE analysis of the human prostate cell line, LNCaP, and discovered that the majority of the genes identified by their system included genes involved in regulation of transcription, splicing, and other bioenergetic processes (Xu et al., 2001).

CANCER GENOME ANATOMY PROJECT

In 1997, the NCI initiated the Cancer Genome Anatomy Project (CGAP) web site (www.ncbi.nlm.nih.gov/cgap). The initial aim of CGAP was to provide a publicly available resource for cancer research investigators, including a comprehensive anno-tated index of genes involved in cancer progression (Strausberg et al., 2000). It is a goal of the CGAP initiative to empower investigators to research the precise roles of these genes in cancer and apply the findings to all aspects of cancer management, including prevention, diagnosis, and treatment. The application of innovative molecular profiling technologies will allow for the development of a complete catalog of genes involved in cancer. The anticipation is that these findings will lead to the definition of a molecular signature or profile that can be used to develop novel cancer prevention and treatment strategies.

A primary component of CGAP includes the Tumor Gene Index (TGI). The TGI is composed of a catalog of human ESTs from a wide variety of normal and tumor tissue. Within this catalog, there is an emphasis on cDNA libraries of five different human cancers: breast, colon, lung, ovary, and prostate. The genes listed in the TGI are categorized by library, tissue, and stage of cancer (Strausberg et al., 2000). Not only are bulk tissue samples examined, but microdissected tumors at various degrees of progression are also studied using LCM technology. Since its inception, CGAP has contributed nearly one million sequences to the EST database, which represent a large number of new human genes available to the public. In prostate cancer alone, the TGI has greatly increased the number of genes that are known to be expressed by the prostate gland from less than 400 to several thousand. Of the new genes annotated in prostate tissue to date, more than a thousand had not been previously observed or annotated in any other human tissue.

There are also many bioinformatic tools that can be used within the CGAP web site, allowing for the direct comparison of two different gene expression libraries. One example includes the SAGE approach to molecular profiling. This is a critical part of the CGAP initiative, and the current annotation can be seen at the SAGEMap web site (www.ncbi.nlm.nih.gov/SAGE/). Associated with the SAGEMap web site are two analytical tools: xProfiler and a "virtual" northern blot. The xProfiler examines the SAGE expression patterns within and between libraries. The "virtual" northern blot allows for the visualization of gene expression levels in a library.

Another analytical tool found within the CGAP web site is the Digital Gene Expression Displayer (DGED). This tool allows for the analysis of differences in gene expression between two pools of libraries. But unlike the xProfiler, which lists every gene in both groups, the DGED finds only the statistically significant differences, based on the sequence odds ratio and Fisher's Exact test. SAGE DGED can be used to com-pare normal and malignant expression profiles from individuals or pools of samples. SAGE expression data from a diverse collection of tissues, including brain, breast, cerebellum, cerebrum, cervix, colon, gastrointestinal tract, heart, kidney, liver, lung, muscle, ovary, pancreas, placenta, prostate, retina, skin, soft tissue, spinal cord, stom-ach, vascular, and whole blood, can be queried using this tool. The bioinformatic tool used to set up DGED analysis is available online and can be seen in Figure 8-2.

Prior to receiving the results of this query, several libraries of interest are displayed that the user can select or deselect for the final analysis. Once the desired libraries, "minimum number of sequences per pool," and p-value filter are specified, the query is submitted to the database for analysis. The SAGE DGED results page contains the Unigene Build number, the total number of sequences or tags in each pool, the total number of libraries in each pool, and a table listing the genes or tags found to be expressed with a statistically significant difference between pool A and pool B

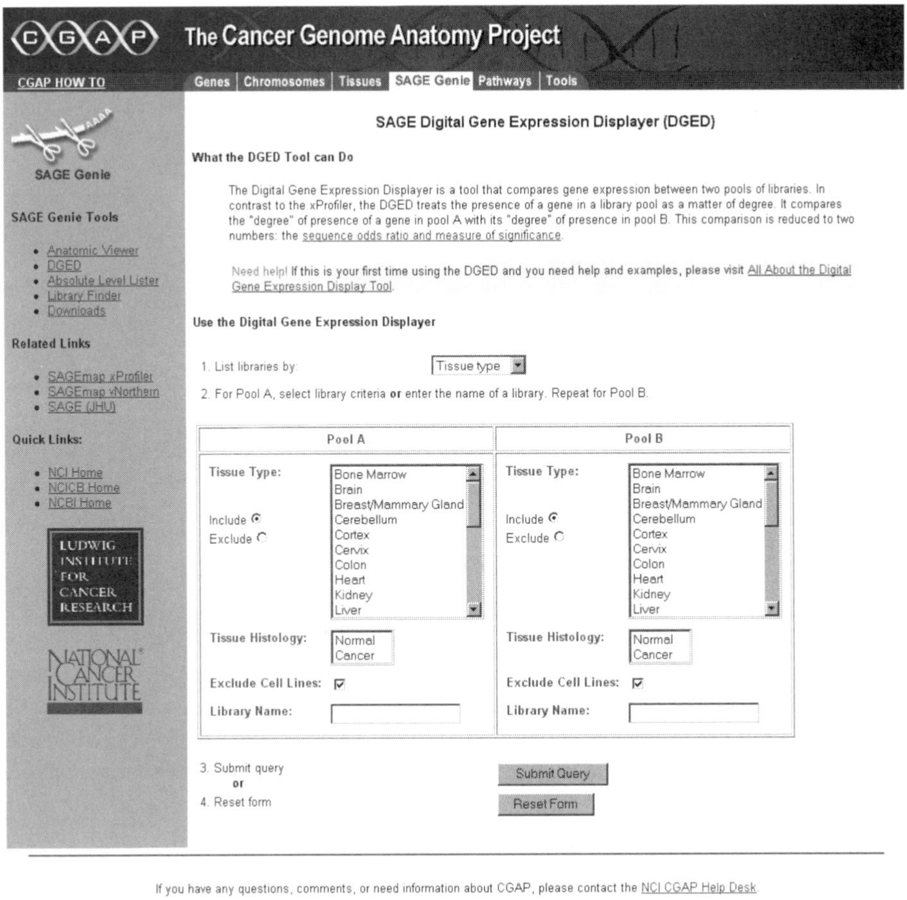

Figure 8-2. The CGAP SAGE Digital Gene Expression Displayer web site. This is the web tool used to set up a gene expression comparison.

(Fig. 8-3). The Tag and Gene columns of the table are hyperlinked to more information about the respective tag or gene. This is a simplified overview of the bioinformatic tools found on the SAGE DGED web site.

Thus far, the CGAP initiative has been very successful in identifying new human genes. Although the complete catalog of human gene alterations is far from complete, these catalogs, even in an unfinished state, can contribute greatly to the identification of molecular profiles and the involvement of genes in the various stages of cancer progression. Further annotation of these genes will be required to gain a better understanding of the molecular profile of cancer and the causal relationships between genotype and phenotype.

Successful profiling of the stages of cancer requires detailed knowledge of protein expression in addition to messenger RNA levels as previously discussed (and genomic DNA sequence variation, as discussed in Chapter 4). There are unique advantages to studying the levels of protein expression in tissue. For the most part, the protein complement is the end product of gene expression and contains the key determinants of cellular phenotype. However, proteins are typically more difficult to work with

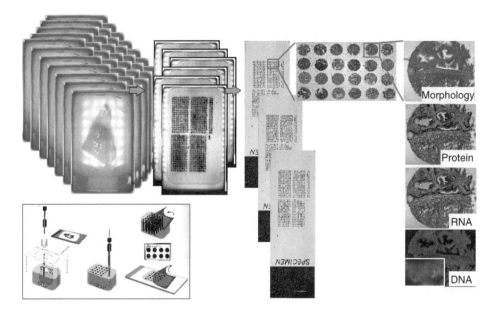

Figure 8-3. Tissue microarrays. Tiny cylinders of tissue (see inset) are acquired from hundreds of different primary tumor blocks and arrayed into several recipient paraffin blocks at high density. Sections from these tissue microarray blocks can then be used for simultaneous in situ analyses of hundreds to thousands of tissue specimens by a variety of molecular analyses, such as H&E staining to ascertain tissue morphology, protein immunostaining or mRNA ISH, or analysis of copy number changes by FISH. (*Source:* Modified from Kallioniemi et al., 2001.) See insert for color representation of this figure.

than nucleic acids. For example, proteins typically undergo important posttranslational modifications that alter their functions. In addition, protein function is dependent on native three-dimensional structure. Any alteration or disruption in native structure may produce artifacts in the results observed during analysis. Unlike DNA, which can be adhered to an array chip in an immobilized fashion, proteins need to retain their native condition for an accurate test of function. This makes the global "proteomic" study of proteins challenging. Nonetheless, the elucidation of protein levels and functions in normal versus tumor cells will ultimately be important for drug discovery and treatment considerations for cancer. Chapter 9 is devoted entirely to oncoproteomics. Two proteomic technologies that have proved useful in tissue microanalysis are discussed here.

SURFACE-ENHANCED LASER DESORPTION AND IONIZATION

SELDI is a new technology for protein analysis that enriches proteins based on their physical properties, such as hydrophobicity (Hutchens and Yip, 1993). Proteomic profiles can be analyzed by applying biological samples to chips that are coated with defined surface affinities. Captured proteins are then analyzed by mass spectroscopy. Laser activation results in ionization and release of proteins from the affinity chip, which then travel with an inverse correlation to their molecular weight. Measurement of the time of flight of the released proteins is represented graphically as peaks, with every peak representing an ionized protein or peptide (Merchant and Weinberger, 2000).

There are two main advantages to this technique: the ability to use a small sample size and the speed with which multiple samples can be studied. SELDI can be used for multiple applications. For example, an antibody affinity-based chip can isolate specific proteins for analysis. The chips may also be used to analyze DNA-protein- and protein-protein-binding interactions.

Through the use of SELDI, scientists at the Food and Drug Administration (FDA) and NCI have determined a serum-based protein fingerprint for the identification of ovarian cancer (Petricoin et al., 2002). The use of a newly developed bioinformatics tool allowed the investigators to identify a protein cluster pattern that correctly identified 50 ovarian cancer cases from a set of 116 masked cases, with a specificity of 95%. In the case of the prostate, studies by our group and others have revealed differences in protein expression patterns between microdissected normal, premalignant, and malignant cells (Wang et al., 2001; Xiao et al., 2001).

TWO DIMENSIONAL POLYACRYLAMIDE GEL ELECTROPHORESIS

A technique developed in the mid-1970s, 2D-PAGE remains a workhorse of proteomic analysis (Klose, 1975; O'Farrell and Goodman, 1976). The advantage of 2D-PAGE is the ability to simultaneously analyze several hundred to a few thousand proteins, based on two physical properties: isoelectric point and molecular weight. This method produces a protein fingerprint of the tissue of interest based on these characteristics. Subsequently, proteins of interest can be excised from the gel and analyzed by mass spectrometry. As discussed in Chapter 9, today 2D-PAGE remains the method of choice for the comparison of protein expression levels of normal versus cancer tissue.

A recent technical study of LCM and 2D-PAGE by Craven et al. indicated that indeed LCM is a useful tool for proteomic research (Craven et al., 2002). LCM has been used in studies of protein expression levels within the prostate gland (Ornstein et al., 2000a,b). Studying LCM isolated prostate cells, Ornstein et al. discovered that prostate-specific antigen (PSA) was found to exist in the unbound form in both normal and cancerous prostate secretory cells. A recent proteomic study of prostate cancer by our laboratory identified 40 tumor-specific changes in protein expression levels in prostate cancer (Ahram et al., 2002). Total cellular proteomes of normal prostate epithelial cells were compared to high-grade prostate cancer cells via tissue microdissection, 2D-PAGE, and subsequent mass spectroscopy (Ahram et al., 2002). Although the significance of the detected protein alterations is still unclear and further studies are necessary to gain a better understanding of these molecular changes, this study illustrates the potential utility of combining phenotypic analysis of tissue sections with global protein measurements.

TISSUE MICROARRAYS

High-throughput screening technologies, such as cDNA microarrays, SAGE, and SELDI, have made it possible to survey thousands of genes and proteins at a time from tissue and cell preparations. The translation of such information to improved diagnostic, prognostic, and therapeutic applications in the clinic requires extensive validation, prioritization, and extension of such raw information. For example, hundreds or even thousands of clinical specimens are required to ascertain the significance of a new diagnostic test or therapeutic target. This is often tedious with conventional molecular pathology technologies, and availability of such tissue resources is often rate limiting.

Tissue microarrays provide a means for rapid, very large-scale molecular analysis of thousands of tissue specimens with thousands of probes for various DNA, RNA, and protein targets. This technique, originally described in 1986 by Battifora, was popularized by Kononen and colleagues (Kononen et al., 1998). Tissue microarrays provide a method for high-throughput molecular profiling of tissue specimens. This technology enables high-throughput molecular analyses of hundreds of tissue specimens or cells in a single experiment. Tissue microarrays are constructed by acquiring cylindrical biopsies from hundreds to thousands of individual tumor tissues into a tissue microarray block, which is then sectioned for probing DNA, RNA, or protein targets (Fig. 8-3). A single immunostaining or in situ hybridization reaction now provides information on all of the specimens on the slide, while subsequent sections can be analyzed with other probes or antibodies.

Tissue microarrays have been constructed for a variety of questions. Multitumor arrays can be used to determine the copy number or expression levels of genes and gene products across different tumor types. Andersen et al. (2000) studied the presence of amplifications of specific genes across a spectrum of different malignancies. This multitumor tissue microarray screening provides an example of the power of tissue microarray analysis in providing a comprehensive screening of molecular alterations not only within a particular tumor type but across all common malignancies. Progression arrays can be used to monitor a gene expression pattern over the course of time or to identify stage-specific markers. Finally, outcome arrays can be used to look for associations between a gene(s) expression and clinical outcome.

Tissue microarrays have been used to study molecular alterations in different stages of tumor progression within a given organ, such as the brain (Tynninen et al., 2000), breast (Kononen et al., 1998), urinary bladder (Nocito et al., 2001, Richter et al., 2000), kidney (Moch et al., 1999) or prostate (Bubendorf et al., 1999a, 1999b). For example, Bubendorf et al. (1999a, 1999b) constructed a prostate cancer progression tissue microarray containing prostate specimens that included all stages of prostate cancer development, starting from normal prostate, benign prostate hyperplasia, prostatic intraepithelial neoplasia, localized clinical cancer, to metastatic and hormone-refractory end-stage cancer. Molecular profiling of such tumor progression arrays revealed sets of genetic alterations and gene expression patterns that are characteristic of a specific stage of cancer progression.

Virtually all kinds of tissues or cell types are compatible with the array format. The range of potential applications thus covers all fields of microscopic analyses of tissues and cells. In the case of cancer research, tissue microarrays significantly facilitate the ability to extend in vitro studies of genes, proteins, and signaling pathways to the in vivo situation. Tissue microarrays also provide access to highly characterized tissues reviewed by expert pathologists, often containing associated clinicopathologic, demographic, or even survival and treatment outcome information. Thus, novel genes discovered through LCM, SAGE, CGAP, DNA microarrays, SELDI, etc., can be linked with clinical endpoints.

LAYERED EXPRESSION SCANNING

Layered expression scanning is a new technology that can be used to analyze both nucleic acid and protein expression levels from biological samples (Englert et al.,

2000). The method permits analysis of mRNA and protein expression patterns using stacked membranes linked to individual capture molecules, such as DNA probes or antibodies, in either a closed or open system (Fig. 8-4). In the open version, the layered expression scanning membranes can be used to make "replicates" of a gel experiment by binding a subset of the target molecules. For example, one RNA can yield at least 10 Northern blot replicates, in which each individual membrane can be subsequently analyzed with a specific gene probe. The closed-layered expression scanning system involves the specific capture of biomolecules based on the coating of the membranes with a specific hybridization molecule—for example, a DNA probe or antibody. The biomolecules from the samples pass through the layers and are captured by the membrane containing the corresponding DNA probe or antibody. Following transfer, the membranes are analyzed, providing both qualitative and quantitative assessment of the target biomolecule. In this application, the membranes permit nontarget molecules to pass through unimpeded; thus the closed system can be utilized with a large number (100 or more) of membranes.

This developing technology allows the investigator to simultaneously analyze the molecular profile of many different platforms, such as tissue sections, microdissected tissue, both 1D and 2D gels, and tissue lysates. The ability to analyze intact tissue sections without the need for tedious removal of cells by microdissection is a significant

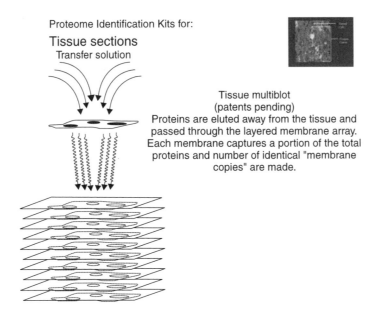

Figure 8-4. Schematic representation of the layered expression scanning technology. A biological sample is placed adjacent to a multilayered set of membranes. The specimen is transferred through the layers as an intact two-dimensional object. The membranes bind a subset of the target molecules, resulting in a series of "replicate" membranes that can be subsequently probed for specific genes or proteins. Alternatively, specific antibodies or DNA molecules are placed on each membrane. The biological sample is prelabeled and passed through the layers; proteins or mRNAs are then captured by their corresponding membrane and the expression level of each is measured.

advantage of this technology over other current methods of molecular profiling. For example, in prostate cancer all of the normal, premalignant, and cancerous cells in a tissue section can be analyzed simultaneously in one experiment using the layered expression scanning technology (Englert et al., 2000).

ETHICAL CONSIDERATIONS

The advancements in tissue microanalysis that allow for new discoveries also raise many ethical questions and concerns. Though these techniques are powerful tools for peering into the molecular profile and genetic makeup of a tissue specimen, it is important to remember that the patient and the patient's rights still must be considered to be of foremost importance. Many questions need to be addressed: Did the patient give consent to use his or her biological sample for genetic analysis? How does access to a patient's genetic information affect his or her ability to maintain health care insurance and employment (Sobel, 1999)? What effect does the knowledge of genetic disease have on the psyche of the patient? It is essential that both the newly gleaned molecular information and the patient's rights and concerns be carefully considered.

FUTURE DIRECTIONS

The amount of molecular profiling data is growing at an exponential rate with the use of the high-throughput techniques described in this chapter and elsewhere in the book. Clearly, it will be important in the future to devise bioinformatic strategies that can synthesize and interpret the dramatic influx of data. Continued development of systems integrating a large amount of biological data with tumor histopathology, pharmacology and outcomes data will be critical in identifying the key elements within a molecular profiling data set that are necessary to successfully impact diagnosis, prognosis, and therapy in the clinic.

REFERENCES

Ahram, M., Best, C. J., Flaig, M. J., Gillespie, J. W., Leiva, I. M., Chuaqui, R. F., Zhou, G., Shu H., Duray, P. H., Linehan, W. M., et al. (2002). Proteomic analysis of human prostate cancer. *Mol Carcinog 33*, 9–15.

Andersen, C. L., Monni, O. M., Kononen, J., Barlund, M., Bucher, C., Hass, P., Nocito, A., Bissig, H., Sauter, G., Kallioniemi, O. P., et al. (2000). High-throughput gene copy number analysis in 4700 tumors: FISH analysis on tissue microarrays identifies multiple tumor types with amplification of the MB-174 gene, a novel amplified gene originally found in breast cancer. *Am J Hum Genet 67*, 448.

Battifora, H. (1986). The multitumor (sausage) tissue block: Novel method for immunohisto-chemical antibody testing. *Lab Invest 55*, 244–248.

Ben-Ezra, J., Johnson, D. A., Rossi, J., Cook, N., and Wu, A. (1991). Effect of fixation on the amplification of nucleic acids from paraffin-embedded material by the polymerase chain reaction. *J Histochem Cytochem 39*, 351–354.

Bonner, R. F., Emmert-Buck, M. R., Cole, K., Pohida, T., Chuaqui, R., Goldstein, S., and Liotta, L. A. (1997). Laser capture microdissection: Molecular analysis of tissue. *Science 278* (5342), 1481–1483.

Bowen, C., Bubendorf, L., Voeller, H. J., Slack, R., Willi, N., Sauter, G., Gasser, T. C., Koivisto, P., Lack, E. E., Kononen, J., et al. (2000). Loss of NKX3.1 expression in human prostate cancers correlates with tumor progression. *Cancer Res 60*, 6111–6115.

Bubendorf, L., Kononen, J., Koivisto, P., Schraml, P., Moch, H., Gasser, T. C., Willi, N., Mihatsch, M. J., Sauter, G., and Kallioniemi, O. P. (1999a). Survey of gene amplifications during prostate cancer progression by high-throughput fluorescence in situ hybridization on tissue microarrays. *Cancer Res 59*, 803–806.

Bubendorf, L., Kolmer, M., Kononen, J., Koivisto, P., Mousses, S., Chen, Y., Mahlamaki, E., Schraml, P., Moch, H., Willi, N., et al. (1999b). Hormone therapy failure in human prostate cancer: Analysis by complementary DNA and tissue microarrays. *J Natl Cancer Inst 91*, 1758–1764.

Cole, K. A., Krizman, D. B., and Emmert-Buck, M. R. (1999). The genetics of cancer—a 3D model. *Nat Genet 21*, 38–41 (supplement).

Craven, R. A., Totty, N., Harnden, P., Selby, P. J., and Banks, R. E. (2002). Laser capture microdissection and two-dimensional polyacrylamide gel electrophoresis. *Am J Pathol 160* (3), 815–822.

Datson, N. A., van der Perk-de Jong, J., van den Berg, M. P., de Kloet, E. R., and Vreugdenhil, E. (1999). MicroSAGE: A modified procedure for serial analysis of gene expression in limited amounts of tissue. *Nucleic Acids Res 27* (5), 1300–1307.

DeRisi, J., Penland, L., Brown, P. O., Bittner, M. L., Meltzer, P. S., Ray, M., Chen, Y., Su, Y. A., and Trent, J. M., (1996). Use of a cDNA microarray to analyse gene expression patterns in human cancer. *Nat Genet. 14*, 457–460.

Duggan, D. J., Bittner, M., Chen, Y., Meltzer, P., and Trent, J. M. (1999). Expression profiling using cDNA microarrays. *Nat Genet. 21*, 10–14.

Emmert-Buck, M. R., Vocke, C. D., Pozzatti, R. O., Duray P. H., Jennings S. B., Florence C. D., Zhnang Z., Bostwick D. G., Liotta, L. A., and Linehan W. M. (1995). Allelic loss on chromosome 8p12-21 in microdissected prostatic intraepithelial neoplasia. *Cancer Res 55* (14), 2959–2962.

Emmert-Buck, M. R., Bonner, R. F., Smith, P. D., Chuaqui, R. F., Zhuang, Z., Goldstein, S. R., Weiss, R. R., and Liotta, L. A. (1996). Laser capture microdissection. *Science 274* (5289), 998–1001.

Emmert-Buck, M. R., Strausberg, R. L., Krizman, D. B., Bonaldo, M. F., Bonner, R. F., Bostwick, D. G., Brown, M. R., Buetow, K. H., Chuaqui, R. F., Cole, K. A., et al. (2000). Molecular profiling of clinical tissues specimens: feasibility and applications. *J Mol Diagn. 2*, 60–66.

Englert, C. R., Baibakov, G. V., and Emmert-Buck, M. R. (2000). Layered expression scanning: Rapid molecular profiling of tumor samples. *Cancer Res 60*, 1526–1530.

Ernst, T., Hergenhahn, M., Kenzelmann, M., Cohen, C. D., Bonrouhi, M., Weninger, A., Klaren, R., Grone, E. F., Wiesel, M., Gudemann, C., et al. (2002). Decrease and gain of gene expression are equally discriminatory markers for prostate carcinoma: a gene expression analysis on total and microdissected prostate tissue. *Am J Pathol. 160*, 2169–2180.

Fend, F., Emmert-Buck, M. R., Chuaqui, R., Cole, K., Lee, J., Liotta, L. A., and Raffeld, M. (1999). Immuno-LCM: Laser capture microdissection of immunostained frozen sections for mRNA analysis. *Am J Pathol 154* (1), 61–66.

Foss, R., Guhathakurta, N., Conran, R. M., and Gutman, P. (1994). Effects of fixative and fixation time on the extraction and polymerase chain reaction amplification of RNA from paraffin-embedded tissue: Comparison of two housekeeping gene mRNA controls. *Diagn Mol Pathol 3*, 148–155.

Gillespie, J. W., Ahram, M., Best, C. J. M., Swalwell, J. I., Krizman, D. B., Petricoin, E. F., III, Liotta, L. A., and Emmert-Buck, M. R. (2001). The role of tissue microdissection in cancer research. *Cancer J 7* (1), 32–39.

Gillespie, J. W., Best, C. J., Bichsel, V. E., Cole, K. A., Greenhut, S. F., Hewitt, S. M., Ahram, M., Gathright, Y. B., Merino, M. J., Strausberg, R. L., Epstein, J. I., Hamilton, S. R., Gannot, G., Baibakova, G. V., Calvat, V. S., Flaig, M. J., Chuaqui, R. F., Herring, J. C., Pfeifer, J., Petricoin, E. F., Linehan, W. M., Durah, P. H., Bova, G. S., and Emmert-Buck, M. R. (2002). Evaluation of non-formalin tissue fixation for molecular profiling studies. *Am J Pathol. 160*, 449–457.

Goldsworthy, S. M., Stockton, P. S., Trempus, C. S., Foley, J. F., and Maronpot, R. R. (1999). Effects of fixation on RNA extraction and amplification from laser capture microdissected tissue. *Mol Carcinogenesis 25*, 86–91.

Golub, T. R., Slonim D. K., Tamayo, P., Huard, C., Gaasenbeek, M., Mesirov, J. P., Coller, H., Loh, M. L., Downing, J. R., Caligiuri, M. A., Bloomfeld, C. D., and Lander, E. S. (1999). Molecular classification of cancer: class discovery and class prediction by gene expression monitoring. *Science 286*, 531–537.

Gopalkrishnan, R. V., Kang, D. C., and Fisher, P. B. (2001). Molecular markers and determinants of prostate cancer metastasis. *J Cell Physiol 189*, 245–256.

Hoos, A. and Cordon-Cardo, C. (2001). Tissue microarray profiling of cancer specimens and cell lines: Opportunities and limitations. *Lab Invest 81* (10), 1331–1338.

Hutchens, T. W. and Yip, T. T. (1993). New desorption strategies for the mass analysis of macromolecules. *Rapid Commun Mass Spectrom. 7*, 576–580.

Kallioniemi, O. P., Wagner, U., Kononen, J., and Sauter, G. (2001). Tissue microarray technology for high-throughput molecular profiling of cancer. *Hum Mol Genet 10*, 657–662.

Klose, J. (1975). Protein mapping by combined isoelectric focusing and electrophoresis of mouse tissues. A novel approach to testing for induced point mutations in mammals. *Humangenetik 26*, 231–243.

Kononen, J., Bubendorf, L., Kallioniemi, A., Barlund, M., Schraml, P., Leighton, S., Torhorst, J., Mihatsch, M. J., Sauter, G., and Kallioniemi, O. P. (1998). Tissue microarrays for high-throughput molecular profiling of tumor specimens. *Nat Med. 4*, 844–847.

Lockhart, D. J., Dong, H., Byrne, M. C., Follettie, M. T., Gallo, M. V., Chee, M. S., Mittmann, M., Wang, C., Kobayashi, M., Horton, H., and Brown, E. L. (1996). Expression monitoring by hybridization to high-density oligonucleotide arrays. *Nat Biotechnol. 14*, 1675–1680.

McGall, G., Labadie, J., Brock, P., Wallraff, G., Nguyen, T., and Hinsberg, W. (1996). Light-directed synthesis of high-density oligonucleotide arrays using semiconductor photoresists. *Proc Natl Acad Sci USA 93*, 13555–13560.

McWilliams, L. J., Roberts, I. S. D., and Davies, D. R. (2002). Problems in grading and staging prostatic carcinoma. *Curr Diagn Pathol 8*, 65–75.

Merchant, M., and Weinberger, S. R. (2000). Recent advancements in surface-enhanced laser desorption/ionization time of flight-mass spectrometry. *Electrophoresis 21*, 1164–1177.

Moch, H., Schraml, P., Bubendorf, L., Mirlacher, M., Kononen, J., Gasser, T., Mihatsch, M. J., Kallioniemi, O. P., and Sauter, G. (1999). High-throughput tissue microarray analysis to evaluate genes uncovered by cDNA microarray screening in renal cell carcinoma. *Am J Pathol. 154*, 981–986.

Nocito, A., Bubendorf, L., Maria Tinner, E., Suess, K., Wagner, U., Forster, T., Kononen, J., Fijan, A., Bruderer, J., Schmid, U., Ackermann, D., Maurer, R., Alund, G., Knonagel, H., Rist, M., Anabitaste, M., Hering, F., Hardmeier, T., Schoenenberger, A. F., Flury, R., Jager, P., Lue Fehr, J., Schraml, P., Moch, H., Mihatsch, M. J., Gasser, T., and Sauter, G. (2001). Microarrays of bladder cancer tissue are highly representative of proliferation index and histological grade. *J Pathol. 194*, 349–357.

O'Farrell, P. Z., and Goodman, H. M. (1976). Resolution of simian virus 40 proteins in whole cell extracts by two-dimensional electrophoresis: Heterogeneity of the major capsid protein. *Cell 9*, 289–298.

Ornstein, D. K., Englert, C., Gillespie, J. W., Paweletz, C. P., Linehan, W. M., Emmert-Buck, M. R., and Petricoin, E. F., (III (2000a). Characterization of intracellular prostate-specific antigen from laser capture microdissected benign and malignant prostatic epithelium. *Clin Cancer Res 6*, 353–356.

Ornstein, D. K., Gillespie, J. W., Paweletz, C. P., Duray, P. H., Herring, J., Vocke, C. D., Topalian, S. L., Bostwick, D. G., Linehan, W. M., Petricoin, E. F., III, and Emmert-Buck, M. R. (2000b). Proteomic analysis of laser capture microdissected human prostate cancer and in vitro prostate cell lines. *Electrophoresis 21*, 2235–2242.

Petricoin, E. F., Ardekani, A. M., Hitt, B. A., Levine, P. J., Fusaro, V. A., Steinberg, S. M., Mills, G. B., Simone, C., Fishman, D. A., Kohn, E. C., and Liotta, L. A. (2002). Use of proteomic patterns in serum to identify ovarian cancer. *Lancet 359*, 572–577.

Ramsay, G. (1998). DNA chips: State of the art. *Nat Biotechnol 16*, 40–44.

Richter, J., Wagner, U., Kononen, J., Fijan, A., Bruderer, J., Schmid, U., Ackermann, D., Maurer, R., Alund, G., Knonagel, H. et al. (2000). High-throughput tissue microarray analysis of cyclin E gene amplification and overexpression in urinary bladder cancer. *Am J Pathol. 157*, 787–794.

Rubin, M. A. (2001). Use of laser capture microdissection, cDNA microarrays, and tissue microarrays in advancing our understanding of prostate cancer. *J Pathol 195*, 80–86.

Schena, M., Shalon, D., Davis, R. W., and Brown, P. (1995). Quantitative monitoring of gene expression patterns with a complementary DNA microarray. *Science 270*, 467–469.

Schena, M., Heller, R. A., Theriault, T. P., Konrad, K., Lachenmeier, E., and Davis, R. W. (1998). Microarrays: biotechnology's discovery platform for functional genomics. *Trends Biotechnol. 16*, 301–306.

Simone, N. L., Remaley, A. T., Charboneau, L., Petricoin, E. F., III, Glickman, J. W., Emmert-Buck, M. R., Fleisher, T. A., and Liotta, L. (2000). Sensitive immunoassay of tissue cell proteins procured by laser capture microdissection. *Am J Pathol 156* (2), 445–452.

Sobel, M. E. (1999). Ethical issues in molecular pathology: Paradigms in flux. *Arch Pathol Lab Med 123*, 1076–1078.

Strausberg, R. L., Buetow, K. H., Emmert-Buck, M. R., and Klausner, R. D. (2000). The Cancer Genome Anatomy Project: Building an annotated gene index. *Trends Genet 16* (3), 103–106.

Tynninen, O., Paetau, A., Von Boguslawski, K., Jaaskelainen, J., Aronen, H. J., and Paavonen T. (2000). p53 expression in tissue microarray of primary and recurrent gliomas. *Brain Pathol 10*, 575–576.

Velculescu, V. E., Zhang, L., Vogelstein, B., and Kinzler, K. W. (1995). Serial analysis of gene expression. *Science 270*, 484–487.

Vogelstein, B., and Kinzler, K. W. (1998). *The Genetic Basis of Human Cancer*. New York: McGraw-Hill.

Waghray, A., Schober, M., Feroze, F., Yao, F., Virgin, J., and Chen, Y. Q. (2001). Identification of differentially expressed genes by serial analysis of gene expression in human prostate cancer. *Cancer Res 61*, 4283–4286.

Wang, S., Diamond, D. L., Hass, G. M., Sokoloff, R., and Vessella, R. L. (2001). Identification of prostate specific membrane antigen (PSMA) as the target of monoclonal antibody 107-1A4 by protein chip, array, surface-enhanced laser desorption/ionization (SELDI) technology. *Int J Cancer 92* (6), 871–876.

Xiao, Z., Adam, B. L., Cazares, L. H., Clements, M. A., Davis, J. W., Schellhammer, P. F., Dalmasso, E. A., and Wright, G. L., Jr. (2001). Quantitation of serum prostate-specific membrane antigen by a novel protein biochip immunoassay discriminates benign from malignant prostate disease. *Cancer Res. 61*, 6029–6033.

Xu, L. L., Su, Y. P., Labiche, R., Segawa, T., Shanmugam, N., McLeod, D. G., Moul, J. W., and Srivastava, S. (2001). Quantitative expression profile of androgen-regulated genes in prostate cancer cells and identification of prostate-specific genes. *Int J Cancer 92* (3), 322–328.

Zhang, L., Zhou, W., Velculescu, V. E., Kern, S. E., Hruban, R. H., Hamilton, S. R., Vogelstein, B., and Kinzler, K. W. (1997). Gene expression profiles in normal and cancer cells. *Science 276*, 1268–1272.

WEB RESOURCES

CGAP:http://www.ncbi.nlm.nih.gov/cgap

Molecular Profiling Initiative: http://www.cgap-mf.nih.gov

SAGEMap:http://www.ncbi.nlm.nih.gov/SAGE/

9

PROTEOMICS IN BLADDER CANCER

Julio E. Celis, Irina Gromova, Fritz Rank, and Pavel Gromov

INTRODUCTION

The behavior of different cell types is largely determined by their unique patterns of protein expression. Proteomic technologies are those capable of analyzing in a parallel fashion the full complement of proteins expressed in cells. We describe several proteomic technologies valuable in basic and clinical oncology to perform early detection and staging of cancer, to classify distinct malignancies, identify novel drug targets, and to inform practitioners which treatments will be most effective for which patients.

Without doubt, genome sequencing is paving the way to a revolution in biology and medicine. We are rapidly moving from the study of single molecules to the analysis of complex biological processes, and the current explosion of new and powerful technologies within gene expression profiling and functional genomics promise to accelerate the application of basic discoveries through translational research into daily clinical practice.

Cancer, which affects a significant fraction of the population, has become a prime target for these new technologies. Indeed, tools for the high-throughput analysis of genes, proteins, and their complex networks are being used to identify markers for the early detection, recurrence, and progression of cancer, response to treatment, development of novel therapies, as well as potential targets for drug discovery (Cunningham, 2000; Srinivas et al., 2001, 2002; Hanash et al., 2002; Petricoin et al.,

Oncogenomics: Molecular Approaches to Cancer, Edited by Charles Brenner and David Duggan
ISBN 0-471-22592-4 © 2004 John Wiley & Sons, Inc.

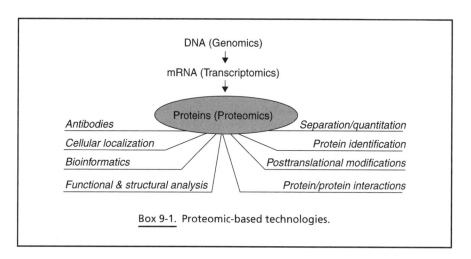

Box 9-1. Proteomic-based technologies.

2002a,b). Molecules being targeted include cell-cycle regulators, growth factors and their receptors, signal transduction components, angiogenesis factors and apoptosis, and DNA repair components (Celis, 2002).

As schematized in Box 9-1, technologies to analyze the proteome are complex and consist of a plethora of techniques to resolve, identify, and characterize protein structure and interactions and to communicate and interlink protein and DNA sequence and mapping information (Celis et al., 1998; Celis and Gromov, 2000; Marshall and Williams, 2002, and references therein). Proteomics can address problems that cannot be approached by DNA analysis—namely, relative abundance of the protein product, posttranslational modifications, compartmentalization, turnover, as well as protein-protein interactions and function. In addition, proteomics is highly relevant to the study of biological fluids (Anderson et al., 1978; Tissot et al., 1991; Kennedy, 2001).

In this chapter, we illustrate the potential of gel-based proteomics to study bladder cancer using fresh tissue biopsies. In particular, we address the problem of cancer heterogeneity by reviewing our strategies to identify (1) tumor subtypes among low-grade papillary transitional cell carcinomas (TCCs; Celis et al., 2002) and (2) metaplastic and premalignant lesions in patients bearing squamous cell carcinomas (SCCs; Celis et al., 1999a, 1999b). Furthermore, we provide a brief description of the principles underlying various proteomic technologies.

BLADDER CANCER

Bladder cancer comprises a broad spectrum of tumors with various histological types that include TCCs, adenocarcinomas, and SCCs (Friedell et al., 1983; Pauli et al., 1983). TCCs are by far the more prevalent tumors and represent nearly 95% of all bladder cancers in the Western Hemisphere (Mostofi et al., 1990). SCCs, in contrast, encompass a small percentage (2–3%) of all bladder lesions diagnosed in Europe and America but are very frequent (80%) in areas of Africa and the Middle East, where *Schistosoma haematobium*, a parasite that induces bladder SCCs in humans, is prevalent (Bryan, 1983; EL-Bolkainy, 1983).

Transitional Cell Carcinomas

TCCs are subdivided into noninvasive papillary and nonpapillary invasive carcinoma types (Friedell et al., 1983; Pauli et al., 1983; Bane et al., 1996) that are believed to originate from different genetic alterations (Heney et al., 1983; Simoneau and Jones, 1994; Spruck et al., 1994). Papillary TCCs correspond to 70% of all TCCs and usually are of low grade and noninvasive at first presentation (Mostofi et al., 1990; Zieger et al., 2000). These lesions begin as localized areas of hyperplasia that later undergo a process of dedifferentiation. Invasive tumors may arise from these lesions, although poorly differentiated neoplasms have a higher tendency to invade and metastasize (Pauli et al., 1983; Cheng et al., 2000).

Papillary TCCs often recur, and of these recurrences, 10–30% will progress to invasive disease. This scenario is in harmony with the notion that bladder cancer is a "field disease" (Slaughter et al., 1953)—that is, the whole bladder urothelium that is in contact with the carcinogen is at risk of developing cancer, although any given lesion is clonal in its origin. Multifocal recurrent papillary tumors provide a unique model system to study the molecular mechanisms underlying the various steps involved in cancer development. They also offer a valuable source of material to search for biomarkers that may form the basis for diagnosis, prognosis, and treatment.

Nonpapillary invasive carcinomas, in contrast, are believed to develop from carcinoma in situ (CIS), a flat lesion of uncertain biological behavior that is often associated with high-grade invasive tumors (Lamm, 1992). CIS neoplasms are usually of high grade (grade III) and are detected late in the disease, often with invasion. Added to the complexity of TCCs is the fact that high-grade tumors (infiltrating or recurrent carcinomas) have a preponderance to undergo metaplasia (squamous and/or glandular; Friedell et al., 1983; Pauli et al., 1983, and references therein) as well as epithelial-mesenchymal transitions (Birchmeier and Birchmeier, 1995). The latter may occur in defined areas as well as in substantial parts of the tumor and may vary from area to area with respect to their degrees of differentiation.

Cytogenetic studies and molecular genetic data have indicated that chromosomes 9 and 17 are frequently altered in TCCs (Perucca et al., 1990; Simoneau and Jones, 1994; Presti et al., 1991), and there is good evidence suggesting that alterations of the tumor suppressor p53 (Sidransky et al., 1991; Simoneau and Jones, 1994; Spruck et al., 1994) are involved in the development and progression of these lesions. It has been shown that chromosome 9 deletions occur early during progression of papillary tumors, leading to a hyperplastic stage, whereas p53 mutations appear later in the process and confer invasive properties. The situation is, however, reversed in CIS, as a large fraction of these lesions harbor p53 mutations. In addition to indicating two divergent pathways of bladder cancer progression, these studies implied that the order in which the genetic changes take place is important in determining the final outcome.

Squamous Cell Carcinomas

SCCs often arise in patients who have a history of many years of chronic inflammation, keratinizing squamous metaplasia, and bladder stones (Bryan, 1983). The histogenesis of SCCs is unclear, although these lesions may arise from (1) extensive squamous differentiation of TCCs—i.e., carcinoma in situ (CIS) or high-grade papillary TCCs—and (2) neoplastic transformation on the basis of squamous metaplasia of the bladder urothelium (Sakamoto et al, 1992; Ostergaard et al., 1997; Celis et al.,

1999a,1999b). SCCs are composed of one cell type closely resembling keratinocytes (Olsen, 1984; Celis et al., 1996a) and exhibit distinct squamous features such as a "pearl" formation and keratohyalin bodies (Olsen, 1984).

Grading of these tumors is subjective and takes into consideration the degree of nuclear polymorphism, nuclear to cytoplasmic ratio, chromatin clumping, as well as the number of mitotic cells (Friedell et al., 1983). These parameters, however, are difficult to evaluate with precision, and, as a result, it is often impossible to distinguish between poorly differentiated TCCs with areas of squamous differentiation and highly undifferentiated SCCs (Friedell et al., 1983). In addition, different areas from the same tumor often show variable degrees of differentiation and/or metaplasia. SCCs are highly malignant and the success of treatment relies heavily on early detection.

PROTEOMIC-BASED DISCOVERY METHODS

Wilkins and colleagues defined the proteome as the complete set of proteins coded by the genome (Wilkins et al., 1996). However, the term has been broadened to include the set of proteins expressed both in space and time. There are two main approaches to proteomics: one is the surrogate model in which all proteins are analyzed in relation to each other (Bravo and Celis, 1982; Garrels, 1983; Taylor et al., 1982), and the other is the cell map model in which only a selected set of proteins, such as complexes and organelles, are analyzed (Celis et al., 1986; Blackstock and Weir, 1999). Ideally, we would like to have separation methods that are able to resolve, in a single map, all of the proteins expressed by a single cell type. This is, however, not possible, and the currently most powerful technique that provides a global profile of a cell proteome is high-resolution two-dimensional polyacrylamide gel electrophoresis (2D-PAGE) (O'Farrell, 1975; O'Farrell et al., 1977; Klose, 1975). 2D-PAGE suffers from various limitations imposed in part by the separation technology itself but also by the lack of sensitive procedures to detect proteins expressed at a wide range of abundances. Approaches based on chromatography-mass spectrometry (Link et al., 1999; Mintz et al., 1999) allow high-throughput but are not yet ready for the study of small and complex tissue samples, such as cancer biopsies (see below).

2D-PAGE-Based Proteomics

Since the mid-1970s, high-resolution 2D-PAGE has been the technique of choice for analyzing the protein composition of a given cell type and for monitoring changes in gene activity through the quantitative and qualitative analysis of the thousands of proteins that orchestrate various cellular functions (Celis and Bravo, 1984, and references therein). 2D-PAGE separates proteins both in terms of their isoelectric points (pI) and molecular weights (M_r), and accordingly, its resolving power is unsurpassed when compared to one-dimensional gel separation techniques. Using the current 2D-PAGE technology, one can (1) separate complex protein mixtures into their individual polypeptide components, (2) compare the protein expression profiles of sample pairs (normal versus transformed cells, cells at different stages of growth or differentiation, etc.; Fig. 9-1), and (3) choose a condition of interest (e.g., the addition of a cytokine or a drug to a given cell type or tissue) and allow the cell or tissue to reveal the global protein behavioral response under conditions where all of the detected proteins

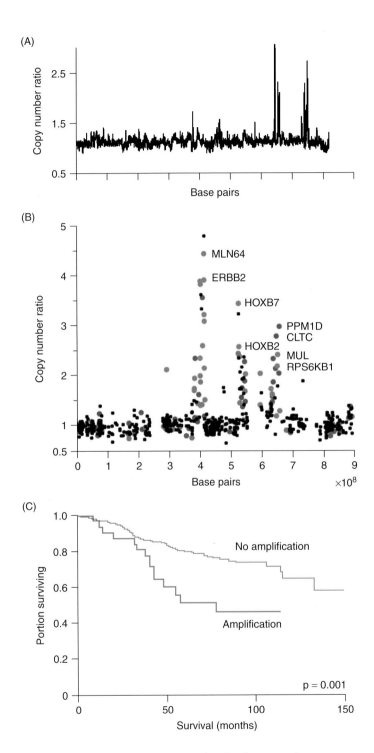

Figure 3-4. See pages 48 and 49 for figure caption.

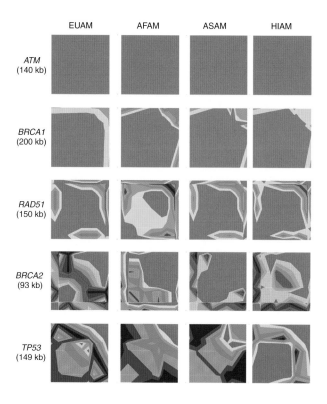

Figure 4-1. See page 68 for figure caption.

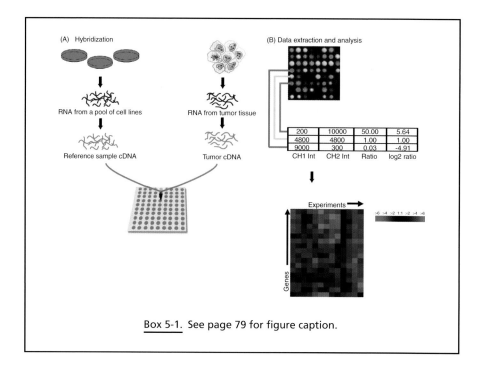

Box 5-1. See page 79 for figure caption.

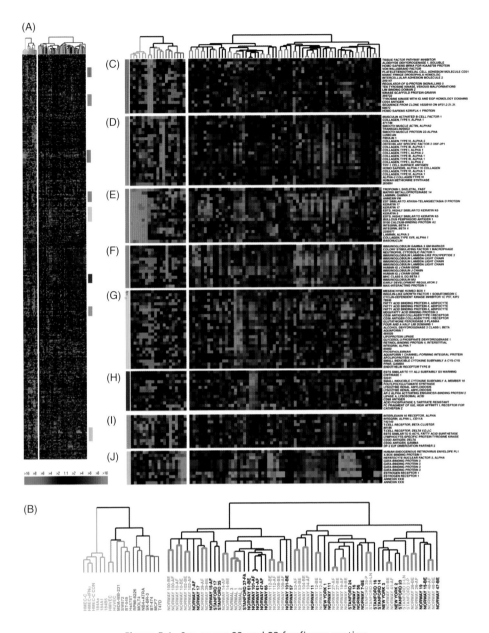

Figure 5-1. See pages 82 and 83 for figure caption.

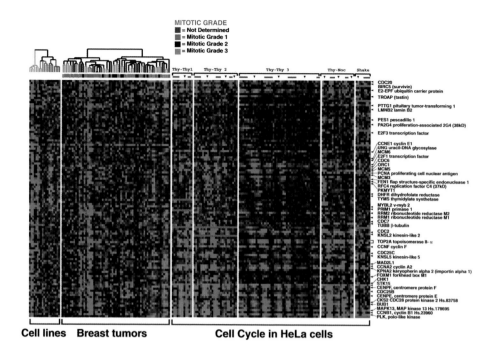

Figure 5-2. See page 84 for figure caption.

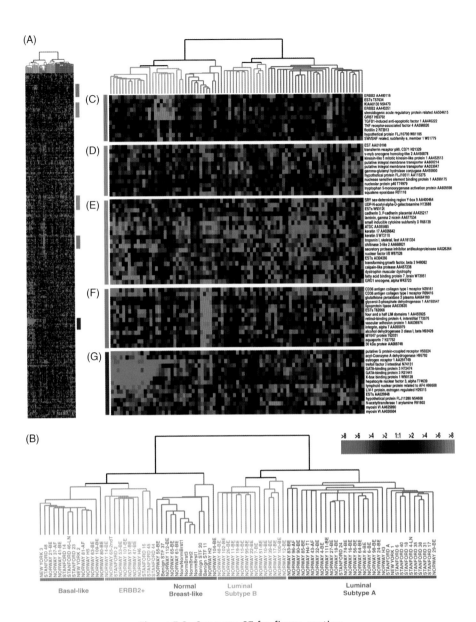

(A)

(C)
ERBB2 AA480116
ESTs T57034
KIAA0130 N56470
ERBB2 AA403351
steroidogenic acute regulatory protein related AA504615
GRB7 H53702
TGFB1-induced anti-apoptotic factor 1 AA446222
TNF receptor-associated factor 4 AA598826
flotillin 2 R72913
hypothetical protein FLJ10700 W81185
SWI/SNF related, subfamily e, member 1 W51779

(D)
EST AA010198
transferrin receptor p90, CD71 N21329
v-myb oncogene homolog-like 2 AA458878
kinesin-like 1 mitotic kinesin-like protein 1 AA452513
putative integral membrane transporter AA600214
putative integral membrane transporter AA033047
gamma-glutamyl hydrolase conjugase AA455800
hypothetical protein FLJ10511 AA115275
nuclease sensitive element binding protein 1 AA599175
nucleolar prctein p40 T74979
tryptophan 5-monooxygenase activation protein AA609598
squalene epoxidase R01118

(E)
SRY sex-determining region Y-box 9 AA400464
UDP-N-acetyl-alpha-D-galactosamine H13686
ESTs W93126
cadherin 3, P-cadherin placental AA425217
laminin, gamma 2 nicein AA677534
small inducible cytokine subfamily D R66139
ATDC AA055485
keratin 17 AA026642
keratin 5 W72110
troponin I, skeletal, fast AA181334
chitinase 3-like 2 AA668821
secretory prctease inhibitor antileukoproteinase AA026264
nuclear factor I/B W87528
ESTs AI304356
transforming growth factor, beta 2 N48092
calpain-like protease AA457238
dystrophin muscular dystrophy
fatty acid binding protein 7, brain W72051
GRO1 oncogene, alpha W42723

(F)
CD36 antigen collagen type I receptor N39161
CD36 antigen collagen type I receptor R09416
glutathione peroxidase 3 plasma AA664180
glycerol-3-phosphate dehydrogenase 1 AA192547
lipoprotein lipase AA633635
ESTs T62068
four and a half LIM domains 1 AA455925
retinol-binding protein 4, interstitial T72076
vascular adhesion protein 1 AA036974
integrin, alpha 7 AA055979
alcohol dehydrogenase 2 class I, beta N93426
MY047 protein T62031
aquaporin 7 R27752
30 kDa protein AA068748

(G)
putative G protein-coupled receptor H50224
acyl-Coenzyme A dehydrogenase H95792
estrogen receptor 1 AA291749
trefoil factor 3 intestinal N74131
GATA-binding protein 3 H72474
GATA-binding protein 3 R31441
X-box binding protein 1 W90128
hepatocyte nuclear factor 3, alpha T74639
lymphoid nuclear protein related to AF4 H99588
LIV-1 protein, estrogen regulated H26315
ESTs AA029948
hypothetical protein FLJ11280 N54608
N-acetyltransferase 1 arylamine R91802
myosin VI AA625890
myosin VI AA030004

(B)

>8 >6 >4 >2 1:1 >2 >4 >6 >8

Basal-like   ERBB2+   Normal
Breast-like

Luminal
Subtype B

Luminal
Subtype A

Figure 5-3. See page 87 for figure caption.

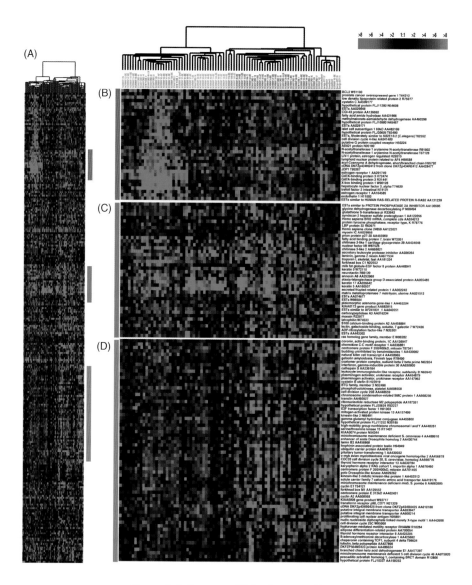

Figure 5-4. See page 88 for figure caption.

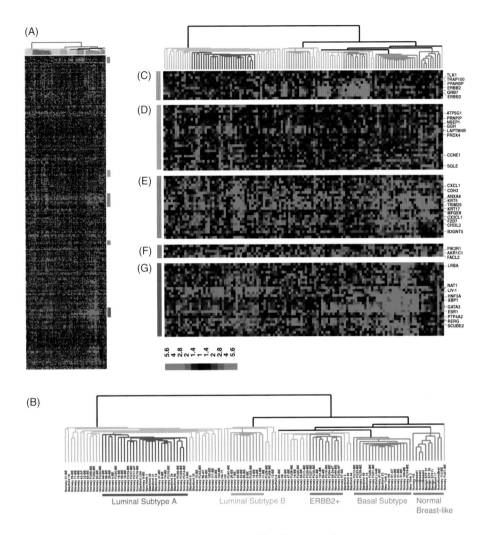

(A)

(C)
TLK1
TRAP100
PPARBP
ERBB2
GRB7
ERBB2

(D)
ATP5G1
PRNPIP
NSEP1
GGH
LAPTM4B
PRDX4

CCNE1

SQLE

(E)
CXCL1
CDH3
ANXA8
KRT5
TRIM29
KRT17
MFGE8
CX3CL1
FZD7
CHI3L2

B3GNT5

(F)
PIK3R1
AKR1C1
FACL2

(G)
LRBA

NAT1
LIV-1
HNF3A
XBP1
GATA3
ESR1
PTP4A2
RERG
SCUBE2

5.6 4 2.8 2 1.4 1 1.4 2 2.8 4 5.6

(B)

Luminal Subtype A   Luminal Subtype B   ERBB2+   Basal Subtype   Normal Breast-like

Figure 5-6. See page 91 for figure caption.

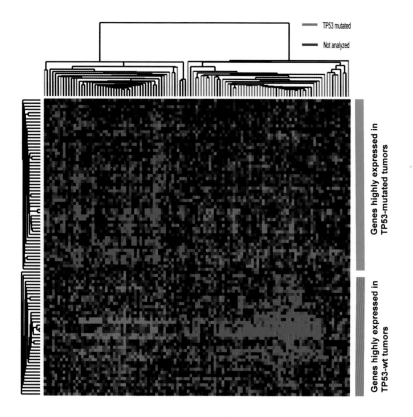

Figure 5-7. See page 93 for figure caption.

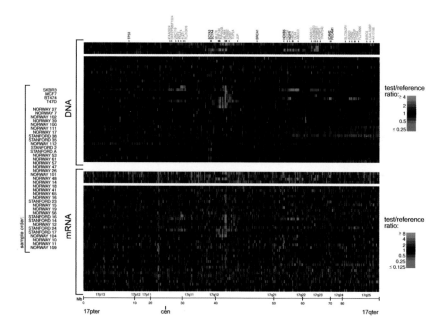

Figure 5-8. See page 94 for figure caption.

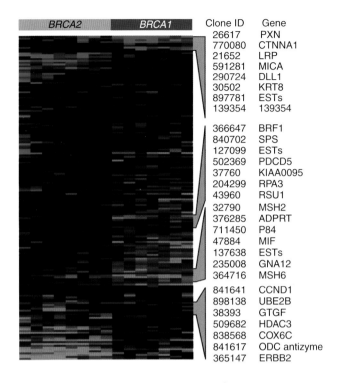

		Clone ID	Gene
BRCA2	BRCA1	26617	PXN
		770080	CTNNA1
		21652	LRP
		591281	MICA
		290724	DLL1
		30502	KRT8
		897781	ESTs
		139354	139354
		366647	BRF1
		840702	SPS
		127099	ESTs
		502369	PDCD5
		37760	KIAA0095
		204299	RPA3
		43960	RSU1
		32790	MSH2
		376285	ADPRT
		711450	P84
		47884	MIF
		137638	ESTs
		235008	GNA12
		364716	MSH6
		841641	CCND1
		898138	UBE2B
		38393	GTGF
		509682	HDAC3
		838568	COX6C
		841617	ODC antizyme
		365147	ERBB2

Figure 6-2. See page 107 for figure caption.

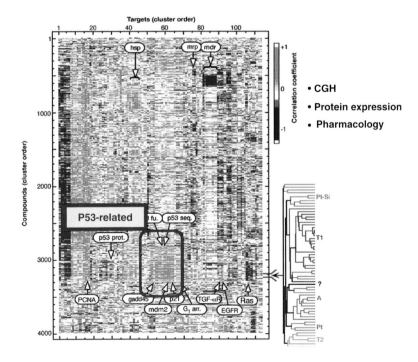

- CGH
- Protein expression
- Pharmacology

Figure 7-1. See page 123 for figure caption.

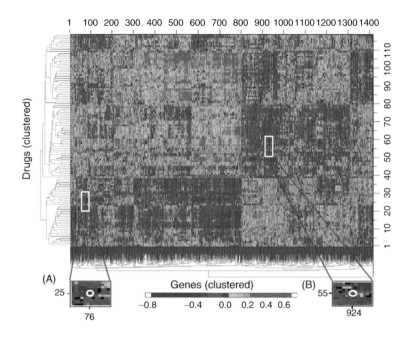

Figure 7-4. See page 128 for figure caption.

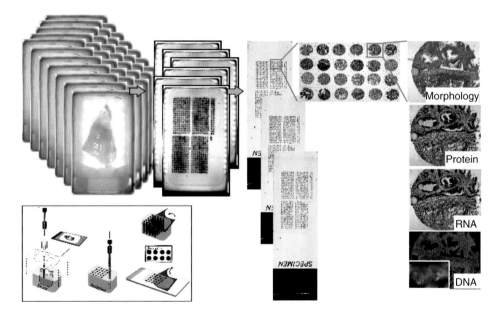

Figure 8-3. See page 148 for figure caption.

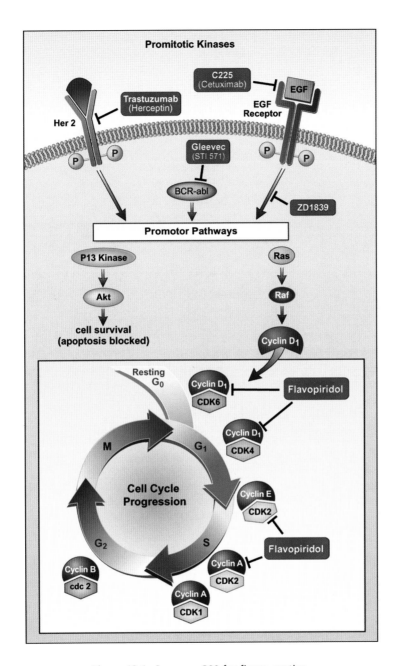

Figure 13-1. See page 300 for figure caption.

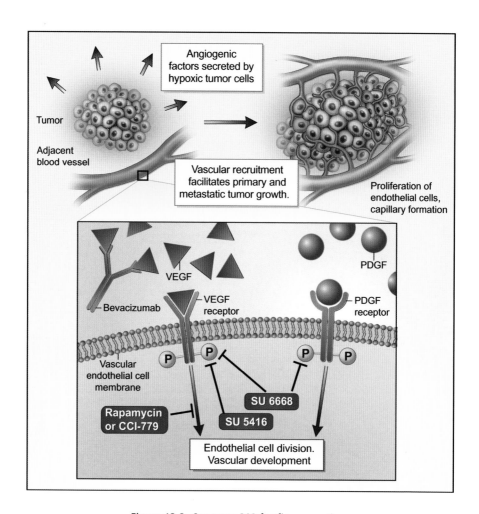

Figure 13-2. See page 302 for figure caption.

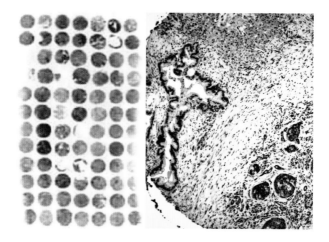

Figure 15-8. See page 353 for figure caption.

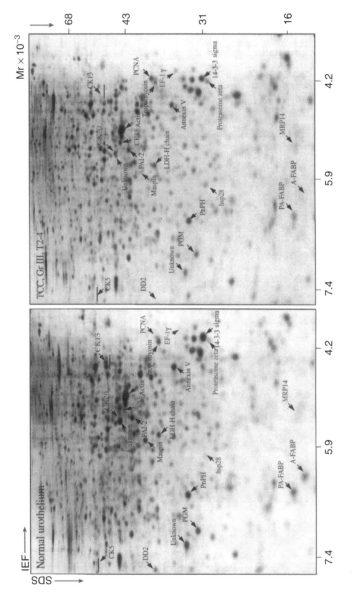

Figure 9-1. Highly deregulated proteins in invasive TCCs. [^{35}S]-methionine-labeled proteins synthesized by normal urothelium and an invasive TCC (grade III, T2–4) were separated by 2D-PAGE (IEF) and visualized by autoradiography. Proteins indicated are up- or down-regulated in the tumor. The position of actin is indicated for reference. (*Source:* From Celis et al., 2002.)

161

can be analyzed qualitatively and quantitatively in relation to each other (Celis and Olsen, 1994).

Protein profiles can be scanned and quantitated to search for protein differences (changes in the levels of preexisting proteins, induction of new products, coregulated polypeptides); interesting targets or molecular signatures can also be identified using additional proteomic technologies such as mass spectrometry (see below) and 2D-PAGE Western blotting (Celis and Gromov, 2000). Furthermore, by carrying out studies in a systematic manner, the information can be stored in comprehensive 2D-PAGE databases that record how genes are regulated in health and disease (see proteomics.cancer.dk; Fig. 9-2; expasy.hcuge.ch/ch2d/2d-index.html). As these databases acquire and organize a critical mass of data, they will become valuable sources of information for expediting the identification of signaling pathways and components that are affected in diseases (Celis et al., 1991a,1991b, 1998; Gromov et al., 2002).

In our laboratory, we have mainly used carrier ampholytes as originally described by O'Farrell and colleagues (1975, 1977) and Klose (1975) to perform proteomic studies of cultured cells and tissues. Even though gels run with carrier ampholytes are difficult to reproduce, we have standardized the technology to a level such that reproducible separations of nearly 4000–5000 [^{35}S]-methionine labeled polypeptides from whole human cell extracts using broad pH gradients can be obtained (Celis et al., 1991a, 1991b, 1998; Celis and Gromov, 2000; see also procedures and videos

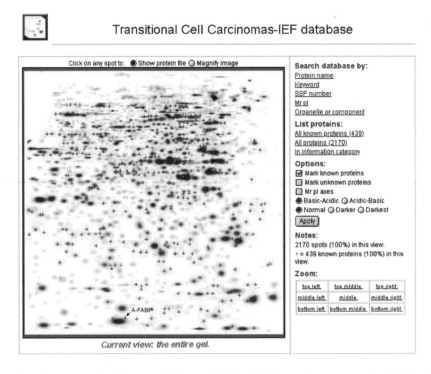

Figure 9-2. Master synthetic image of human bladder TCC proteins separated by IEF 2D-PAGE as shown at www.proteomics.cancer.dk. Proteins flagged with a cross correspond to identified proteins. By clicking on any spot, it is possible to open a file that contains protein information available in the database (proteomics.cancer.dk) as well as other links to other related web sites.

at proteomics.cancer.dk). Clearly, this number is still considerably short of the total number of proteins that may be present in a eukaryotic cell. Missing polypeptides are either not resolved by the pH gradient (too acidic or too basic), do not enter the gel due to solubilization problems and/or size, or are present in too low abundance to be detected with the current detection procedures.

Beyond sample preparation and gel standardization, the problem of detection, remains as many interesting proteins are present in very low copy numbers. For *known* low-abundance proteins for which there are highly specific antibodies available, detection does not pose a problem, as we have shown that 2D-PAGE immunoblotting in combination with enhanced chemoluminescence can detect as few as 100–500 molecules per cell in unfractionated cellular extracts (Celis and Gromov, 2000). The latter is exemplified in Figure 9-3, which shows an ECL-developed 2D-gel Western blot of crude keratinocyte extract reacted with antibodies raised against p21$^{\text{H-ras}}$, a protein that is known to be expressed in about 20,000 molecules per cell (Scheele et al., 1995). The corresponding area of the ^{35}S-methionine autoradiogram is shown for comparison. The amplitude of the intensities of the various p21$^{\text{H-ras}}$ spots shown in Figure 9-3 indicate that the low-abundance product marked with a small arrow may be present in no more than 500 molecules per cell. This technology reveals, in addition, the extent of the modification(s) and can effectively complement mass spectrometry and metabolic labeling with specific radioactive precursors to determine the nature of the modifications. Similarly, using blot overlay procedures, it may be possible to detect low-abundance proteins that bind to a particular radiolabeled ligand. Figure 9-4 shows blots of human keratinocyte proteins reacted with ^{32}P-labeled GTP (Gromov and Celis, 1994).

Everyday research, however, requires detection techniques that can be applied routinely to a large number of resolved proteins whose abundance may span through 7 or 8 orders of magnitude. Clearly, the sensitivity of silver nitrate and Coomassie Blue staining is inadequate, and only metabolic labeling with specific isotopes may reveal enough proteins to warrant proteomic projects. Furthermore, using phosphorimaging

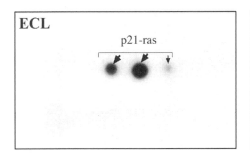
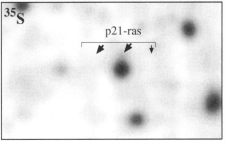

Figure 9-3. 2D-gel ECL immunodetection of p21$^{H\text{-}ras}$ and their modified variants expressed in human keratinocytes. Left: 2D-gel Western blot of human keratinocyte proteins reacted with a monoclonal antibody against p21$^{\text{H-ras}}$ and developed using the ECL procedure. Right: A corresponding autoradiograph of [^{35}S]-methionine-labeled proteins obtained from the same blot (see left). The positions of the p21$^{\text{H-ras}}$ spots are indicated with arrows. (*Source*: From Gromov et al., 2002.)

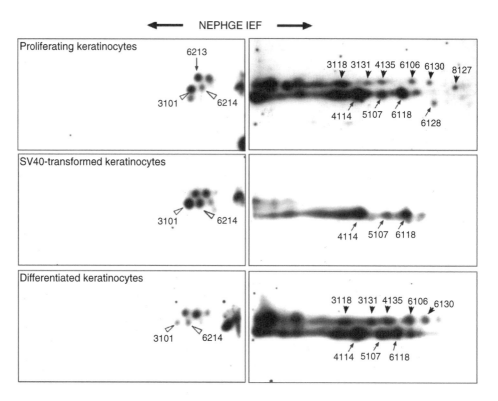

Figure 9-4. Small GTP-binding proteins expressed normal proliferating, SV40-transformed (K14), and differentiated human keratinocytes as revealed by the $[\alpha^{32}P]$GTP overlay technique. Proteins were separated by 2D-PAGE (IEF and NEPHGE), electroblotted onto a nitrocellulose membrane, and overlayed with 1 μCi of $[\alpha^{32}P]$GTP/ml. Only fractions of the 2D-gel blot ^{32}P-autoradiographs are shown. Some small GTP-binding proteins are indicated with their SSP numbers as recorded in the 2-D human keratinocyte database (proteomics.cancer.dk). Closed arrowheads show GTP-binding proteins that are elevated in differentiated keratinocytes and strongly down-regulated in transformed cells. Open arrowheads indicate three proteins upregulated in SV-40 transformed cells. (*Source*: From Gromov and Celis, 1994.)

technology, it is possible to enhance the sensitivity and linearity of detection. Limitations of the radiolabeling approach include (1) lack of labeling of some proteins due to low turnover, (2) problems associated with safety regulations and disposal, and (3) difficulties in obtaining fresh human biopsy material for labeling experiments. Ideally, one would like to have a highly sensitive fluorescence-based protein detection technique able to support all types of studies irrespective of the sample or the end point of the analysis. Preferably, the dye should not alter the molecular weight and pI of the proteins if it is to be added prior to electrophoresis and should support quantitative studies involving proteins that have extreme differences in their copy numbers. SYPRO Orange and SYPRO Red (Steinberg et al., 1996) offer some advantages over silver staining include wide linear range, short staining time and the fact that the gels do not need to be fixed prior to staining. More sensitive fluorescent dyes produced by Oxford Glyco Science (www.ogs.com/proteome/home.html) are not yet generally available.

Considerable improvements in 2D-gel technology have been made in an effort to overcome some of its limitations (Görg et al., 2000; Hanash, 2000, and references therein). In particular, immobilized pH gradients (IPGs: wide and narrow pH gradients) provide more reproducible focusing patterns, avoid some of the problems associated with carrier ampholytes (e.g., cationic drift), allow higher protein loading, and offer enhanced resolution in the first dimension. Görg and colleagues have considerably improved the separation of very basic proteins (Görg, 1999) using IPGs of very basic pH range, and isoelectric prefractionation has been used to enrich for proteins with basic pIs (Zuo and Speicher, 2000). Appropriate extraction procedures in combination with pre-gel fractionation have been utilized to enhance the separation and visualization of integral membrane proteins (Santoni et al., 2000). Additional developments include the use of very narrow pH gradients (Wildgruber et al., 2000; Zuo and Speicher, 2002).

Protein Arrays

Protein arrays provide a promising parallel, multiplex approach to carry out high-throughput screening for gene expression as well as broad studies of protein-targeting interactions (Cahill, 2001; Kodadek, 2001; Templin et al., 2002). To date, there are two main types of protein microarray-based technologies, which differ mainly on the type of molecules that are immobilized on the surface array. In the protein function array format (Kodadek, 2001), a repertoire of proteins is deposited on a surface in a regular manner and is tested for binding with specific ligands such as proteins, antibodies, hormones, nucleotides, nucleic acids, metal ions, etc. Several applications of peptide-based microarrays for high-throughput protein function screening, such as the identification of protein kinase substrates, have recently been described (MacBeath and Schreiber, 2000; Lesaicherre et al., 2002).

In the protein-detecting array format, a set of probes is spotted on the surface of the array to capture interacting proteins. The most promising application of this type of chip is to profile gene expression using antibodies (Jenkins and Pennington, 2001; Wilson and Nock, 2002; Bussow et al., 2001, and references therein). This type of array is based on the classical overlay immunoblotting technology in which specific antibodies are spotted on the immobilized matrix and probed with a protein mixture of interest such as protein extracts from cells or tissues or biological fluids. Antibody arrays can be used for large-scale and high-throughput protein analyses provided that a large amount of highly specific antibodies or derivatives—for example, a repertoire of Ig variable-chain fragments—are available (Hayhurst and Georgiou, 2001). Array-reading systems for the detection of protein complexes are based on fluorescence, chemoluminescence, mass spectrometry, radioactivity, and electrochemistry.

High-throughput protein expression and antibody screening on high-density filters and microarrays has recently been achieved using the PROfusion covalent mRNA-protein fission technology (Roberts and Szostak, 1997; Liu et al., 2000; Weng et al., 2002). The approach is based on the generation of comprehensive mRNA-protein fusion libraries prepared en masse by in vitro translation from highly complex, tissue-specific mRNA samples (Hammond et al., 2001). Cell-free protein synthesis on a microchip using different expression systems may provide a valuable tool for the miniaturization of proteome-scale protein-targeting interaction studies as well as for linking transcriptome and proteome data (Tabuchi et al., 2002). These types of protein microarrays link recombinant proteins to clones identified by DNA hybridization or sequencing, and as a result they provide a connection between nucleic acid–based and proteomic databases (Bussow et al., 2001).

Miniaturized and paralleled binding assays such as those previously described can be highly sensitive, extremely precise, as well as easily quantitated; however, they suffer from drawbacks such as (1) weak or uneven binding of some proteins to the immobilizing matrix, (2) loss of reactivity of complex-forming components, and (3) problems in re-creating the specific microenvironment in which proteins exist in vivo. A few of the most important challenges for the full implementation of protein microarrays relates to the acquisition of large sets of high-affinity and highly specific protein capture reagents, optimization of conditions for protein-targeting interactions, as well as data validation (Kodadek, 2002; Zhu and Snyder, 2001, and references therein).

One effective format for high-throughput profiling of protein expression is provided by the surface-enhanced laser desorption/ionization (SELDI) ProteinChip technology developed by Ciphergen Biosystems (Fung et al., 2001; Weinberger et al., 2002; Fung and Enderwick, 2002, and references therein) introduced in Chapter 8. The technology is based on the retentate chromatography of proteins from a chemically modified surface on a biochip. Coupled with mass spectrometry, this technology allows on-chip protein characterization of the affinity-bound proteins. The technology has shown great potential for the early detection of cancer by revealing biomarker patterns in fluids such as serum, urine, and nipple fluid aspirates (Weinberger et al., 2002; Fung and Enderwick, 2002). Cancers studied so far include ovary, prostate, bladder, breast, neck, and head (Paweletz et al., 2001; von Eggeling, et al., 2000; Adam et al., 2002; Li et al., 2002).

A publication by Petricoin and co-workers (Petricoin et al., 2002b) illustrated the power of the technology by using an artificial intelligence–based algorithm to identify a protein cluster pattern in serum for ovarian cancer. The same approach has been successfully applied to the study of prostate and breast cancer (Adam et al., 2002; Paweletz et al., 2001). At present, there is much discussion concerning the numbers of features required for a protein cluster or pattern and there is also concern as to the reproducibility of the results when using samples collected from different sites.

Mass Spectrometry-Based Protein Identification and High-Throughput Gel-Free Proteomics

Until the late 1980s, the identification and characterization of proteins was mainly performed by direct Edman N-terminal amino acid microsequencing of purified proteins or microsequence analysis of the digested peptides separated by RP-HPLC (Matsudaira, 1987; Aebersold et al., 1987; Rasmussen et al., 1992). Protein sequencing requires a large amount of starting material for analysis; as a result, only the abundant proteins ($>10^5$ copies per cell) can be identified. Using this procedure on a relatively large scale (Bauw et al., 1989) and in collaboration with Vanderkerckhove's laboratory in Ghent, we established the first 2D-gel protein databases that laid out the principles of modern proteomics (Celis et al., 1990, 1991b; Rasmussen et al., 1991). Today, current developments in protein identification are being fueled by developments in large-scale genome sequencing and bioinformatics as well as by improvements in mass spectrometry.

Ionization techniques that allow production of gas-phase molecular ions of proteins or peptides from the liquid phase—electrospray ionization (ESI; Fenn et al., 1989)—or the solid phase—matrix-assisted laser desorption ionization (MALDI; Karas and Hil-lenkamp, 1988)—were developed in the late 1980s. ESI and MALDI can be used in combination with a variety of mass analyzers—namely, time-of-flight (ToF; Ver-entchikov et al., 1994), single or triple quadruple (Fenn et al., 1989), ion trap (McLuckey et al., 1994; Arnott et al., 1998), the newly developed hybrid quadruple/time-of-flight instrument (Qq-TOF/Q/TOF; Morris et al., 1996; Shevchenko et al., 1997), and Fourier transform ion cyclotron resonance (FTCIR) (Buchanan and Hettich, 1993; Li et al., 1994).

Both MALDI-ToF-MS and ESI-MS technologies are the methods of choice when a systematic comparison of multiple clinical samples is required. These methods are highly complementary, but MALDI-ToF–MS is more straightforward and sensitive. It almost exclusively produces singly charged ions, can tolerate relatively high buffer and salt concentrations in the analyte mixture, and is usually the first method of choice in any protein study (Shevchenko et al., 1996; Jensen et al., 1998). The method is often used in cancer proteomics for the analysis of gel-separated proteins or for proteins transferred to nitrocellulose membranes followed by immuno- or specific overlay assay detection (Klarskov and Naylor, 2002). The later approach is very promising, since most proteins are often found as multiple forms on two-dimensional gels due to posttranslational processing and chemical modifications (phosphorylation, glycosylation, methylation, acetylation, myristoylation, palmitoylation, sulfation, ubiquitination, etc.; Wilkins et al., 1999; Fryksdale et al., 2002; Mann et al., 2002). Modified forms can also be characterized by combining MS approaches with a number of biochemical procedures (Pandey and Mann, 2000, and references therein).

MALDI-ToF-MS and ESI-MS technologies are highly dependent on gene and protein bioinformatics, as the precise mass of any given protein, peptide, or ion fragment is a unique feature that can be matched with the theoretically calculated mass obtained from sequence information available in protein, EST, or genomic databases. There are two main approaches that are used for protein identification and characterization: peptide mass fingerprinting (PMF) and tandem mass spectrometry. In our laboratory, the position of the protein of interest is determined by superimposing of unstained dried gel containing [^{35}S]methionine-labeled material with the corresponding autoradiogram. Proteins are then excised from the gel and digested with a sequence-specific protease that produces a set of peptides that serve as a unique fingerprint (Fig. 9-5; Patterson and Aebersold, 1995; Pappin, 1997).

The experimentally obtained peptide masses are compared to the calculated peptide masses resulting from the theoretical digestion of every full-length protein sequence entry present in protein, cDNA, or genomic databases. The list of the potential matching candidates is usually scored by taking into account the species of origin, the accuracy of the measurement, the number of matching peptides, and the degree of amino acid coverage in the predicted protein, with the top-scoring protein retrieved as a possible candidate. A peptide mass accuracy as high as several parts per million can be achieved using modern MALDI-ToF MS, permitting the identification of several components in a single digestion mixture (Jensen et al., 1996, 1997).

If the protein cannot be identified unambiguously by PMF, higher resolution mass and sequence information of selected peptides can be obtained either by ESI-MS or MALDI-ToF-PSD. In our laboratory, we use the Bruker MALDI-ToF-MS instrument (Biflex and Reflex IV), which is equipped with a variable-voltage reflector and allows protein identification by PMF and direct sequencing using Post-Source-Decay (PSD)

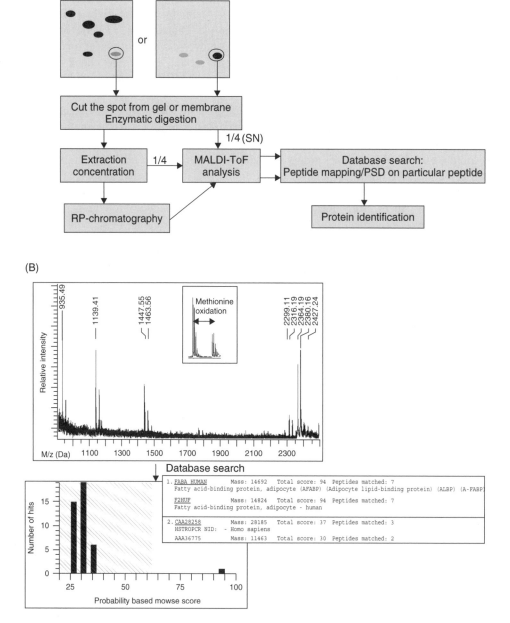

Figure 9-5. (A) Strategy for identifying proteins using MALDI-ToF. (B) Identification of proteins excised from 2-D gels followed by in situ digestion and MALDI-ToF analysis. The upper panel shows the MALDI-ToF mass spectrum. The pick list provides the input data for protein identification obtained by searching the MCDB database with the MASCOT software. The lower panels present the identification probability plot from the database search. Probability scores greater then 57 are considered significant ($p < 0.05$).

fragmentation (Fig. 9-5). The latter allows the analysis of the metastable decomposition of peptides that occur in a field-free region of the mass spectrometer (Spengler et al., 1992; Kaufmann, 1995). Despite the complexity of the PSD fragmentation pattern (Gevaert and Vandekerckhove, 2000), this method is very attractive as the sample can be analyzed both by PMF and PSD in the same experiment. Keough et al. have demonstrated that N-terminal modification of tryptic peptides facilitates the MS/MS fragmentation and selectively enhances detection of a single-fragment ion series. This observation has opened the door for the use of the MALDI-ToF-PSD method for de novo sequencing, as well as for the fast identification of posttranslational modifications (Keough et al., 2002).

Modern mass spectrometers can routinely analyze peptides even at the femtomole level (Wilm et al., 1996; Stensballe and Jensen, 2001) with a mass accuracy of 1 Da per 1000 to 10,000 Da (Takach et al., 1997; Clauser et al., 1999; Gobom et al., 2002). A number of innovations have been developed that minimize starting material, extending sensitivity to the low attomole range. These innovations make use of nanoliter bed volume reversed-phase columns of different configurations alone or in combination with prestructured sample supports (Schuerenberg et al., 2000; Johnson et al., 2001).

ESI-MS is the method of choice to generate direct sequence information from small proteins or peptides using triple quadrupole or ESI ion trap instruments due to its ability to produce multiple charged ions (Chapman, 1996) and to interface with liquid-phase separation techniques such as high-performance liquid chromatography (HPLC) and capillary electrophoresis. Micro-ESI-MS as well as nano-ESI-MS are often used for the de novo sequencing of proteins derived from species whose sequences are only partly present in databases. MALDI-ToF and ESI-MS have been combined lately in the new hybrid quadruple/time-of-flight instrument, Qq-TOF, which has several of the advantages of ESI-MS—i.e., ability to acquire tandem mass spectra with a very high-mass resolution—and MALDI-ToF-MS—i.e., to record all ions simultaneously, thus increasing sensitivity of measurement (Morris et al., 1996; Shevchenko et al., 1997).

Rapid advances in MS hardware and software have made possible the development of shotgun proteomics, which analyzes total digest of complex samples rather than individual proteins (Yates et al., 1996; Washburn et al., 2001). The approach couples multidimensional microcapillary liquid chromatography (LC-MS-MS) with automated ESI-MS-MS, allowing the automated, large-scale identification of proteins in a gel-free environment (Link et al., 1999). The method has very high sensitivity, mass accuracy and resolution (Quenzer et al., 2001; Martin et al., 2000; Aebersold and Goodlett, 2001).

It should be noted that MS analysis of digested protein mixtures separated by multiple LC-HPLC cannot differentiate the origin of peptides—that is, from the intact protein, splice variants, modified forms, and/or degradation products. The development of the isotope-coded affinity tag (ICAT) technology has, in addition, enabled the concurrent identification and comparative quantitative analysis of proteins present in both cell extracts and fluids by mass spectrometry (Gygi et al., 1999). So far, the technology has been used for the analysis of biological fluids (Croubels et al., 2002; Taylor et al., 2002; Berna et al., 2002) and cultured cells (Zappacosta et al., 2002; Ho et al., 2002). Further increases in sensitivity will be required for shotgun MS methods to analyze small tissue biopsies such as those described in Chapter 8.

PROTEOMIC APPROACHES TO THE STUDY OF BLADDER CANCER HETEROGENEITY

Identification of Cancer Heterogeneity Among Low-Grade Papillary TCCs: Correlation with Recurrence

The biological relevance of low-grade papillary tumors is underlined by the fact that about 70% of the bladder lesions are diagnosed as superficial (Ta, T1) at first presentation (Zieger et al., 2000). These tumors have a high frequency of recurrence (>60%), and about 10–15% of them will progress to life-threatening malignancies (Cheng et al., 2000). Currently, it is not possible to assess with certainty the biological behavior of these tumors based on clinical or morphological criteria alone; as a result, it is urgent to identify early and accurate biomarkers that may predict recurrence, progression, and response to treatment. Also, it is important to distinguish those lesions that have no significant effect on the life expectancy of the patient, as all tumor-bearing patients are diagnosed with cancer—a fact that has practical and economic implications as well as a profound psychological effect on the patient (Harnden et al., 1999). To be able to predict which patients with low-grade papillary tumors will develop recurrences and/or progress to invasive disease is one of the major challenges we face today; thus, more research should be directed at early diagnosis.

Our strategy for identifying cancer heterogeneity among low-grade papillary TCCs encompasses a blind and systematic study of the proteomic profiles of hundreds of fresh biopsy specimens from both normal and tumor origin (Celis et al., 2002). First, we identify major proteins that are differentially expressed in invasive lesions (Gr III, T2–4) as compared to normal urothelium, and thereafter we use specific antibodies against these proteins to immunostain cryostatic sections of low-grade papillary tumors diagnosed as having the same grade of atypia and stage (Gr I, Ta). Invasive TCCs, rather than low-grade papillary TCCs, are chosen to generate the protein markers, as these lesions are expected to harbor proteomic alterations associated with recurrence and progression. Areas of tumor heterogeneity may comprise only a small proportion of low-grade tumors; as a result, neither down- nor upregulated protein markers may be detected under these conditions.

Figure 9-1 shows representative proteome expression profiles of fresh biopsies of normal urothelium and a Gr III, T2–4 invasive tumor (Celis et al., 2002). Some deregulated polypeptides that showed variations of at least twofold in 40% of the invasive tumors analyzed are indicated in Figure 9-1. Upregulated proteins included elongation factor 1, Hsp28, CKs 18 and 20, PCNA, the proteasome subunit, and MRP14. Downregulated proteins included A-FABP, annexin V, high-affinity bile-binding protein (DD2), CKs 5 and 13, lactate dehydrogenase H chain (LDH H), maspin, plasminogen activator inhibitor 2 (PAI-2), PA-FABP, phosphoglycerate kinase, purine nucleoside phosphorylase (PnPH), a tropomyosin isoform, and 14-3-3, (stratifin). The identity of these proteins was determined by mass spectrometry and/or 2D-PAGE immunoblotting.

Tumor heterogeneity among 30 low-grade papillary TCCs collected during a period of 5 years was revealed by indirect immunofluorescence of cryostat sections reacted with a panel of antibodies consisting of probes against CKs 5, 13, 18, and 20. This panel was supplemented with markers of squamous metaplasia (CKs 7, 8, and 14), as these lesions are a rather common feature of invasive TCCs (Harnden and Southgate,

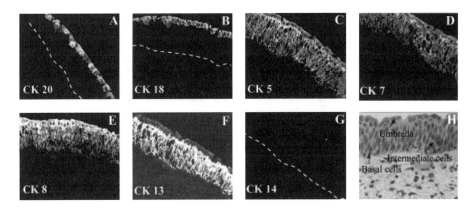

Figure 9-6. Immunofluorescence staining of formaldehyde fixed cryostat sections from normal urothelium reacted with the panel of antibodies against keratins (A–G). Hemotoxylin staining of normal urothelium (H). (*Source*: From Celis et al., 2002.)

1997; Southgate et al., 1999). It should be stressed that the rate-limiting step in the procedure is the preparation of specific antibodies that react both in immunoblots and immunofluorescence. So far, antibodies against only a few of the deregulated proteins have been obtained that satisfy rigorous specificity tests.

Of the 30 low-grade papillary tumors analyzed by immunofluorescence, only 4 displayed identical staining patterns as normal urothelium (Fig. 9-6). With the exception of type 1, the rest could be grouped into five major types that shared aberrant staining with the CK20 antibody (Fig. 9-7). As expected, the size of the areas showing heterogeneity varied from tumor to tumor, but most tumors exhibited only one major type of heterogeneity. Type 1 heterogeneity ($n = 4$) showed preferred staining of the umbrella cells with the CK8 antibody (Fig. 9-7A), while type 2 ($n = 11$) was typified by the staining of the basal and intermediate layers with the CK20 antibody as previously described by Southgate's group (Harnden et al., 1999; Fig. 9-7B). Type 3 heterogeneity ($n = 7$) was characterized by predominant staining of the basal cell layer with the CK5 antibody (Fig. 9-7C), whereas type 4 ($n = 1$) showed areas of CK7-negative cells (Fig. 9-7D). Type 5 heterogeneity ($n = 3$), in contrast, showed loss of staining of the basal cells with the CK20 antibody (Fig. 9-7E), although in one lesion the basal cells reacted positively with CK14 (Fig. 9-7F; type 5B), suggesting early events in squamous differentiation.

Recurrences were experienced by 29% of the patients, but none progressed to invasive disease during the follow-up period. Patients harboring phenotypic alterations in the basal, proliferative compartment (types 3 and 5) showed the highest number of recurrences (4/7 and 2/3, respectively), and all type 3 lesions progressed to a higher degree of dedifferentiation. Though a long-term prospective study involving a larger sample size is required to assess the biological potential of these lesions, we believe that this approach implemented with a larger battery of antibodies will prove instrumental for revealing early phenotypic changes in different types of cancer. Currently, we are carrying out a systematic analysis of low-grade noninvasive and invasive TCCs in an effort to determine the incidence of the various protein expression changes at various stages of cancer development.

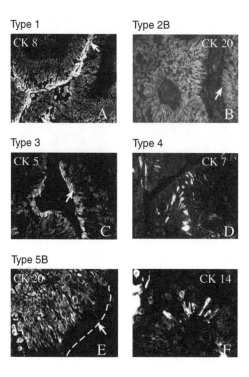

Figure 9-7. Tumor heterogeneity types. Immunofluorescence staining of formaldehyde fixed cryo-stat sections from selected urothelial papillomas showing various types of tumor heterogeneity. (*Source*: From Celis et al., 2002.)

Identification of Metaplastic Lesions in SCC-Bearing Patients

A major aim of our research on bladder SCCs has been to reveal premalignant lesions and markers that may identify individuals at risk of developing the disease (Celis et al., 2000a, and references therein). This goal is being pursued systematically by blind analysis of the proteome expression profiles of fresh tumors and random biopsies as well as urothelial tissue from patients who have undergone removal of the bladder due to invasive disease (cystectomy). Because bladder cancer is a field disease (Slaughter et al., 1953)—that is, a large part of the urothelium is at risk of developing disease—we surmised that this material could be invaluable for dissecting some of the steps involved in the squamous differentiation of the bladder urothelium. The presence of extensive areas of squamous metaplasia in bladder SCCs is often associated with poorly differentiated and invasive tumors, and is considered an unfavorable prognostic factor (Sakamoto et al., 1992).

The approach first makes use of proteomic technologies to reveal and identify proteins that are differentially expressed in pure SCCs and normal urothelium, much in the same way as it has been described previously for low-grade papillary tumors. Thereafter, specific antibodies against the differentially expressed proteins are used to stain serial cryostatic sections of cystectomy biopsies from SCC-bearing patients in a process that we have termed *immunowalking*—that is, walking from a morphologically normal-looking urothelium toward the tumor (Celis et al., 1999a, 1999b).

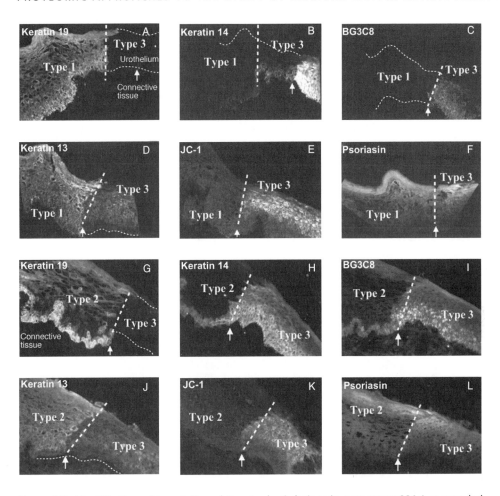

Figure 9-8. Identification of type 1, 2, and 3 metaplastic lesions in cystectomy 884-1 as revealed by staining with CK19 antibodies. Serial cryostat sections of cystectomy 884-1 were reacted with antibodies against proteins differentially expressed by the normal urothelium and the SCCs. (A–F) and (G–L) correspond to serial sections of two different areas of cystectomy 884-1 in which all three lesion types are represented. White arrows indicate reference points for comparison. (*Source*: From Celis et al., 1999a.)

Immunofluorescence analysis of SCC cystectomy biopsies using antibodies specific for some of the proteins differentially expressed in SCCs has so far revealed at least three types of nonkeratinizing metaplastic lesions that can be readily distinguished based on the expression of CK19 (Fig. 9-8). Type 1 metaplasias express CK19 in all cell layers (Fig. 9-8A, left part) but show variable staining with CK14 and BG3C8 antibodies depending on the intensity of the CK19 staining of the basal cells (not shown). These lesions do not express CKs 7, 8, 18, and 20 (not shown). Type 2 lesions express CK19 and CK14 mainly in the basal proliferative compartment (Fig. 9-8G and H, left part). Type 3 lesions are characterized by lack of staining with the CK19 antibody and by the basal and suprabasal expression of CK14 (Fig. 9-8A and G; here shown next to type 1 and 2 lesions). The basal cells in the type 3 lesions shown in

Figure 9-8D and J (right part) do not express CK13, suggesting that the tumor, which is also CK13 negative (not shown, but see Celis et al., 1999a), most likely arose from the expansion of the basal cell compartment. These lesions may be considered as direct precursors of the tumor.

Clearly, there is much work to be done to derive specific markers that may identify premalignant lesions early during the disease course; nevertheless, these studies have shown that it is possible to use proteomic approaches in combination with immunohisto-chemistry to unravel some of the steps involved in the transformation from transitional to stratified squamous epithelia. This approach is currently being used in combination with laser microdissection (Bonner et al., 1997) discussed in Chapter 8 to gain further insight into the proteome alterations that precede cancer.

CONCLUSIONS

To date there have been hundreds of reports illustrating the power of proteomics in the study of cancer (Celis and Olsen, 1994; Celis and Gromov, 2000b; Pucci-Minafra et al., 2002; Harris et al., 2002, and references therein). Most of these studies, however, have been carried out using cultured cells, which we know undergo important alterations due to changes in environmental and growth conditions (Celis et al., 1999c). There are, however, several reports on proteomic studies carried out with tissue biopsies from various types of cancer. These include breast (Franzen et al., 1996; Wulfkuhle et al., 2001), colon (Stulik et al., 1997, 2001; Lawrie et al., 2001), prostate (Ahram et al., 2002; Meehan et al., 2002; Alaiya et al., 2000), and ovarian (Jones et al., 2002; Alaiya et al., 2002) cancer. In addition, there have been several reports on leukemia and

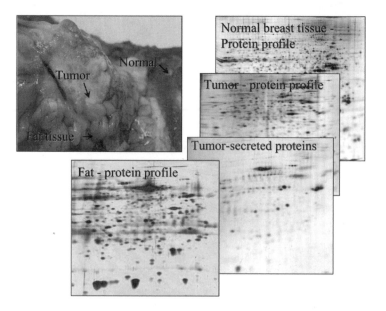

Figure 9-9. Proteome profiles of fresh breast tissue biopsies obtained shortly after surgery. 2D gels of fat proteins have been stained with silver nitrate, while the others correspond to an autoradiogram of [^{35}S]-methionine-labeled samples.

hematological malignancies (Melhem et al., 1991, 1997). In general, these studies are aimed at characterizing proteomic alterations, including posttranslational modifications that take place during tumor progression.

In our laboratory, we have applied proteomics to the study of fresh tissue biopsies in bladder (Celis, 2002; Celis et al., 1996b, 1999a,1999b), colon (unpublished observations), and kidney cancer (unpublished observations), and have recently started a collaboration with clinicians, oncologists, surgeons, and pathologists to study breast cancer using fresh tissue biopsies and biological fluids. A pilot study has so far shown that it is possible to obtain protein profiles of very small fresh tissue biopsies from tumors, normal tissue, metastasis, as well as fat obtained shortly after surgery (Fig. 9-9). This clinical oncoproteomic project seeks to develop (1) new molecular noninvasive diagnostics able to detect cancer at a very early stage, (2) improved methodology to determine the stage of breast cancer and to prognose the outcome, and (3) individualized breast cancer therapy based on defined molecular signatures.

ACKNOWLEDGMENTS

The work was supported by a grant from the Danish Cancer Society.

REFERENCES

Adam, B. L., Qu, Y., Davis, J. W., Ward, M. D., Clements, M. A., Cazares, L. H., Semmes, O. J., Schellhammer, P. F., Yasui, Y., Feng, Z., Wright, G. L. Jr. (2002). Serum protein fingerprinting coupled with a pattern-matching algorithm distinguishes prostate cancer from benign prostate hyperplasia and healthy men. *Cancer Res 62*, 3609–3614.

Aebersold, R., and Goodlett, D. R. (2001). Mass spectrometry in proteomics. *Chem Rev 101*, 269–295.

Aebersold, R. H., Leavitt, J., Saavedra, R. A., Hood, L. E., and Kent, S. B. (1987). Internal amino acid sequence analysis of proteins separated by one- or two-dimensional gel electrophoresis after in situ protease digestion on nitrocellulose. *Proc Natl Acad Sci USA 84*, 6970–6974.

Ahram, M., Best, C. J., Flaig, M. J., Gillespie, J. W., Leiva, I. M., Chuaqui, R. F., Zhou, G., Shu, H., Duray, P. H., Linehan, W. M., Raffeld, M., Ornstein, D. K., Zhao, Y., Petricoin, E. F. III, and Emmert-Buck, M. R. (2002). Proteomic analysis of human prostate cancer. *Mol Carcinogenesis 33*, 9–15.

Alaiya, A., Roblick, U., Egevad, L., Carlsson, A., Franzen, B., Volz, D., Huwendiek, S., Linder, S., and Auer, G. (2000). Polypeptide expression in prostate hyperplasia and prostate adenocarcinoma. *Anal Cell Pathol 21*, 1–9.

Alaiya, A. A., Franzen, B., Hagman, A., Dysvik, B., Roblick, U. J., Becker, S., Moberger, B., Auer, G., and Linder, S. (2002). Molecular classification of borderline ovarian tumors using hierarchical cluster analysis of protein expression profiles. *Int J Cancer 98*, 895–899.

Anderson, N. G., Matheson, A., and Anderson, N. L. (2001). Back to the future: The human protein index (HPI) and the agenda for post-proteomic biology. *Proteomics 1*, 3–12.

Anderson, N. L., Eisler, W. J., and Anderson, N. G. (1978). Analytical techniques for cell fractions. XXIII. A stable thermal gradient device for heat denaturation studies on proteins. *Anal Biochem 91*, 441–445.

Arnott, D., Henzel, W. J., and Stults, J. T. (1998). Rapid identification of comigrating gel-isolated proteins by ion trap-mass spectrometry. *Electrophoresis 19*, 968–980.

Bane, B. L., Rao, J. Y., and Hemstreet, G. P. (1996). Pathology and staging of bladder cancer. *Semin Oncol 23*, 546–570.

Bauw, G., Van Damme, J., Puype, M., Vandekerckhove, J., Gesser, B., Ratz, G. P, Lauridsen, J. B., and Celis, J. E. (1989). Protein-electroblotting and -microsequencing strategies in generating protein data bases from two-dimensional gels. *Proc Natl Acad Sci USA 86*, 7701–7705.

Berna, M., AcKermann, B., Rutherborles, K., and Glass, S. (2002). Determination of olanzapine in human blood my liquid chromatography-tandem mass spectrometry. *J chromatogr B Analyt Technol Biomed Life 767*, 163–168.

Birchmeier, W., and Birchmeier, C. (1995). Epithelial-mesenchymal transitions in development and tumor progression. In *Epithelial-Mesenchymal Interactions in Cancer*, I. D. Goldberg and E. M. Rosen (eds.). Basel: Berkhaeuser Verlag, pp. 1–15.

Blackstock, W. P., and Weir, M. P. (1999). Proteomics: Quantitative and physical mapping of cellular proteins. *Trends Biotechnol 17*, 121–127.

Bonner, R. F., Emmert-Buck, M., Cole, K., Pohida, T., Chuaqui, R., Goldstein, S., and Liotta, L. A. (1997). Laser capture microdissection: Molecular analysis of tissue. *Science 278*, 1481–1483.

Bravo, R., and Celis, J. E. (1982). Up-dated catalogue of HeLa cell proteins: Percentages and characteristics of the major cell polypeptides labeled with a mixture of 16 14C-labeled amino acids. *Clin Chem 28*, 766–781.

Bryan, G. T. (1983). Etiology and pathogenesis of bladder cancer. In *The Pathology of Bladder Cancer*, vol. 1 G. T. Bryan and S. M. Cohen (eds.)., Boca Raton, FL: CRC Press, pp. 1–11.

Buchanan, M. V., and Hettich, R. L. (1993). Fourier transform mass spectrometry of high-mass biomolecules. *Anal Chem 65*, 245A–259A.

Bussow, K., Konthur, Z., Lueking, A., Lehrach, H., and Walter, G. (2001). Protein array technology. Potential use in medical diagnostics. *Am J Pharmacogenomics 1*, 37–43.

Cahill, D. J. (2001). Protein and antibody arrays and their medical applications. *J Immunol Methods 250*, 81–91

Celis, J. E. (2002). A new start in Madrid: Symposium on basic and translational cancer research. *EMBO Rep 3*, 718–723.

Celis, J. E., and Bravo, R. (eds.) (1984). *Two-Dimensional Gel Electrophoresis of Proteins: Methods and Applications*. New York: Academic Press.

Celis, J. E., and Gromov, P. (2000). High-resolution two-dimensional gel electrophoresis and protein identification using western blotting and ECL detection. *EXS 88*, 55–67.

Celis, J. E., and Olsen, E. (1994). A qualitative and quantitative protein database approach identifies individual and groups of functionally related proteins that are differentially regulated in simian virus 40 (SV40) transformed human keratinocytes: An overview of the functional changes associated with the transformed phenotype. *Electrophoresis 15*, 309–344.

Celis, J. E., Bravo, R., Arenstorf, H. P., and LeStourgeon, W. M. (1986). Identification of proliferation-sensitive human proteins amongst components of the 40 S hnRNP particles. Identity of hnRNP core proteins in the HeLa protein catalogue. *FEBS Lett 194*, 101–109.

Celis, J. E., Cruger, D., Kiil, J., Dejgaard, K., Lauridsen, J. B., Ratz, G. P., Basse, B., Celis, A., Rasmussen, H. H., Bauw, G., et al. (1990). A two-dimensional gel protein database of non-cultured total normal human epidermal keratinocytes: Identification of proteins strongly up-regulated in psoriatic epidermis. *Electrophoresis 11*, 242–254.

Celis, J. E., Rasmussen, H. H., Leffers, H., Madsen, P., Honore, B., Gesser, B., Dejgaard, K., and Vandekerckhove, J. (1991a). Human cellular protein patterns and their link to genome DNA sequence data: Usefulness of two-dimensional gel electrophoresis and microsequencing. *FASEB J 5*, 2200–2208.

Celis, J. E., Leffers, H., Rasmussen, H. H., Madsen, P., Honore, B., Gesser, B., Dejgaard, K., Olsen, E., Ratz, G. P., Lauridsen, J. B., et al. (1991b). The master two-dimensional gel database of human AMA cell proteins: Towards linking protein and genome sequence and mapping information (update 1991). *Electrophoresis 12*, 765–801.

Celis, J. E., Rasmussen, H. H., Vorum, H., Madsen, P., Honore, B., Wolf, H., and Orntoft, T. F. (1996a). Bladder squamous cell carcinomas express psoriasin and externalize it to the urine. *J Urol 155*, 2105–2112.

Celis, J. E., Ostergaard, M., Basse, B., Celis, A., Lauridsen, J. B., Ratz, G. P., Andersen, I., Hein, B., Wolf, H., Orntoft, T. F., and Rasmussen, H. H. (1996b). Loss of adipocyte-type fatty acid binding protein and other protein biomarkers is associated with progression of human bladder transitional cell carcinomas. *Cancer Res 56*, 4782–4790.

Celis, J. E., Ostergaard, M., Jensen, N. A., Gromova, I., Rasmussen, H. H., and Gromov, P. (1998). Human and mouse proteomic databases: Novel resources in the protein universe. *FEBS Lett 430*, 64–72.

Celis, J. E., Celis, P., Ostergaard, M., Basse, B., Lauridsen, J. B., Ratz, G., Rasmussen, H. H., Orntoft, T. F., Hein, B., Wolf, H., and Celis, A. (1999a). Proteomics and immunohistochemistry define some of the steps involved in the squamous differentiation of the bladder transitional epithelium: A novel strategy for identifying metaplastic lesions. *Cancer Res 59*, 3003–3009.

Celis, J. E., Ostergaard, M., Celis, P., Rasmussen, H. H., and Wolf, H. (1999b). Proteomics in bladder cancer research: Protein profiling of bladder squamous cell carcinomas. *BioRadiations 101*, 24–27.

Celis, J. E., Rasmussen, H. H., Celis, P., Basse, B., Lauridsen, J. B., Ratz, G., Hein, B., Ostergaard, M., Wolf, H., Orntoft, T., and Celis, J. E. (1999c). Short-term culturing of low-grade superficial bladder transitional cell carcinomas leads to changes in the expression levels of several proteins involved in key cellular activities. *Electrophoresis 20*, 355–361.

Celis, J. E., Wolf, H., and Ostergaard, M. (2000a). Bladder squamous cell carcinoma biomarkers derived from proteomics. *Electrophoresis 21*, 2115–2121.

Celis, J. E., Kruhoffer, M., Gromova, I., Frederiksen, C., Ostergaard, M., Thykjaer, T., Gromov, P., Yu, J., Palsdottir, H., Magnusson, N., and Orntoft, T. F. (2000b). Gene expression profiling: Monitoring transcription and translation products using DNA microarrays and proteomics. *FEBS Lett 480*, 2–16.

Celis, J. E., Celis, P., Palsdottir, H., Ostergaard, M., Gromov, P., Primdahl, H., Orntoft, T. F., Wolf, H., Celis, A., and Gromova, I. (2002). Proteomic strategies to reveal tumor heterogeneity among urothelial papillomas. *Mol Cell Proteomics 1*, 269–279.

Chapman, J. R. (1996). *Methods in Molecular Biology: Protein and Peptide Analysis by Mass Spectrometry*. Totowa, NJ: Humana Press, pp. 9–29.

Cheng, L., Neumann, R. M., Nehra, A., Spotts, B. E., Weaver, A. L., and Bostwick, D. G. (2000). Cancer heterogeneity and its biologic implications in the grading of urothelial carcinoma. *Cancer 88*, 1663–1670.

Clauser, K. R., Baker, P., and Burlingame, A. L. (1999). Role of accurate mass measurement (+/−10 ppm) in protein identification strategies employing MS or MS/MS and database searching. *Anal Chem 71*, 2871–2882.

Croubels, S., Cherlet, M., and De Backer, P. (2002). Quantitative analysis of diclazuril in animal plasma by liquid chromatography/electrospray ionization mass spectrometry. *Rapid Commun Mass Spectrom 16*, 1463–1469.

Cunningham, M. J. (2000). Genomics and proteomics: The new millennium of drug discovery and development. *J Pharmacol Toxicol Methods 44*, 291–300.

EL-Bolkainy, M. N. (1983). Schistosomasis and bladder cancer. In *The Pathology of Bladder Cancer*, vol. I, G. T. Bryan and S. M. Cohen (eds.). Boca Raton, FL: CRC Press, pp. 57–90.

Eickhoff, H., Konthur, Z., Lueking, A., Lehrach, H., Walter, G., Nordhoff, E., Nyarsik, L., and Bussow, K. (2002). Protein array technology: The tool to bridge genomics and proteomics. *Adv Biochem Eng Biotechnol 77*, 103–112.

Fenn, J. B., Mann, M., Meng, C. K., Wong, S. F., and Whitehouse, C. M. (1989). Electrospray ionization for mass spectrometry of large biomolecules. *Science 246*, 64–71.

Franzen, B., Auer, G., Alaiya, A. A., Eriksson, E., Uryu, K., Hirano, T., Okuzawa, K., Kato, H., and Linder, S. (1996). Assessment of homogeneity in polypeptide expression in breast carcinomas shows widely variable expression in highly malignant tumors. *Int J Cancer 69*, 408–414.

Friedell, G. H., Nagy, G. K., and Cohen, S. M. (1983). Pathology of human bladder cancer and related lesions. In *The Pathology of Bladder Cancer*, vol I, G. T. Bryan and S. M. Cohen (eds.). Boca Raton, FL: CRC Press, pp. 11–42.

Fryksdale, B. G., Jedrzejewski, P. T., Wong, D. L., Gaertner, A. L., and Miller, B. S. (2002). Impact of deglycosylation methods on two-dimensional gel electrophoresis and matrix assisted laser desorption/ionization–time of flight–mass spectrometry for proteomic analysis. *Electrophoresis 23*, 2184–2193.

Fung, E. T., Thulasiraman, V., Weinberger, S. R., and Dalmasso, E. A. (2001). Protein biochips for differential profiling. *Curr Opin Biotechnol 12*, 65–69.

Fung, E. T., and Enderwick, C. (2002). ProteinChip clinical proteomics: Computational challenges and solutions. *Biotechniques 34–8*, 40–41.

Garrels, J. I. (1983). Quantitative two-dimensional gel electrophoresis of proteins. *Methods Enzymol 100*, 411–423.

Gevaert, K., and Vandekerckhove, J. (2000). Protein identification methods in proteomics. *Electrophoresis 21*, 1145–1154.

Gobom, J., Mueller, M., Egelhofer, V., Theiss, D., Lehrach, H., and Nordhoff, E. (2002). A calibration method that simplifies and improves accurate determination of peptide molecular masses by MALDI-TOF MS. *Anal Chem 74*, 3915–3923.

Görg, A. (1999). IPG-Dalt of very alkaline proteins. *Methods Mol Biol 12*, 197–209.

Görg, A., Obermaier, C., Boguth, G., Harder, A., Scheibe, B., Wildgruber, R., and Weiss, W. (2000). The current state of two-dimensional electrophoresis with immobilized pH gradients. *Electrophoresis 21*, 1037–1053.

Gromov, P. S., and Celis, J. E. (1994). Several small GTP-binding proteins are strongly down-regulated in simian virus 40 (SV40) transformed human keratinocytes and may be required for the maintenance of the normal phenotype. *Electrophoresis 15*, 474–481.

Gromov, P., Ostergaard, M., Gromova, I., and Celis, J. E. (2002). Human proteomic databases: A powerful resource for functional genomics in health and disease. *Prog Biophys Mol Biol 80*, 3–22.

Gygi, S. P., Rist, B., Gerber, S. A., Turecek, F., Gelb, M. H., and Aebersold, R. (1999). Quantitative analysis of complex protein mixtures using isotope-coded affinity tags. *Nat Biotechnol 17*, 994–999.

Hammond, P. W., Alpin, J., Rise, C. E., Wright, M., and Kreider, B. L. (2001). In vitro selection and characterization of Bcl-X(L)-binding proteins from a mix of tissue-specific mRNA display libraries. *J Biol Chem 276*, 20898–20906.

Hanash, S. M. (2000). Biomedical applications of two-dimensional electrophoresis using immobilized pH gradients: Current status. *Electrophoresis 21*, 1202–1209.

Hanash, S. M., Madoz-Gurpide, J., and Misek, D. E. (2002). Identification of novel targets for cancer therapy using expression proteomics. *Leukemia 16*, 478–485.

Harnden, P., and Southgate, J. (1997). Cytokeratin 14 as a marker of squamous differentiation in transitional cell carcinomas. *J Clin Pathol 50*, 1032–1033.

Harnden, P., Mahmood, N., and Southgate, J. (1999). Expression of cytokeratin 20 redefines urothelial papillomas of the bladder. *Lancet 353*, 974–977.

Harris, R. A., Yang, A., Stein, R. C., Lucy, K., Brusten, L., Herath, A., Parekh, R., Waterfield, M. D., O'Hare, M. J., Neville, M. A., Page, M. J., and Zvelebil. M. J. (2002). Cluster analysis of an extensive human breast cancer cell line protein expression map database. *Proteomics 2*, 212–223.

Hayhurst, A., and Georgiou, G. (2001). High-throughput antibody isolation. *Curr Opin Chem Biol. 5*, 683–689.

Heney, N. M., Ahmed, S., Flanagan, M. J., Frable, W., Corder, M. P., Hafermann, M. D., and Hawkins, I. R. (1983). Superficial bladder cancer: Progression and recurrence. *J Urol 130*, 1083–1086.

Ho, Y., Gruhler, A., Heilbut, A., Bader, G. D., Moore, L., Adams, S. L., Millar, A., Taylor, P., Bennett, K., Boutilier, K., Yang, L., Wolting, C., Donaldson, I., Schandorff, S., Shewnarane, J., Vo, M., Taggart, J., Goudreault, M., Muskat, B., Alfarano, C., Dewar, D., Lin, Z., Michalickova, K., Willems, A. R., Sassi, H., Nielsen, P. A., Rasmussen, K. J., Andersen, J. R., Johansen, L. E., Hansen, L. H., Jespersen, H., Podtelejnikov, A., Nielsen, E., Crawford, J., Poulsen, V., Sorensen, B. D., Matthiesen, J., Hendrickson, R. C., Gleeson, F., Pawson, T., Moran, M. F., Durocher, D., Mann, M., Hogue, C. W., Figeys, D., and Tyers, M. (2002). Systematic identification of protein complexes in *Saccharomyces cerevisiae* by mass spectrometry. *Nature 415*, 180–183.

Issaq, H. J., Veenstra, T. D., Conrads, T. P., and Felschow, D. (2002). The SELDI-TOF MS approach to proteomics: Protein profiling and biomarker identification. *Biochem Biophys Res Commun 292*, 587–592.

Jenkins, R. E., and Pennington, S. R. (2001). Arrays for protein expression profiling: Towards a viable alternative to two-dimensional gel electrophoresis? *Proteomics 1*, 13–29.

Jensen, O. N., Podtelejnikov, A., and Mann, M. (1996). Delayed extraction improves specificity in database searches by matrix-assisted laser desorption/ionization peptide maps. *Rapid Commun Mass Spectrom 10*, 1371–1378.

Jensen, O. N., Podtelejnikov, A. V., and Mann, M. (1997). Identification of the components of simple protein mixtures by high-accuracy peptide mass mapping and database searching. *Anal Chem 69*, 4741–4750.

Jensen, O. N., Larsen, M. R., and Roepstorff, P. (1998). Mass spectrometric identification and microcharacterization of proteins from electrophoretic gels: strategies and applications. *Proteins suppl 2*, 74–89.

Johnson, T., Bergquist, J., Ekman, R., Nordhoff, E., Schurenberg, M., Kloppel, K. D., Muller, M., Lehrach, H., and Gobom, J. (2001). A CE-MALDI interface based on the use of prestructured sample supports. *Anal Chem 73*, 1670–1675.

Jones, M. B., Krutzsch, H., Shu, H., Zhao, Y., Liotta, L. A., Kohn, E. C., and Petricoin, E. F., III. (2002). Proteomic analysis and identification of new biomarkers and therapeutic targets for invasive ovarian cancer. *Proteomics 2*, 76–84.

Karas, M., and Hillenkamp, F. (1988). Laser desorption ionization of proteins with molecular masses exceeding 10,000 daltons. *Anal Chem 60*, 2299–2301.

Kaufmann, R. (1995). Matrix-assisted laser desorption ionization (MALDI) mass spectrometry: A novel analytical tool in molecular biology and biotechnology. *Biotechnology 41*, 155–175.

Kennedy, S. (2001). Proteomic profiling from human samples: The body fluid alternative. *Toxicol Lett 120*, 379–384.

Keough, T., Lacey, M. P., and Youngquist, R. S. (2002). Solid-phase derivatization of tryptic peptides for rapid protein identification by matrix-assisted laser desorption/ionization mass spectrometry. *Rapid Commun Mass Spectrom 16*, 1003–1015.

Klarskov, K., and Naylor, S. (2002). India ink staining after sodium dodecyl sulfate polyacrylamide gel electrophoresis and in conjunction with Western blots for peptide mapping by matrix-assisted laser desorption/ionization time-of-flight mass spectrometry. *Rapid Commun Mass Spectrom 16*, 35–42.

Klose J. (1975). Protein mapping by combined isoelectric focusing and electrophoresis of mouse tissues. A novel approach to testing for induced point mutations in mammals. *Humangenetik 26*, 231–243.

Kodadek, T. (2001). Protein microarrays: Prospects and problems. *Chem Biol 8*, 105–115.

Kodadek, T. (2002). Development of protein-detecting microarrays and related devices. *Trends Biochem Sci 27*, 295–300.

Lamm, D. L. (1992). Carcinoma in situ. *Urol Clin North Am 19*, 499–508.

Lawrie, L. C., Curran, S., McLeod, H. L., Fothergill, J. E., and Murray, G. I. (2001). Application of laser capture microdissection and proteomics in colon cancer. *Mol Pathol 54*, 253–258.

Lesaicherre, M. L., Uttamchandani, M., Chen, G. Y., and Yao S. Q. (2002). Antibody-based fluorescence detection of kinase activity on a peptide array. *Bioorg Med Chem Lett 12*, 2085–2088.

Li, J., Zhang, Z., Rosenzweig, J., Wang, Y. Y., and Chan, D. (2002). Proteomics and bioinformatics approaches for identification of serum biomarkers to detect breast cancer. *Clin Chem 48*, 1296–1304.

Li, Y., McIver, R. T., Jr., and Hunter, R. L. (1994). High-accuracy molecular mass determination for peptides and proteins by Fourier transform mass spectrometry. *Anal Chem 66*, 2077–2083.

Link, A. J., Eng, J., Schieltz, D. M., Carmack, E., Mize, G. J., Morris, D. R., Garvik, B. M., and Yates, J. R., III. (1999). Direct analysis of protein complexes using mass spectrometry. *Nat Biotechnol 17*, 676–682.

Liu, R., Barrick, J. E., Szostak, J. W., and Roberts, R. W. (2000). Optimized synthesis of RNA-protein fusions for in vitro protein selection. *Methods Enzymol 318*, 268–293.

MacBeath, G., and Schreiber, S. L. (2000). Printing proteins as microarrays for high-throughput function determination. *Science 289*, 1760–1763.

Mann, M., and Wilm, M. (1994). Error-tolerant identification of peptides in sequence databases by peptide sequence tags. *Anal Chem 66*, 4390–4399.

Mann, M., Ong, S. E., Gronborg, M., Steen, H., Jensen, O. N., and Pandey, A. (2002). Analysis of protein phosphorylation using mass spectrometry: Deciphering the phosphoproteome. *Trends Biotechnol 20*, 261–268.

Marshall, T., and Williams, K. M. (2002). Proteomics and its impact upon biomedical science. *Br J Biomed Sci. 59*, 47–64.

Martin, S. E., Shabanowitz, J., Hunt, D. F., and Marto, J. A. (2000). Subfemtomole MS and MS/MS peptide sequence analysis using nano-HPLC micro-ESI Fourier transform ion cyclotron resonance mass spectrometry. *Anal Chem 72*, 4266–4274.

Matsudaira, P. (1987). Sequence from picomole quantities of proteins electroblotted onto polyvinylidene difluoride membranes. *J Biol Chem 262*, 10035–10038.

McLuckey, S. A., Van Berkel, G. J., Goeringer, D. E., and Glish, G. L. (1994). Ion trap mass spectrometry. Using high-pressure ionization. *Anal Chem 66*, 737A–743A.

Meehan, K. L., Holland, J. W., and Dawkins, H. J. (2002). Proteomic analysis of normal and malignant prostate tissue to identify novel proteins lost in cancer. *Prostate 50*, 54–63.

Melhem, R. F., Zhu, X. X., Hailat, N., Strahler, J. R., and Hanash, S. M. (1991). Characterization of the gene for a proliferation-related phosphoprotein (oncoprotein 18) expressed in high amounts in acute leukemia. *J Biol Chem 266*, 17747–17753.

Melhem, R., Hailat, N., Kuick, R., and Hanash, S. M. (1997). Quantitative analysis of Op18 phosphorylation in childhood acute leukemia. *Leukemia 11*, 1690–1695.

Mintz, P. J., Patterson, S. D., Neuwald, A. F., Spahr, C. S., and Spector, D. L. (1999). Purification and biochemical characterization of interchromatin granule clusters. *EMBO J 18*, 4308–4320.

Morris, H. R., Paxton, T., Dell, A., Langhorne, J., Berg, M., Bordoli, R. S., Hoyes, J., and Bateman, R. H. (1996). High sensitivity collisionally-activated decomposition tandem mass spectrometry on a novel quadrupole/orthogonal-acceleration time-of-flight mass spectrometer. *Rapid Commun Mass Spectrom 10*, 889–896.

Mostofi, F. K., Davis, C. J., Jr., and Sesterhenn, I. A. (1990). Current understanding of pathology of bladder cancer and attendant problems. *J Occup Med 32*, 793–796.

O'Farrell, P. H. (1975). High resolution two-dimensional electrophoresis of proteins. *J Biol Chem 250*, 4007–4021.

O'Farrell, P. Z., Goodman, H. M., and O'Farrell, P. H. (1977). High resolution two-dimensional electrophoresis of basic as well as acidic proteins. *Cell 12*, 1133–1141.

Olsen, S. (ed.) (1984). *Tumors of the Kidney and the Urinary Tract. Color Atlas and Textbook*. Copenhagen: Munksgaard.

Ostergaard, M., Rasmussen, H. H., Nielsen, H. V., Vorum, H., Orntoft, T. F., Wolf, H., and Celis, J. E. (1997). Proteome profiling of bladder squamous cell carcinomas: Identification of markers that define their degree of differentiation. *Cancer Res 57*, 4111–4117.

Pandey, A., and Mann, M. (2000). Proteomics to study genes and genomes. *Nature 405*, 837–846.

Pappin, D. J. (1997). Peptide mass fingerprinting using MALDI-TOF mass spectrometry. *Methods Mol Biol 64*, 165–173.

Patterson, S. D., and Aebersold, R. (1995). Mass spectrometric approaches for the identification of gel-separated proteins. *Electrophoresis 16*, 1791–1814.

Pauli, B. U., Alroy, J., and Weinstein, R. S. (1983). The ultrastructure and pathobiology of urinary bladder cancer. In *The Pathology of Bladder Cancer*, vol. II, G. T Bryan and S. M. Cohen (eds.). Boca Raton, FL: CRC Press, pp. 41–140.

Paweletz, C. P., Trock, B., Pennanen, M., Tsangaris, T., Magnant,. C., Liotta, L. A., and Petricoin, E. F., III. (2001). Proteomic patterns of nipple aspirate fluids obtained by SELDI-TOF: Potential for new biomarkers to aid in the diagnosis of breast cancer. *Dis Markers 17*, 301–307.

Perucca, D., Szepetowski, P., Simon, M. P., and Gaudray, P. (1990). Molecular genetics of human bladder carcinomas. *Cancer Genet Cytogenet 49*, 143–156.

Petricoin, E. F., Zoon, K. C., Kohn, E. C., Barrett, J. C., and Liotta, L. A. (2002a). Clinical proteomics: Translating benchside promise into bedside reality. *Nat Rev Drug Discov 1*, 683–695.

Petricoin, E. F., Ardekani, A. M., Hitt, B. A., Levine, P. J., Fusaro, V. A., Steinberg, S. M., Mills, G. B., Simone, C., Fishman, D. A., Kohn, E. C., and Liotta, L. A. (2002b). Use of proteomic patterns in serum to identify ovarian cancer. *Lancet 359*, 572–577.

Presti, J. C., Jr, Reuter, V. E., Galan, T., Fair, W. R., and Cordon-Cardo, C. (1991). Molecular genetic alterations in superficial and locally advanced human bladder cancer. *Cancer Res 51*, 5405–5409.

Pucci-Minafra, I., Fontana, S., Cancemi, P., Basirico, L., Caricato, S., and Minafra, S. (2002). A contribution to breast cancer cell proteomics: Detection of new sequences. *Proteomics 2*, 919–927.

Quenzer, T. L., Emmett, M. R., Hendrickson, C. L., Kelly, P. H., and Marshall, A. G. (2001). High sensitivity Fourier transform ion cyclotron resonance mass spectrometry for biological analysis with nano-LC and microelectrospray ionization. *Anal Chem 73*, 1721–1725.

Rasmussen, H. H., Van Damme, J., Puype, M., Gesser, B., Celis, J. E., and Vandekerckhove, J. (1991). Microsequencing of proteins recorded in human two-dimensional gel protein databases. *Electrophoresis 12*, 873–882.

Rasmussen, H. H., van Damme, J., Puype, M., Gesser, B., Celis, J. E., and Vandekerckhove, J. (1992). Microsequences of 145 proteins recorded in the two-dimensional gel protein database of normal human epidermal keratinocytes. *Electrophoresis 13*, 960–969.

Roberts, R. W., and Szostak, J. W. (1997). RNA-peptide fusions for the in vitro selection of peptides and proteins. *Proc Natl Acad Sci USA 94*, 12297–12302.

Sakamoto, N., Tsuneyoshi, M., and Enjoji, M. (1992). Urinary bladder carcinoma with a neoplastic squamous component: A mapping study of 31 cases. *Histopathology 21*, 135–141.

Santoni, V., Molloy, M., and Rabilloud, T. (2000). Membrane proteins and proteomics: Un amour impossible? *Electrophoresis 21*, 1054–1070.

Scheele, J. S., Rhee, J. M., and Boss, G. R. (1995). Determination of absolute amounts of GDP and GTP bound to Ras in mammalian cells: Comparison of parental and Ras-overproducing NIH 3T3 fibroblasts. *Proc Natl Acad Sci USA 92*, 1097–1100.

Schuerenberg, M., Luebbert, C., Eickhoff, H., Kalkum, M., Lehrach, H., and Nordhoff, E. (2000). Prestructured MALDI-MS sample supports. *Anal Chem 72*, 3436–3442.

Shevchenko, A., Wilm, M., Vorm, O., Jensen, O. N., Podtelejnikov, A. V., Neubauer, G., Shevchenko, A., Mortensen, P., and Mann, M. (1996). A strategy for identifying gel-separated proteins in sequence databases by MS alone. *Biochem Soc Trans 24*, 893–896.

Shevchenko, A., Chernushevich, I., Ens, W., Standing, K. G., Thomson, B., Wilm, M., and Mann, M. (1997). Rapid "de novo" peptide sequencing by a combination of nanoelectrospray, isotopic labeling and a quadrupole/time-of-flight mass spectrometer. *Rapid Commun Mass Spectrom 11*, 1015–1024.

Sidransky, D., Von Eschenbach, A., Tsai, Y. C., Jones, P., Summerhayes, I., Marshall, F., Paul, M., Green, P., Hamilton, S. R., Frost, P., et al. (1991). Identification of p53 gene mutations in bladder cancers and urine samples. *Science 252*, 706–709.

Simoneau, A. R., and Jones, P. A. (1994). Bladder cancer: The molecular progression to invasive disease. *World J Urol 12*, 89–95.

Slaughter, D. P., Southwick, H. W., and Smejkal, W. (1953). "Field cancerization" in oral stratified squamous epithelium. *Cancer 6*, 963–968.

Southgate, J., Harnden, P., and Trejdosiewicz, L. K. (1999). Cytokeratin expression patterns in normal and malignant urothelium: A review of the biological and diagnostic implications. *Histol Histopathol 14*, 657–664.

Spengler, B., Kirsch, D., Kaufmann, R., and Jaeger, E. (1992). Peptide sequencing by matrix-assisted laser-desorption mass spectrometry. *Rapid Commun Mass Spectrom 6*, 105–108.

Spruck, C. H., III, Ohneseit, P. F., Gonzalez-Zulueta, M., Esrig, D., Miyao, N., Tsai, Y. C., Lerner, S. P., Schmutte, C., Yang, A. S., Cote, R., et al. (1994). Two molecular pathways to transitional cell carcinoma of the bladder. *Cancer Res 54*, 784–788.

Srinivas, P. R., Srivastava, S., Hanash, S., and Wright, G. L. (2001). Proteomics in early detection of cancer. *Clin Chem 47*, 1901–1911.

Srinivas, P. R., Verma, M., Zhao, Y., and Srivastava, S. (2002). Proteomics for cancer biomarker discovery. *Clin Chem 48*, 1160–1169.

Steinberg, T. H., Haugland, R. P., and Singer, V. L. (1996). Applications of SYPRO orange and SYPRO red protein gel stains. *Anal Biochem 239*, 238–245.

Stensballe, A., and Jensen, O. N. (2001). Simplified sample preparation method for protein identification by matrix-assisted laser desorption/ionization mass spectrometry: In-gel digestion on the probe surface. *Proteomics 1*, 955–966.

Stulik, J., Kovarova, H., Macela, A., Bures, J., Jandik, P., Langr, F., Otto, A., Thiede, B., and Jungblut, P. (1997). Overexpression of calcium-binding protein calgranulin B in colonic mucosal diseases. *Clin Chim Acta 265*, 41–55.

Stulik, J., Hernychova, L., Porkertova, S., Knizek, J., Macela, A., Bures, J., Jandik, P., Langridge, J. I., and Jungblut, P. R. (2001). Proteome study of colorectal carcinogenesis. *Electrophoresis 22*, 3019–3025.

Tabuchi, M., Hino, M., Shinohara, Y., and Baba, Y. (2002). Cell-free protein synthesis on a microchip. *Proteomics 2*, 430–435.

Takach, E. J., Hines, W. M., Patterson, D. H., Juhasz, P., Falick, A. M., Vestal, M. L., and Martin, S. A. (1997). Accurate mass measurements using MALDI-TOF with delayed extraction. *J Protein Chem 16*, 363–369.

Taylor, J., Andersson, N. L., Scandora, A. E., Jr., Willard, K. E., and Anderson, N. G. (1982). Design and implementation of a prototype human protein index. *Clin Chem 28*, 861–866.

Taylor, R. L., Machacek, D., and Singh, R. J. (2002). Validation of a high-throughput liquid chromatography-tandem mass spectrometry method for urinary cortisol and cortisone. *Clin Chem 48*, 1511–1519.

Templin, M. F., Stoll, D., Schrenk, M., Traub, P. C., Vohringer, C. F., and Joos, T. O. (2002). Protein microarray technology. *Trends Biotechnol 20*, 160–166.

Tissot, J. D., Schneider, P., James, R. W., Daigneault, R., and Hochstrasser, D. F. (1991). High-resolution two-dimensional protein electrophoresis of pathological plasma/serum. *Appl Theor Electrophor 2*, 7–12.

Verentchikov, A. N., Ens, W., and Standing, K. G. (1994). Reflecting time-of-flight mass spectrometer with an electrospray ion source and orthogonal extraction. *Anal Chem 66*, 126–133.

von Eggeling, F., Davies, H., Lomas, L., Fiedler, W., Junker, K., Claussen, U., and Ernst, G. (2000). Tissue-specific microdissection coupled with ProteinChip array technologies: Applications in cancer research. *Biotechniques 29*, 1066–1070.

Washburn, M. P., Wolters, D., and Yates, J. R., III. (2001). Large-scale analysis of the yeast proteome by multidimensional protein identification technology. *Nat Biotechnol 19*, 242–247.

Weinberger, S. R., Dalmasso, E. A., and Fung, E. T. (2002). Current achievements using ProteinChip Array technology. *Curr Opin Chem Biol 6*, 86–91.

Weng, S., Gu, K., Hammond, P. W., Lohse, P., Rise, C., Wagner, R. W., Wright, M. C., and Kuimelis, R. G. (2002). Generating addressable protein microarrays with PROfusion covalent mRNA-protein fusion technology. *Proteomics 2*, 48–57.

Wildgruber, R., Harder, A., Obermaier, C., Boguth, G., Weiss, W., Fey, S. J., Larsen, P. M., and Görg, A. (2000). Towards higher resolution: Two-dimensional electrophoresis of *Saccharomyces cerevisiae* proteins using overlapping narrow immobilized pH gradients. *Electrophoresis 21*, 2610–2616.

Wilkins, M. R., Sanchez, J. C., Gooley, A. A., Appel, R. D., Humphery-Smith, I., Hochstrasser, D. F., and Williams, K. L. (1996). Progress with proteome projects: Why all proteins expressed by a genome should be identified and how to do it. *Biotechnol Genet Eng Rev 13*, 19–50.

Wilkins, M. R., Gasteiger, E., Gooley, A. A., Herbert, B. R., Molloy, M. P., Binz, P. A., Ou, K., Sanchez, J. C., Bairoch, A., Williams, K. L., and Hochstrasser, D. F. (1999). High-throughput mass spectrometric discovery of protein post-translational modifications. *J Mol Biol 289*, 645–657.

Wilm, M., Shevchenko, A., Houthaeve, T., Breit, S., Schweigerer, L., Fotsis, T., and Mann, M. (1996). Femtomole sequencing of proteins from polyacrylamide gels by nano-electrospray mass spectrometry. *Nature 379*, 466–469.

Wilson, D. S., and Nock, S. (2002). Functional protein microarrays. *Curr Opin Chem Biol 6*, 81–85.

Wulfkuhle, J. D., McLean, K. C., Paweletz, C. P., Sgroi, D. C., Trock, B. J., Steeg, P. S., and Petricoin, E. F., III. (2001). New approaches to proteomic analysis of breast cancer. *Proteomics 1*, 1205–1215.

Yates, J. R., III, McCormack, A. L., Link, A. J., Schieltz, D., Eng, J., and Hays, L. (1996). Future prospects for the analysis of complex biological systems using micro-column liquid chromatography-electrospray tandem mass spectrometry. *Analyst 121*, 65R–76R.

Zappacosta, F., Huddleston, M. J., Karcher, R. L., Gelfand, V. I., Carr, S. A., and Annan, R. S. (2002). Improved sensitivity for phosphopeptide mapping using capillary column HPLC and micro ion spray mass spectrometry: Comparative phosphorylation site mapping from gel-derived proteins. *Anal Chem 74*, 3221–3231.

Zhu, H., and Snyder, M. (2001). Protein arrays and microarrays. *Curr Opin Chem Biol 5*, 40–45.

Zieger, K., Wolf, H., Olsen, P. R., and Hojgaard, K. (2000). Long-term follow-up of noninvasive bladder tumours (stage Ta): Recurrence and progression. *BJU Int 85*, 824–828.

Zuo, X., and Speicher, D. W. (2000). A method for global analysis of complex proteomes using sample prefractionation by solution isoelectrofocusing prior to two-dimensional electrophoresis. *Anal Biochem 284*, 266–278.

Zuo, X., and Speicher, D. W. (2002). Comprehensive analysis of complex proteomes using microscale solution isoelectrofocusing prior to narrow pH range two-dimensional electrophoresis. *Proteomics 2*, 58–68.

Section III

MODEL SYSTEMS

10

CHEMICAL AND GENETIC METHODS TO VALIDATE TARGETS IN NONMAMMALIAN ORGANISMS

Tia M. Maiolatesi and Charles Brenner

INTRODUCTION

Toward the goal of having available genotype-specific cancer drugs for most of the common cancer genotypes, there is a need to develop varied cell culture-based, fungal and animal assays. Though murine experiments and clinical trials remain the penultimate and the ultimate tests for drugs, respectively, neither is suitable for early-stage drug discovery. Genetic tricks and advantages in generation times and throughput make nonmammalian screens and selections compelling for early-stage drug discovery, validation and mechanism-of-action studies.

As has been amply illustrated in Chapters 2 through 9, there are numerous ways to profile tumors, and for a small number of cancer genotypes there are targeted therapeutics. However, not all oncoproteins are therapeutically useful targets. Additionally, as shown in Chapter 14, some proteins that are unaltered in cancer cells turn out to be genotype-specific targets for reasons that were not immediately obvious. To sift through the vast numbers of molecules that have become *potential targets* as a result of genetic and genomic work, there is a pressing need for chemical and genetic methods to *validate targets*. This chapter critically reviews seven chemical and genetic themes for

Oncogenomics: Molecular Approaches to Cancer, Edited by Charles Brenner and David Duggan
ISBN 0-471-22592-4 © 2004 John Wiley & Sons, Inc.

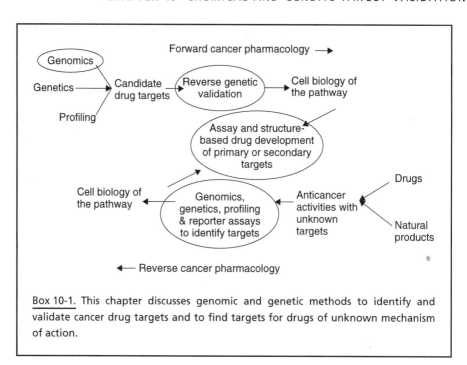

Box 10-1. This chapter discusses genomic and genetic methods to identify and validate cancer drug targets and to find targets for drugs of unknown mechanism of action.

target validation. A summary of the key concepts in this chapter illustrating the initial steps in "forward" and "reverse" cancer pharmacology is illustrated in Box 10-1.

It is a testament to the power of molecular biology and genetics that what is now considered "forward," i.e., molecularly targeted, pharmacology has become the routine orientation for drug discovery only within the last generation. One of us (C.B.) recalls a high school trip to the Boehringer Ingelheim laboratories in Ridgefield, Connecticut, in the late 1970s. Chemists there logged the synthesis of new compounds that were fed to mice for assays of analgesia. The assays consisted of placing mice on a hot plate and recording the time before the mice hopped off. Compounds that scored positive in such assays had no known target and no known mechanism of action. Though many companies retain banks of compounds that were synthesized without a target and many scientists are interested in natural products that work in mysterious ways, the targeted orientation pervades current academic and industrial cancer pharmacology efforts. Thus, although a century of pharmacology history was written with drugs with initially unknown targets used to dissect biological processes, we now consider this to be the "reverse" approach to pharmacology and consider the targeted approach to be "forward."

In deference to the long history of pharmacology, three things should be said in defense of drug discovery that was or is done without a known target. First, targeted pharmacology is frequently equated with "rational" drug design. While structure-based approaches and directed medicinal chemistry are clearly rational, pure combinatorial chemistry and high-throughput screening are not particularly rational, but they can be effective in identifying lead compounds. The goal of cancer pharmacology is not the most rational process but discovery of the most efficacious compounds while conserving time and resources.

Second, while a primary assay based on analgesia in mice sounds primitive, it does not produce hits on compounds that will fail to be bioavailable. Thus, while animal-based screens historically produced hits without targets, these hits had already passed some of the most stringent bottlenecks in drug discovery that relate to absorption, distribution, metabolism, and excretion (ADME). The lesson is that a hit is only as good as the assay that produces it. Astute people in drug discovery get this point. For this reason, there has been impressive growth related to in vitro and in silico screening for ADME parameters. At the same time, we are seeing a resurgence of interest in animal-based screens that incorporate sensitized genetic backgrounds and specific phenotypic scoring.

Third, every pharmacologist knows that drugs can have unintended secondary or even primary targets. As Prendergast documents in Chapter 14, farnesyl transferase inhibitors (FTIs) were developed "rationally" to target tumors expressing Ras onco-proteins, and these compounds do provide a therapeutic window against transformed cells. However, the therapeutic effects of FTIs do not correlate well with the presence of Ras mutations and appear to be mediated by blocking membrane association of RhoB. The great thing about the convergent nature of research today is that once a drug's *true targets* are identified, genetic and structural approaches to drug development can accelerate cycles of medicinal chemistry and evaluation.

THEME 1: THE POWER OF PHARMACOLOGY: DRUGS THEMSELVES PROVE THAT DRUGS ARE FEASIBLE

The *MYC* oncogene holds an honored seat in the history of molecular oncology. Insertions in the vicinity of *c-MYC* illustrated the variety of ways in which oncogenes can be activated by retroviral mutagenesis (Duesberg et al., 1977; Payne, 1982; Westaway, 1984). Discovery of translocations (Dalla-Favera, 1982) and amplifications (Alitalo, 1983) involving *MYC* in human cancers, discovery of the DNA-binding properties of Myc (Ramsay, 1986), and development of cellular assays for structure-function analysis of oncoproteins (Stone, 1987) are among the huge contributions to cancer biology that have their roots in *MYC*.

The fact that *MYC* is activated early and often in the development of tumors did not by itself prove that *MYC* gene activity is required for the continued transformed phenotype of tumors, but once again the *MYC* people were among the first to address this. By generating transgenic mice that conditionally express *MYC* in lymphocytes and develop osteosarcomas, investigators were able to examine the effect of turning off *MYC* in established tumors. Remarkably, tumors regressed with *MYC* gene inactivation and resumption of expression of *MYC* led to apoptosis rather than regrowth of tumors (Jain, 2002). Thus, Myc is a genetically validated target for genotype-specific cancer chemotherapy.

Independently, another approach was taken to block Myc function in cancer that simultaneously produced a lead compound and validated Myc as a cancer target. Myc is a basic helix-loop-helix zipper protein that binds DNA with its basic domain and dimerizes via the helix-loop-helix zipper domain. All known oncogenic functions of Myc depend on heterodimerization with Max, another basic helix-loop-helix zipper protein (Blackwood and Eisenman, 1991; Grandori, 2000). This approach suggested that disruption of the Myc-Max dimer might be a way to fight *MYC*-transformed cells.

By constructing fusions of Myc and Max to fluorescent proteins that exhibit fluorescent resonance energy transfer, it was possible to screen combinatorial chemical libraries for dimerization inhibitors (Berg, 2002). The best compounds that were obtained not only blocked dimerization but also transformation of chick embryo fibroblasts (Berg, 2002). Though the cellular transformation assay blocked by Myc-Max dimerization inhibitors (Berg, 2002) is not as physiologically relevant as the murine model in which *MYC* was genetically validated (Jain, 2002), it is important to note that neither approach depended on the other and the results are completely complementary.

There are useful lessons in the experience with *MYC*. Academic researchers have discovered nearly all of the known oncoproteins that are now considered attractive cancer targets. Historically, university researchers have approached industrial researchers with the hope that companies would commit high-throughput screens to find inhibitors. Typically, companies respond with two requests. First, the companies would like to see the target genetically or chemically validated before they commit themselves to search for inhibitors. Second, the companies would like to see an assay that is amenable to high-throughput screening. Companies tend to enter the drug discovery process later rather than sooner, being willing to pay up for a lead compound or an extensively validated target rather than to be involved prior to experiments that might show that the target does not allow pharmacological discrimination of tumor from normal. In this respect the big pharmaceutical companies are more like investment banks than research enterprises. Flush with cash from sales of approved drugs, they prefer to acquire technology to *develop* new drugs rather than to take on high-risk *research* projects on their own. As conservative investors, pharmaceutical companies do not care which target is chosen for development as long as they perceive a favorable reward-to-risk ratio. University researchers, in contrast, are funded to complete *specific aims* on *specific molecules* in which we are personally and intellectually invested. Whereas the pharmaceutical community might have balked at Myc in 2001 as a target that was not genetically validated for maintenance of the malignant phenotype and not obviously "druggable," the results of the 2002 genetic (Jain et al., 2002) and chemical (Berg et al., 2002) validation experiments (both NIH funded) ensure that substantial public and private resources will be invested to develop Myc-targeted drugs in coming years.

THEME 2: MICROARRAY-BASED TARGET DISCOVERY IN CELL LINES

As we discussed at the outset, there are large stores of compounds that were synthesized without a target or derived from natural products that have promising activities in cellular or animal assays or in human population-based studies. Though chemists can synthesize variants of any compound, most modern medicinal chemistry efforts are tightly linked to biochemical and structural assays with the compound's presumed biological target. When compounds are thought to act by altering mRNA levels, microarray analysis can be used to identify candidate gene expression targets.

Cationic porphyrins were developed as compounds that bind G-quadruplexes in human telomeres. However, the relationship between telomere binding and activity in xenograft tumor inhibition broke down and it became clear that certain porphyrins such as TMPyP4 might have a mechanism of action that does not involve binding telomeres. Microarray experiments showed that transcriptional repression of *c-MYC* might be the mechanism of action of this compound (Grand et al., 2002). As compounds such as epigallocatechin-3-gallate, which is thought to be the cancer chemopreventive active ingredient in green tea, appear to have transcriptional effects (Dashwood et al., 2002), we anticipate that microarray analysis will be a key tool to dissect mechanism of action of many natural products.

A program to discover the targets and mechanism of action of retinoic acid is being conducted by Dmitrovsky and co-workers. All-*trans* retinoic acid (RA) causes remission in individuals with acute promyelocytic leukemia who possess a translocation-induced fusion of the *PML* gene with the *RARα* gene; function of RA has been linked to proteolytic degradation of Pml-RARα (Dragnev et al., 2000). To dissect the mechanism for RA-dependent cancer prevention, microarray analysis was performed and a number of genes were identified as RA responsive (Tamayo et al., 1999). Critically, though, good programs do not end but rather begin with microarray analysis. Cloning the Ube11 promoter showed that Ube11, a ubiquitin-activating enzyme E1-like protein, is transcriptionally induced by RA and that ectopic Ube11 expression results in RA-independent Pml-RARα degradation (Kitareewan et al., 2002). This is precisely the point at which reverse cancer pharmacology can turn around and go forward. Now, a cellular screen for inducers of the *UBEL1* promoter can be conducted as a moderately high-throughput primary screen with a secondary screen for induction of Pml-RARα degradation.

THEME 3: NUCLEIC ACID–BASED TARGET VALIDATION

Because cancer is a disease of escape, it is difficult to imagine that gene therapy approaches will succeed in altering the genetic content of 100% of tumor cells. However, nucleic acid–based approaches including viral gene delivery, antisense, and other "knock-down" strategies have critical roles in validating gene products as targets, if only to motivate development of small molecule inhibitors. The *AML1/MTG8* fusion gene is produced as a result of a t(8;21) translocation that is associated with more than 10% of new cases of acute myeloid leukemia. When the fusion gene was knocked down with siRNA, leukemic cell lines with this translocation gained differentiation markers and lost clonogenicity, suggesting that sustained expression of the fusion protein is required to maintain the malignant phenotype (Heidenreich et al., 2002). This type of analysis is going to be extremely common. It has to be remembered, though, that the data are only as good as the assay: cell lines and tumors are two different things.

THEME 4: DRUG-INDUCED HAPLOINSUFFICIENCY CAN IDENTIFY TARGETS

A consortium of researchers constructed a set of baker's yeast strains containing targeted deletions of nearly every gene (Shoemaker, 1996; Winzeler, 1999 ; Giaever, 2002; Steinmetz, 2002). For the set of genes that encode essential functions, haploid deletion mutants are not available, but heterozygous diploids are available. The beauty of the yeast deletion project was in the design: Though every deletion marker confers G418 resistance, the strains can be mixed and followed by oligonucleotide bar-code hybridization. Oligonucleotide bar codes are unique 20mers that were integrated adjacent to the disrupting G418 resistance markers between common pairs of PCR primers that can be used to amplify the unique tags. Consequently, researchers can grow a pool of bar-coded disruption strains under any condition, prepare fluorescently labeled target DNA by amplifying bar codes from the pool, and determine by array hybridization which strains have growth advantages or disadvantages (Shoemaker et al., 1996; Winzeler et al., 1999; Giaever et al., 2002; Steinmetz et al., 2002). The consortium reasoned that in many cases sensitivity to a drug may be conferred by reduced levels of a specific gene product such that in a pool of yeast strains heterozygous for many different genes the strain containing a single copy of the target, rather than two, may be at the greatest growth disadvantage (Giaever et al., 1999). In other cases, depending on the way in which the drug and target work, the most resistant strain might identify the drug target. As the majority of compounds with unknown targets are in private hands, it is our impression that many such experiments are being done by biotechnology companies under contracts with pharmaceutical firms. Because publishing the identity of a target enables competition, it is reasonable to expect that these experiments are being done and are remaining corporate secrets. Additionally, once a drug target is identified by altered sensitivity or resistance, it is straightforward to examine the gene expression consequences of a drug in the presence and in the absence of the primary target (Marton et al., 1998) in order to determine whether there are secondary consequences of a drug's application.

THEME 5: SYNTHETIC LETHALS: HOW TO COPE WITH LOSSES

Losses of tumor suppressor genes (TSGs) are as important as activation of oncogenes in initiation and progression of cancer. However, while oncoproteins themselves can be considered candidate molecular targets, losses of TSGs do not suggest a particular target for elimination of cancer cells. As reviewed in Chapter 1, activated oncogenes typically arise as dominant alleles of growth-promoting genes while mutations in tumor suppressor genes in cancer are loss-of-function alleles that are recessive at the cellular level. Because cancer is a disease of escape, it is difficult to imagine that a tumor suppressor gene could be added back to 100% of tumor cells.

Considering this problem, Hartwell and co-workers suggested that the problem of identifying specific targets to eliminate cells with missing genetic information is similar to a yeast geneticist's synthetic lethal screen (Hartwell et al., 1997). In a synthetic lethal screen, researchers start with a viable mutant strain containing a known mutation of

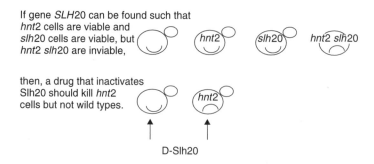

Figure 10-1. A search for synthetically lethal genes is, in principal, a search for drug targets for cells with missing genetic information.

interest. Typically, to uncover additional genes that interact in an essential pathway, the geneticist mutagenizes the singly mutant strain to generate a library of double mutants. A second mutation is of interest if, combined with the first mutation, it leads to an inviable strain—the two mutations are then said to be synthetically lethal. In addition to providing pathway information about both genes, synthetic lethal screens enable structure-function studies to be done on each gene product. Moreover, as illustrated in Figure 10-1, the synthetic lethal relationship suggests that a small molecule targeted to one gene product will kill a cell with a mutation in the other gene product.

Model organisms are important because a variety of tricks and tools are available to conduct synthetic lethal screens. In budding yeast, Boone and co-workers have developed methods to perform synthetic lethal screens in a comprehensive way (Tong et al., 2001). Though the technology is not as well established, methods have recently been developed to screen human cultured cells for synthetic lethal mutations (Simons et al., 2001). Should synthetic lethal screens be performed successfully in model systems or human cells, we would have candidate drug targets for tumors missing genetic information. Small molecules would then be developed against these targets and tested against tumors with the indicated tumor suppressor gene losses.

THEME 6: FLY GENETICS IS COMPLEMENTARY TO HUMAN GENETICS AND MAMMALIAN CELL BIOLOGY IN IDENTIFYING TARGETS

Tuberous sclerosis is a relatively common autosomal-dominant disorder characterized by benign hamartomas in multiple organs and an increased risk of renal cell carcinoma (Cheadle et al., 2000). The hamartomas consist of masses of differentiated but giant cells with loss of heterozygosity in either the *TSC1* or the *TSC2* gene (Consortium, 1993; Green et al., 1994; van Slegtenhorst et al., 1997), and renal malignancies can result from losses in *TSC2* as well (van Slegtenhorst et al., 1997). Cowden's disease is another multiple hamartomatous syndrome with frequent development of breast, renal, and other malignancies due to loss of the *PTEN* gene (Li et al., 1997; Steck et al., 1997; Liaw et al., 1997). Experiments done in mammalian cell lines established that losses in the lipid phosphatase activity of Pten activate the phospholipid-dependent protein kinase, Akt (Myers et al., 1998; Li and Sun, 1998; Furnari et al., 1998; Haas-Kogan et al., 1998; Wu et al., 1998), thereby suggesting that Akt ought to be considered a specific target for combating all of the neoplastic and preneoplastic diseases involving *PTEN* mutations.

As noted, tuberous sclerosis mutations and Cowden's mutations have similar consequences in humans. Similar effects on eye development were observed in flies bearing loss-of-function mutations in homologs of *TSC1, TSC2,* and *PTEN* (Ito and Rubin, 1999; Huang et al., 1999; Goberdhan et al., 1999). Considering the "holy grail" nature of identifying a specific target for chemotherapeutic elimination of cancer cells that arise from losses of genetic information, one would love to know whether Akt can be considered a target for losses in *TSC1* and *TSC2* in addition to *PTEN*. Epistasis experiments were performed in fly eyes to determine how these genes interact in the fly development pathway. While overexpression of the fly Tsc1,2 complex rescued the lethality of insulin receptor overexpression (indicating that Tsc1 and Tsc2 function somewhere downstream of insulin receptor), inactivating mutations in Akt (small cells) plus Tsc1 (big cells) displayed the Tsc1 phenotype (Potter et al., 2001). Failure to suppress the Tsc1 phenotype with Akt mutation strongly suggests that Tsc1 and Tsc2 function *downstream* of Akt such that inhibiting Akt will neither restore function nor kill cells with *TSC1* or *TSC2* mutations (Potter et al., 2001). All is not lost, however. Further work in flies suggests that the Akt-phosphorylation-dependent function of Tsc1, Tsc2 is to inhibit the TOR-S6 kinase pathway (Potter et al., 2002). Because TOR and S6 kinase are downstream of Tsc1 and Tsc2 and potentially are constitutively active in patients with tuberous sclerosis mutations, these are attractive kinase targets. Kinases as oncology targets are discussed extensively in Chapter 13.

THEME 7: ZEBRAFISH MODELS CAN BE USED TO IDENTIFY MODIFIER GENES AND SCREEN FOR CHEMOPREVENTIVE AGENTS

Chapters 11 and 12 deal with the oncogenomics of the house mouse, with Chapter 11 describing mostly reverse genetic methods to model human cancers in *Mus* and Chapter 12 describing mostly forward screens to define loci that affect the penetrance of tumors in hereditary syndromes. While in vitro systems, yeast, worms, flies, and cell lines have all proven to be valuable for drug screens and genetic screens and selections, the mouse reigns supreme as host of the penultimate tests of disease and treatment hypotheses (the ultimate being human clinical trials). As stated earlier, data are only as good as the assays that produce them. The most quantitative enzyme-based screen might identify hits that have subnanomolar inhibitory constants yet have no possibility of bioavailability. Cell culture–based screens might poorly represent the physiology of tumor cells, and fungal or invertebrate screens could either produce fabulous insights into tumor biology or reveal unfortunate differences between humans and other eukaryotes. However, once an organism has the body plan and the complexity of a mammal, it is usually a good bet that the genetic circuits are fully conserved with humans, that general ADME parameters are conserved (though the kinetics of specific steps are going to be different in our smaller friends), and that well-modeled diseases will produce sound proving grounds for drug trials. Though other vertebrate systems such as birds and rats have their proponents, they are generally more costly and time-consuming than the mouse and less technologically advanced in terms of genetic manipulation.

And then came the zebrafish *Danio rerio*. Fish have long been subjects of forward genetic screens for developmental mutants. More recently, reverse genetic methods have been applied, particularly with morpholino antisense knock-down technology. Because knocking in gene expression is usually easier than knocking down or knocking down gene expression, investigating the consequences of oncogene transformation is relatively straightforward. Germ-line transgenic fish have now been developed in which the *MYC* oncogene, marked by green fluorescent protein, is expressed from a high-level cell-type-specific promoter (Langenau et al., 2003). This system allows visualization of the entire process of clonal neoplastic transformation, migration, and metastasis. It is anticipated that such fish will be used to screen for drugs that block any step in this process and that modifier screens will be performed to find mutations that suppress *MYC* transformation.

CONCLUSIONS

No reader should come away thinking that we wish to challenge the ultimacy of the human clinical trial or the penultimacy of murine models for testing drug treatments.

It should be equally clear that in vitro systems, cell lines, and model organisms such as yeast, worms, flies, and zebrafish are indispensable components of the target discovery, validation, and drug discovery enterprise. Indispensability flows from two essential characteristics. First, these systems are less costly than human trials. Second, these systems contain advantages in design and quantitative analysis that allow us to discover true modes of action and to refine our hypotheses.

Resources and time are limited and in need of intelligent allocation. Too many times we have seen drug companies perform trials on drugs soon to be approved for specific neoplasias against patients with diseases such as end-stage lung cancer without sufficient justification from model studies. To test such hypotheses is to consume tremendous resources with little likelihood of positive outcomes. We not only burn resources on such studies, we burn the goodwill of the patient community that has entrusted us for improvements in care. James J. Cramer, the investment guru, has said, "Hope is not a valid investment hypothesis." Similarly, we argue that hope is not a valid basis for clinical testing and we urge oncology researchers to use all genetic and pharmacological tools to their greatest advantage.

REFERENCES

Alitalo, K., Schwab, M., Lin, C. C., Varmus, H. E., and Bishop, J. M. (1983). Homogeneously staining chromosomal regions contain amplified copies of an abundantly expressed cellular oncogene (c-myc) in malignant neuroendocrine cells from a human colon carcinoma. *Proc Natl Acad Sci USA 80*, 1707–1711.

Berg, T., Cohen, S. B., Desharnais, J., Sonderegger, C., Maslyar, D. J., Goldberg, J., Boger, D. L., and Vogt, P. K. (2002). Small-molecule antagonists of Myc/Max dimerization inhibit Myc-induced transformation of chicken embryo fibroblasts. *Proc Natl Acad Sci USA 99*, 3830–3835.

Blackwood, E. M., and Eisenman, R. N. (1991). Max: a helix-loop-helix zipper protein that forms a sequence-specific DNA-binding complex with Myc. *Science 251*, 1211–1217.

Cheadle, J. P., Reeve, M. P., Sampson, J. R., and Kwiatkowski, D. J. (2000). Molecular genetic advances in tuberous sclerosis. *Hum Genet 107*, 97–114.

Consortium, T. E. C. T. S. (1993). Identification and characterization of the tuberous sclerosis gene on chromosome 16. *Cell 75*, 1305–1315.

Dalla-Favera, R., Bregni, M., Erikson, J., Patterson, D., Gallo, R. C., and Croce, C. M. (1982). Human c-myc oncogene is located on the region of chromosome 8 that is translocated in Burkitt lymphoma cells. *Proc Natl Acad Sci USA 79*, 7824–7827.

Dashwood, W. M., Orner, G. A., and Dashwood, R. H. (2002). Inhibition of betacatenin/Tcf activity by white tea, green tea, and epigallocatechin-3-gallate (EGCG): minor contribution of $H(2)O(2)$ at physiologically relevant EGCG concentrations. *Biochem Biophys Res Commun 296*, 584–588.

Dragnev, K. H., Rigas, J. R., and Dmitrovsky, E. (2000). The retinoids and cancer prevention mechanisms. *Oncologist 5*, 361–368.

Duesberg, P. H., Bister, K., and Vogt, P. K. (1977). The RNA of avian acute leukemia virus MC29. *Proc Natl Acad Sci USA 74*, 4320–4324.

Furnari, F. B., Huang, H. J., and Cavenee, W. K. (1998). The phosphoinositol phosphatase activity of PTEN mediates a serum-sensitive G1 growth arrest in glioma cells. *Cancer Res 58*, 5002–5008.

Giaever, G., Chu, A. M., Ni, L., Connelly, C., Riles, L., Veronneau, S., Dow, S., Lucau-Danila, A., Anderson, K., Andre, B., et al. (2002). Functional profiling of the Saccharomyces cerevisiae genome. *Nature 418*, 387–391.

Giaever, G., Shoemaker, D. D., Jones, T. W., Liang, H., Winzeler, E. A., Astromoff, A., and Davis, R. W. (1999). Genomic profiling of drug sensitivities via induced haploinsufficiency. *Nat Genet 21*, 278–283.

Goberdhan, D. C., Paricio, N., Goodman, E. C., Mlodzik, M., and Wilson, C. (1999). Drosophila tumor suppressor PTEN controls cell size and number by antagonizing the Chico/PI3-kinase signaling pathway. *Genes Dev 13*, 3244–3258.

Grand, C. L., Han, H., Munoz, R. M., Weitman, S., Von Hoff, D. D., Hurley, L. H., and Bearss, D. J. (2002). The cationic porphyrin TMPyP4 down-regulates c-MYC and human telomerase reverse transcriptase expression and inhibits tumor growth in vivo. *Mol Cancer Ther 1*, 565–573.

Grandori, C., Cowley, S. M., James, L. P., and Eisenman, R. N. (2000). The Myc/Max/Mad network and the transcriptional control of cell behavior. *Annu Rev Cell Dev Biol 16*, 653–699.

Green, A. J., Smith, M., and Yates, J. R. (1994). Loss of heterozygosity on chromosome 16p13.3 in hamartomas from tuberous sclerosis patients. *Nat Genet 6*, 193–196.

Haas-Kogan, D., Shalev, N., Wong, M., Mills, G., Yount, G., and Stokoe, D. (1998). Protein kinase B (PKB/Akt) activity is elevated in glioblastoma cells due to mutation of the tumor suppressor PTEN/MMAC. *Curr Biol 8*, 1195–1198.

Hartwell, L. H., Szankasi, P., Roberts, C. J., Murray, A. W., and Friend, S. H. (1997). Integrating genetic approaches into the discovery of anticancer drugs. *Science 278*, 1064–1068.

Heidenreich, O., Krauter, J., Riehle, H., Hadwiger, P., John, M., Heil, G., Vornlocher, H. P., and Nordheim, A. (2002). AML1/MTG8 Oncogene Suppression by Small Interfering RNAs Supports Myeloid Differentiation of t(8;21)-positive Leukemic Cells. Blood.

Huang, H., Potter, C. J., Tao, W., Li, D. M., Brogiolo, W., Hafen, E., Sun, H., and Xu, T. (1999). PTEN affects cell size, cell proliferation and apoptosis during Drosophila eye development. *Development 126*, 5365–5372.

Ito, N. and Rubin, G. M. (1999). gigas, a Drosophila homolog of tuberous sclerosis gene product-2, regulates the cell cycle. *Cell 96*, 529–539.

Jain, M., Arvanitis, C., Chu, K., Dewey, W., Leonhardt, E., Trinh, M., Sundberg, C. D., Bishop, J. M., and Felsher, D. W. (2002). Sustained loss of a neoplastic phenotype by brief inactivation of MYC. *Science 297*, 102–104.

Kitareewan, S., Pitha-Rowe, I., Sekula, D., Lowrey, C. H., Nemeth, M. J., Golub, T. R., Freemantle, S. J., and Dmitrovsky, E. (2002). UBE1L is a retinoid target that triggers PML/RARalpha degradation and apoptosis in acute promyelocytic leukemia. *Proc Natl Acad Sci USA 99*, 3806–3811.

Langenau, D. M., Traver, D., Ferando, A. A., Kutok, J. L., Aster, J. C., Kanki, J. P., Lin, S., Prochownik, E., Trede, N. S., Zon, L. I., and Look, A. T. (2003). Myc-induced T cell leukemia in transgenic zebrafish. *Science 299*, 887–890.

Li, D. M., and Sun, H. (1998). PTEN/MMAC1/TEP1 suppresses the tumorigenicity and induces G1 cell cycle arrest in human glioblastoma cells. *Proc Natl Acad Sci USA 95*, 15406–15411.

Li, J., Yen, C., Liaw, D., Podsypanina, K., Bose, S., Wang, S. I., Puc, J., Miliaresis, C., Rodgers, L., McCombie, R., et al. (1997). PTEN, a putative protein tyrosine phosphatase gene mutated in human brain, breast, and prostate cancer. *Science 275*, 1943–1947.

Liaw, D., Marsh, D. J., Li, J., Dahia, P. L., Wang, S. I., Zheng, Z., Bose, S., Call, K. M., Tsou, H. C., Peacocke, M., et al. (1997). Germline mutations of the PTEN gene in Cowden disease, an inherited breast and thyroid cancer syndrome. *Nat Genet 16*, 64–67.

Marton, M. J., DeRisi, J. L., Bennett, H. A., Iyer, V. R., Meyer, M. R., Roberts, C. J., Stoughton, R., Burchard, J., Slade, D., Dai, H., et al. (1998). Drug target validation and identification of secondary drug target effects using DNA microarrays. *Nat Med 4*, 1293–1301.

Myers, M. P., Pass, I., Batty, I. H., Van der Kaay, J., Stolarov, J. P., Hemmings, B. A., Wigler, M. H., Downes, C. P., and Tonks, N. K. (1998). The lipid phosphatase activity of PTEN is critical for its tumor supressor function. *Proc Natl Acad Sci USA 95*, 13513–13518.

Payne, G. S., Bishop, J. M., and Varmus, H. E. (1982). Multiple arrangements of viral DNA and an activated host oncogene in bursal lymphomas. *Nature 295*, 209–214.

Potter, C. J., Huang, H., and Xu, T. (2001). Drosophila Tsc1 functions with Tsc2 to antagonize insulin signaling in regulating cell growth, cell proliferation, and organ size. *Cell 105*, 357–368.

Potter, C. J., Pedraza, L. G., and Xu, T. (2002). Akt regulates growth by directly phosphorylating Tsc2. *Nat Cell Biol 4*, 658–665.

Ramsay, G., Stanton, L., Schwab, M., and Bishop, J. M. (1986). Human proto-oncogene N-myc encodes nuclear proteins that bind DNA. *Mol Cell Biol 6*, 4450–4457.

Shoemaker, D. D., Lashkari, D. A., Morris, D., Mittmann, M., and Davis, R. W. (1996). Quantitative phenotypic analysis of yeast deletion mutants using a highly parallel molecular barcoding strategy. *Nat Genet 14*, 450–456.

Simons, A. H., Dafni, N., Dotan, I., Oron, Y., and Canaani, D. (2001). Genetic synthetic lethality screen at the single gene level in cultured human cells. *Nucleic Acids Res 29*, E100.

Steck, P. A., Pershouse, M. A., Jasser, S. A., Yung, W. K., Lin, H., Ligon, A. H., Langford, L. A., Baumgard, M. L., Hattier, T., Davis, T., et al. (1997). Identification of a candidate tumour suppressor gene, MMAC1, at chromosome 10q23.3 that is mutated in multiple advanced cancers. *Nat Genet 15*, 356–362.

Steinmetz, L. M., Scharfe, C., Deutschbauer, A. M., Mokranjac, D., Herman, Z. S., Jones, T., Chu, A. M., Giaever, G., Prokisch, H., Oefner, P. J., and Davis, R. W. (2002). Systematic screen for human disease genes in yeast. *Nat Genet 31*, 400–404.

Stone, J., de Lange, T., Ramsay, G., Jakobovits, E., Bishop, J. M., Varmus, H., and Lee, W. (1987). Definition of regions in human c-myc that are involved in transformation and nuclear localization. *Mol Cell Biol 7*, 1697–1709.

Tamayo, P., Slonim, D., Mesirov, J., Zhu, Q., Kitareewan, S., Dmitrovsky, E., Lander, E. S., and Golub, T. R. (1999). Interpreting patterns of gene expression with self-organizing maps: methods and application to hematopoietic differentiation. *Proc Natl Acad Sci USA 96*, 2907–2912.

Tong, A. H., Evangelista, M., Parsons, A. B., Xu, H., Bader, G. D., Page, N., Robinson, M., Raghibizadeh, S., Hogue, C. W., Bussey, H., et al. (2001). Systematic genetic analysis with ordered arrays of yeast deletion mutants. *Science 294*, 2364–2368.

van Slegtenhorst, M., de Hoogt, R., Hermans, C., Nellist, M., Janssen, B., Verhoef, S., Lindhout, D., van den Ouweland, A., Halley, D., Young, J., et al. (1997). Identification of the tuberous sclerosis gene TSC1 on chromosome 9q34. *Science 277*, 805–808.

Westaway, D., Payne, G., and Varmus, H. E. (1984). Proviral deletions and oncogene base-substitutions in insertionally mutagenized c-myc alleles may contribute to the progression of avian bursal tumors. *Proc Natl Acad Sci USA 81*, 843–847.

Winzeler, E. A., Shoemaker, D. D., Astromoff, A., Liang, H., Anderson, K., Andre, B., Bangham, R., Benito, R., Boeke, J. D., Bussey, H., et al. (1999). Functional characterization of the S. cerevisiae genome by gene deletion and parallel analysis. *Science 285*, 901–906.

Wu, X., Senechal, K., Neshat, M. S., Whang, Y. E., and Sawyers, C. L. (1998). The PTEN/MMAC1 tumor suppressor phosphatase functions as a negative regulator of the phosphoinositide 3-kinase/Akt pathway. *Proc Natl Acad Sci USA 95*, 15587–15591.

11

MOUSE MODELS OF CANCER

Debrah M. Thompson, Louise van der Weyden, Patrick J. Biggs,
Yeun-Jun Chung, and Allan Bradley

INTRODUCTION

Mouse models of cancer have both enhanced and driven research into the molecular basis of human cancers. Using selected examples, we illustrate the role of mouse models, from conventional transgenics and gene targeting approaches to recent conditional or inducible systems designed to more precisely the stochastic nature of cancer and to mimic the human multistage process model of malignant transformation. We finish with a discussion of some of the latest tools for analysis of genetic changes during tumorigenesis.

The use of the house mouse *Mus musculus* in modeling human cancer has spanned just over a century. Fueled by the desire for valid models of human cancer, mouse models have been generated to experimentally test the discoveries of the molecular mechanisms of cancer. As a result, increasingly sophisticated methods for more accurate modeling have developed since the 1980s. An overview of the types of mouse models and analyses that are performed with them is provided in Box 11-1.

Molecular Mechanisms of Cancer: Oncogenes

Principal insights into the molecular mechanisms involved in cancer began with studies of animal tumor viruses, particularly retroviruses. In 1911, Rous demonstrated that viral

Oncogenomics: Molecular Approaches to Cancer, Edited by Charles Brenner and David Duggan
ISBN 0-471-22592-4 © 2004 John Wiley & Sons, Inc.

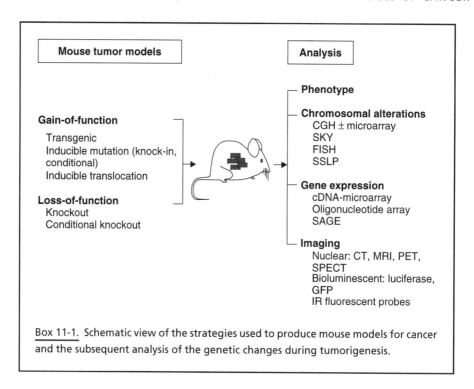

Box 11-1. Schematic view of the strategies used to produce mouse models for cancer and the subsequent analysis of the genetic changes during tumorigenesis.

infection could cause sarcomas in chickens (reprinted in Rous, 1983). Transforming RNA viruses, such as the Rous sarcoma virus (RSV), carry an oncogene—in this case, *v-SRC*—which can cause unregulated cell growth. In 1976, it was recognized that viral *SRC* was derived from a normal, nontransforming chicken gene (*c-SRC*), which had become part of the viral genome at some point in the past (Stehelin et al., 1976). RSV transforms through the nonessential, cell-derived, and mutated oncogene it carries, which is driven by the strong promoter in the long terminal repeats (LTRs) of the virus. However, retroviruses can also transform cells by modifying the activity of endogenous genes. The insertion of a provirus into a cellular gene may cause transformation through mutation, or the viral LTR promoter may cause activation of the gene. For example, in tumors arising in mouse strains that carry mouse mammary tumor virus (MMTV), the provirus is often found to be inserted in the mouse oncogene *Wnt-1* (Nusse et al., 1984, 1991).

While transforming retroviruses carry a modified version of an endogenous gene, DNA tumor viruses possess essential genes that can also transform cells. For example, the polyomavirus simian virus 40 (SV40) transforms through the action of its large T-antigen (Tag, or tumor antigen) gene product, which interacts with endogenous, host-derived regulatory proteins such as the retinoblastoma protein (RB1) and p53 (Lane and Crawford, 1979). The papillomavirus E6 and adenovirus E1B oncoproteins also inactivate p53, albeit through different mechanisms (Scheffner et al., 1990; Yew et al., 1994). Similarly, RB1 is bound by the papillomavirus E7 and adenoviral E1A oncoproteins (DeCaprio et al., 1988). Thus, studies with transforming viruses contributed to the realization that losses in endogenous genes can also cause uncontrolled cell growth.

Molecular Mechanisms of Cancer: Tumor Suppressor Genes

The existence of negative factors in human cancer was postulated before the discovery of oncogenes, but the principal lines of evidence demonstrating the existence of tumor suppressor genes (TSGs) came later. Studies showed that fusions of tumorigenic and nontumorigenic cells resulted in a nontumorigenic cell, and that this suppression depended on the presence of certain chromosomes (Harris et al., 1969). Working from a very different perspective, Knudson developed the two-hit hypothesis while studying familial retinoblastoma. Using statistical methods, he predicted that two mutations or "hits" were required for tumorigenesis in this syndrome (Knudson, 1971). Therefore, in familial cancers, tumors may result from an initial germ-line mutation of one TSG allele, with loss of the second allele due to another event, such as a somatic mutation or chromosomal rearrangement. This process is known as loss of heterozygosity (LOH; reviewed in Knudson, 2000). In the case of sporadic cancer, both mutations are somatically acquired. Many TSGs responsible for human cancer syndromes have now been cloned, principally by positional cloning. Today, TSGs are typically divided into two broad classes based on their mechanism of action: "gatekeepers," genes that inhibit the growth of tumors or promote apoptosis, and "caretakers," which regulate cellular processes that repair genetic lesions and maintain the overall genetic integrity of each cell (Kinzler and Vogelstein, 1997).

Mouse Modeling Techniques

Before the rediscovery of Mendel's laws in 1900, mice were not extensively used in biological research, though mouse fanciers collected and bred the animals. In 1901, William Castle from Harvard began using some of these mouse strains to test Mendel's laws. Clarence Little recognized that mice used in scientific studies should have genetically homogeneous backgrounds and generated the first inbred strains by performing at least 20 generations of brother-sister matings. Some of these inbred strains showed a high incidence of certain cancers—for example, the 129 strain was prone to testicular cancer (Stevens, 1970). Thus, mouse strains with a genetic predisposition to cancer were the first real cancer models.

Investigations of mutagenic agents identified a variety of chemical and physical methods that could be used reliably to induce or enhance tumorigenesis in these mouse strains, though little was known about the specific genetic targets of these various agents. To move beyond these genetically uncharacterized, stochastic methods, techniques to stably and precisely introduce specific mutations into the mouse genome were needed. Transgenic mouse and embryonic stem (ES) cell technologies have met this need.

Transgenesis, the stable introduction of an exogenous gene into the germ line of an organism (usually by pronuclear injection), was first demonstrated in 1981 (Gordon and Ruddle, 1981). The first transgenic mouse models of cancer overexpressed viral oncogenes. More recently, models have been generated in which the activity of a transgene can be controlled temporally and spatially. This has enabled the production of mouse models that more accurately reflect the cascade of genetic events that characterize human malignancies.

The isolation of pluripotent ES cells and the development of mice carrying endogenous genes modified by homologous recombination were important developments that have played key roles in improving cancer models (Evans and Kaufman, 1981; Thomas

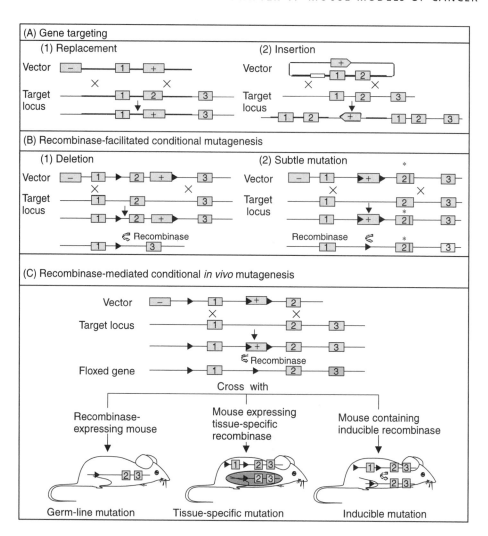

Figure 11-1. Gene-targeting strategies in vitro and in vivo. (A) Integration patterns of targeting vectors by replacement or insertion. (1) Exon 2 of the target gene is replaced with the positive selection marker (+) by homologous recombination. (2) Homologous recombination of the insertion vector with the target locus results in the insertion of the whole vector and duplication of exons 1 and 2. (−) and the thick line represent the negative selection marker and homology to the target locus, respectively. (B) Recombinase-facilitated conditional mutagenesis. Conditional gene targeting exploits the unique properties of site-specific recombinases, most commonly Cre from bacteriophage P1, or Flp from the yeast *Saccharomyces cerevisiae*. Both have short, unique recognition sequences (filled triangle): *loxP* and frt (FLP recognition target), respectively. (1) DNA between two such sites in *cis* is deleted upon action of the recombinase. (2) A subtle mutation (asterisk) was introduced by homologous recombination and subsequent recombinase facilitated removal of the selection marker. (C) Recombinase-mediated in vivo conditional mutation. Most conditional targeting vectors follow the 3-*loxP* design, in which both the targeted region and a selectable marker are flanked by *loxP* sites. The removable selection marker is used in the initial targeting but is normally removed in cell culture before mice are generated. Recombination to generate the inactive allele can be done by crossing conditional mice to mice expressing whole-body, tissue-specific, or inducible recombinase.

and Capecchi, 1987). ES cell technology allows for replacement or deletion of a specific gene, a chromosomal region, or even a single nucleotide. Although it is beyond the scope of this review to detail the methods for generating ES cell targeting vectors, detailed practical advice can be found in Hasty et al. (2000). Virtually any change in the genome can be generated in ES cells, which can be injected into host embryos and implanted in a recipient host mother. Resulting chimeras are mated to produce progeny that carry the desired change in their genome. Consequently, knockout and knock-in mice have both contributed immensely to cancer research (Fig. 11-1).

Conditional Mutations

Optimally, a mouse model should reflect the biological, genetic, etiological, and therapeutic aspects of a particular human cancer. High penetrance and short latency of tumorigenesis are desirable because of the short mouse life span. While no model will accurately reflect all criteria, better models address more of them (Hann and Balmain, 2001). A common criticism of mouse models of human familial lesions is that the tumor spectra do not always mirror those of the human (Jacks, 1996). Conditional models of both oncogenic activation and tumor suppressor mutations have gained popularity for their ability to more precisely model the random nature of tumorigenesis (Fig. 11-1).

OVEREXPRESSION OF ONCOGENES

Transgenic Mouse Models of Cancer

A Summary of Transgenic Mouse Models. The experimental paradigm of a transgenic model is simple. Based on the expression pattern of its gene, a promoter is chosen to drive expression of an oncogene. Overexpression of the oncogene from this promoter may then generate a tumorigenic phenotype in tissues where the gene is expressed. The construct is usually microinjected into the pronuclei of fertilized eggs. Carrier animals are bred to ensure germ-line transmission of the construct, and multiple independent lines are studied, as different transgenic lines will have different integration sites. Hundreds of different lines of transgenic mice have been generated to model human cancer; hence, it is not possible to mention all that has been accomplished in this field. A sample of the kinds of promoters, genes, and phenotypes are shown in Table 11-1. Some web sites that describe and list the models are included in the web addresses at the end of the chapter. We have selected a few examples to illustrate how these models can be used.

The RIP-Tag Model of Insulinoma. Insulinomas are benign or malignant tumors originating from the β-cells in the islets of Langerhans in the pancreas. These tumors serve as a good model of multistep carcinogenesis because clearly defined stages can be observed. Hanahan developed the RIP-Tag model in 1985, in which the rat insulin II promoter (RIP) is used to drive transcription of SV40 Tag in β-cells (Hanahan, 1985). Tumors derived from the insulin-producing β-cells were seen in transgenic mice at 12 weeks of age. Subsequent work investigating the multistage nature of the model demonstrated angiogenic activity within a subset of hyperplastic islets before tumor formation (Folkman et al., 1989). These hyperplastic islets were neovascularized at a frequency that correlated with subsequent tumor incidence. These were some of

TABLE 11-1. Selected Transgenic Models of Cancer

Organ System Modeled	Viral Element/Gene	Promoter/ Gene	Phenotype	Comments	References
Brain	SV40 Tag	Brain-specific (1B) *FGF1* promoter	Brain tumors in pontine gray, rostral to fourth ventricle.		Chiu et al., 2001
Brain	HPV16 E6 and E7	*β-actin* promoter	Neuroepithelial tumors by 2.5 months. 71% developed fatal brain tumors by 10 months.	Choroid plexus and pituitary carcinomas also seen.	Arbeit et al., 1993
Breast	SV40 Tag	C3(1) component of rat *PSBP* promoter	Mammary hyperplasia by 3 months. Adenocarcinoma by 6 months (100% of animals).	Rat *PSBP* was thought to be prostate specific; hence, expression in the breast was unexpected.	Maroulakou et al., 1994
Breast	MMTV LTR	*c-Myc*	Adenocarcinoma developed during pregnancy.	Various portions of the *c-Myc* promoter were used in the fusion.	Stewart et al., 1984
Breast	MMTV LTR	*c-Myc*	Locally invasive mammary tumors as well as testicular, lymphocytic (B cell and T cell), and mast cell tumors.	*c-Myc* expressed in a variety of tissues, but only developed tumors in a subset of these tissues.	Leder et al., 1986
Breast	*WAP*	*c-Myc*	*WAP-Myc* transgene expressed during lactation. Adenocarcinoma seen as early as 2 months after expression.	*WAP* and *β-casein* also expressed.	Schoenenberger et al., 1988
Breast	MMTV LTR	*Cyclin D1*	Abnormal mammary gland proliferation and adenocarcinoma.	Proliferative changes coincided with transgene expression at sexual maturity.	Wang et al., 1994

Tissue	Promoter	Transgene	Phenotype	Notes	Reference
Breast	MMTV LTR	Wnt-1 (originally called Int-1)	Mammary glands of males and virgin females grossly hyperplastic. Mammary and (less frequently) salivary adenocarcinomas occur by 1 year.	Wnt-1 RNA expressed at high levels in mammary and salivary glands of male and female mice and in male reproductive organs.	Tsukamoto et al., 1988
Cervix	HPV16 E6 and E7	Human keratin 14 promoter/enhancer	Transgenic mice treated with slow-release pellets of 17β-estradiol. Squamous carcinomas seen in a multistage pathway in vagina and cervix.	Expression of HPV transgenes in untreated transgenic mice was detectable only during estrus.	Arbeit et al., 1996
Hypothalamus	SV40 Tag	Rat gonadotropin-releasing hormone (GnRH)	Hypothalamus-specific tumors.	Tumors used to make specific cell lines that produce Tag and GnRH.	Mellon et al., 1992
Liver	SV40 Tag	Albumin, expressed in hepatocytes	Multifocal hepatocellular carcinomas at 5 months.	Morphological and enzymatic variation around lesions. Some H-ras point mutations (probably a late event).	Kitagawa et al., 1991
Liver	SV40 Tag	Human α-1-antitrypsin	Hepatic neoplasias seen by 6 months.	Carcinomas of stomach and pancreas, and kidney hyperplasia also seen.	Butel et al., 1990
Prostate (the TRAMP model)	SV40 Tag	Prostate-specific rat probasin promoter	Progression from mild PIN to multinodular malignant neoplasia seen after 10 weeks (resembling human disease).	Model has been used to evaluate chemotherapeutics (toremifene, α-difluoromethylornithine, flutamide, R-flurbiprofen) and examine the role of diet in prostate cancer risk (genistein, green tea polyphenols).	Greenberg et al., 1995; Gupta et al., 2000, 2001; Mentor-Marcel et al., 2001; Raghow et al., 2000, 2002; Wechter et al., 2000

(*continued*)

TABLE 11-1 (*continued*)

Organ System Modeled	Viral Element/Gene	Promoter/ Gene	Phenotype	Comments	References
Prostate	SV40 Tag	C3(1) component of *PSBP*	Human prostatic intraepithelial neoplasia progressing to invasive carcinoma. Lung metastases.		Maroulakou et al., 1994
Salivary gland	SV40 Tag	Tet-op promoter in a tetracycline-responsive system	Extensive ductal hyperplasia by 4 months.	Reversal of hyperplasia with removal of teracycline, seen at 4 months (but not 7 months).	Ewald et al., 1996; Furth et al., 1998
Skin	HPV16 E6 and E7	Human *keratin 14* promoter/enhancer	Hyperplasia, papillomatosis, and dysplasia appeared at multiple epidermal and squamous mucosal sites, including ear and truncal skin, face, snout and eyelids, and anus. Ears were the most consistently affected site (with 100% penetrance).	Absence of E1 or E2 function did not influence the severity of the phenotype that eventually developed in these transgenic mice. Phenotype also progressed through discernible stages.	Arbeit et al., 1994
Thyroid	*RET/PTC* oncogene	Bovine *thyroglobulin*	Bilateral thyroid cancers similar to human papillary thyroid cancers seen within 3 weeks.	Low-copy transgenes developed tumors slower than high-copy transgenes. Cellular abnormalities seen in thyroid before birth.	Cho et al., 1999

the first studies showing the importance of angiogenesis in the carcinogenic process, highlighting a potential therapeutic intervention point.

In a large screen of growth factors, receptors, and oncogenes, it was shown that there was a correlation of the initial proliferative switch with the focal activation of various growth factors such as insulin-like growth factor II (Igf2; Christofori et al., 1994). Indeed, RIP-Tag $Igf2^{-/-}$ mice showed reduced cellular and tumor growth, thereby causally implicating Igf2 in the signaling pathway (Christofori et al., 1994). Similarly, *fibroblast growth factor receptor 4* (*Fgfr4*) was activated in cell lines derived from RIP-Tag tumors but not from those derived from hyperplastic islets (Olson et al., 1998). However, in contrast to *Igf2*, neither gain-of-function nor loss-of-function alleles of *Fgfr4* appeared to affect the well-characterized tumorigenesis pathway (Olson et al., 1998), suggesting that *Fgfr4* is a marker for, but not causal in, β-cell transformation. More recently, the RIP-Tag model has been used to investigate the role of L-selectin in metastasis, because L-selectin directs the extravasation of lymphocytes to the lymph nodes. Metastasis in the RIP-Tag model usually targets the liver and not the lymph nodes. Transgenic mice in which L-selectin expression was targeted to endogenous primary insulinomas through the use of a RIP-L-selectin cDNA transgene showed an increased frequency of metastases to the lymph nodes in cells expressing L-selectin on their surface, indicating that vascularized islet carcinomas shed tumor cells into the bloodstream (Qian et al., 2001).

Alongside attempts to understand the angiogenic aspects of the RIP-Tag model, genome-wide efforts to find genes involved in the multistage nature of the model have also been pursued. RIP-Tag was one of the first transgenic models on which detailed LOH analyses were performed to locate TSGs involved in the progression to end-stage insulinomas and carcinomas. Two regions of 3 and 30 Mb were found on mouse chromosomes 9 and 16, respectively. LOH was not detected in the regions of the genome where the TSGs *Rb1* and *p53*—known to interact with Tag—are found (Dietrich et al., 1994). This confirmed that the mode of action of Tag in this model is likely via p53 and Rb1 sequestration, and that additional genetic hits in these TSGs are not required. However, the depletion of functional p53 may allow mutations and LOH to occur in other genes that contribute to tumorigenesis. Using the technique of comparative genomic hybridization (CGH) to DNA microarrays (see Chapter 3), the region on chromosome 16 has been narrowed down to 3 Mb and chromosomal locations for three TSGs and two oncogenes were identified (Hodgson et al., 2001).

Neu/c-ERBB2 Models of Breast Cancer. The protein target of herceptin, which is discussed in Chapter 13, *c-ERBB2* is a member of the epidermal growth factor family, and is amplified and overexpressed in 20–40% of human breast tumors (Slamon et al., 1987, 1989). *c-ERBB2* amplification correlates with a poor prognosis in a variety of tumor types; thus, mouse models overexpressing *c-ERBB2* have been generated. The first mouse models of *c-ERBB2* amplification expressed a mutated form of *Neu* containing point mutations that increased Neu tyrosine kinase activity (Bargmann and Weinberg, 1988) from the MMTV LTR (Bouchard et al., 1989; Muller et al., 1988). In contrast to mice carrying MMTV/*c-Myc* (which stochastically develop mammary tumors), MMTV-*Neu* mice developed mammary adenocarcinomas that involved the entire epithelium in each gland (Muller et al., 1988). Because the tumors arose synchronously, it was suggested that expression of the activated *Neu* was sufficient to induce transformation in the mammary gland (Muller et al., 1988).

Subsequent studies using a normal version of *neu* (without the activating point mutation) under the control of the MMTV promoter/enhancer concluded that expression of wild-type *neu* was not sufficient for induction of malignant transformation of the mammary epithelial cells, as *neu* was also expressed in adjacent mammary epithelium (Guy et al., 1992). Focal mammary tumors that metastasized to the lung showed a longer latency when wild-type *neu* was used compared with an activated version (Guy et al., 1992). The wild-type *neu* in these tumors was subsequently shown to be activated by somatic mutations within the transgene; small, transforming, in-frame deletions were found in the extracellular region proximal to the transmembrane domain (Siegel et al., 1994).

The downstream targets of Neu-mediated signal transduction have been investigated in this model. The activity of c-Src, a tyrosine kinase showing elevated activity in breast cancers, was six- to eightfold higher in tumor extracts than in the surrounding normal epithelium, due to an elevation in its specific activity rather than an increase in c-Src protein levels (Muthuswamy et al., 1994).

The relatively long tumor latency in the model carrying a wild-type *neu* (>200 days) suggests that other mutations are required for tumorigenesis. The murine equivalent of the most common human *p53* mutation in breast cancer (R175H) was used to generate $p53^{R172H}$/MMTV-*Neu* bitransgenic mice (Li et al., 1997). These mice showed a shorter tumor latency (~150 days) and had no activating deletions in the *Neu* transgene, suggesting a cooperative role for *p53* in *Neu*-mediated tumorigenesis (Li et al., 1997).

Most transgenic models do not accurately recapitulate the physiological events in cancer, since they rely on promoters that provide strong, uniform expression of an oncogene. However, cancer is characterized by genetic changes that occur in a more stochastic manner. In an effort to better mimic these genetic changes, conditional mouse models have been used. In the case of *neu*, a floxed (*fl*anked by *lox P* sites) *neomycin phosphotransferase* cassette was placed upstream of an activated cDNA under the control of the endogenous *Neu* promoter (Andrechek et al., 2000). When interbred with *MMTV-Cre* mice, the offspring (now expressing the activated *Neu*) exhibited accelerated mammary epithelial development. However, expression from the endogenous promoter was not sufficient to initiate carcinogenesis. Tumors were eventually seen after a long latency period (~450 days), with a correlation between tumor progression and an elevation in *Neu* transcript and protein levels. There was amplification (from 2 to 22 copies) of the activated *neu* oncogene relative to the wild-type allele (Andrechek et al., 2000), indicating that a certain level of activated *neu* is required for oncogenic conversion in mammary epithelial cells.

Modeling Translocations in Leukemias and Lymphomas

Chromosomal translocations are involved in the genesis of many types of human tumors, altering expression of oncogenes and tumor suppressor genes or by generating novel fusion genes (reviewed in Mitelman et al., 1997; Rabbitts, 1994). This phenomenon is particularly common in leukemia (Rowley, 1998). For example, the Philadelphia chromosome, a translocation of human chromosomes 9 and 22, associated with 95% of chronic myelogenous leukemia (CML) and a subset of acute lymphoblastic leukemia, involves c-*ABL* on chromosome 9q34 and *BCR* on chromosome 22q11, which fuse to form *BCR-ABL*. There are variable breakpoints within the two genes, and three different products can be formed, p185[BCR-ABL], p210[BCR-ABL], and p230$^{BCR-ABL}$, which are preferentially associated with different leukemias (Wong and Witte, 2001). Initial studies modeling the Philadelphia chromosome in the mouse used retroviral transduction of the *c-Abl* oncogene. Noticeable differences between strains made interpretation of the data complex (reviewed in Wong and Witte, 2001). More recent studies utilized a set of conditional transgenic lines expressing a *Bcr-Abl* fusion construct, which mimics the human CML p210 translocation, under the control of tetracycline in the tet-repressor system (Gossen and Bujard, 1992; for a good review of the tet-repressor system, see Baron and Bujard, 2000). Withdrawal of tetracycline after birth resulted in expression of the *Bcr-Abl* fusion, and, depending on the transgenic line used, lethal leukemia developed in 3–11 weeks. Tumor regression could be induced by readdition of tetracycline (Huettner et al., 2000), indicating that *Bcr-Abl* expression is required for maintenance of the transformed phenotype and validating Brc-Abl as a leukemia drug target (see Chapter 13 for more on Gleevec as a drug that targets kinases related to activated Abl).

Burkitt's lymphoma (BL) is characterized by translocations involving c-*MYC* on human chromosome 8q24 and most frequently the immunoglobulin heavy-chain locus on chromosome 14q32. Initial efforts to make transgenic BL mice placed c-*MYC* under IgH or IgL regulatory control. However, the phenotype of these mice was more consistent with lymphoblastic leukemia than BL (Adams et al., 1985). A more accurate mouse model for BL has been described in which c-*MYC* derived from a BL patient was fused to elements of an alternative immunoglobulin locus, Igλ (Kovalchuk et al., 2000). These transgenic mice showed a phenotype very similar to that seen in human BL, although their reaction to treatment regimens has yet to be reported. A novel pharmacological strategy targeted at *c-Myc*-overexpressing tumors is described in Chapter 10.

Acute promyelocytic leukemia (APL) is characterized by translocations involving the retinoic acid receptor α (*RARα*) on human chromosome 17q11, and, most usually, a gene called *promyelocytic leukemia (PML)* on chromosome 15q22 (although genes on other chromosomes have also been shown to be reciprocal partners in the translocation, such as *PLZF* (also known as *ZNF145*) on chromosome 11q23; He et al., 2000; Pandolfi, 2001). PML and PLZF have been studied most extensively in the mouse. *PML-RARα* transgenic mice develop retinoic acid (RA)–responsive APL similar to that seen in human APL (He et al., 1997), whereas *PLZF-RARα* transgenic mice develop a RA-resistant leukemia more like that seen in human CML (He et al., 1998). Interactions of the gene products can also have an effect, as can be seen from phenotypic modification in double transgenic mice. For example, the presence of the *RARα-PLZF* in mice bitransgenic for both *RARα-PLZF* and *PLZF-RARα* changed the disease to one with characteristics of APL, rather than the CML seen with *PLZF-RARα* alone (He et al., 2000). Experiments designed to dissect the mechanism of RA-responsive APL are described in Chapter 10.

Two groups have reported conditional systems that model leukemia-related translocations. Buchholz et al. were interested in t(8;21) involved in human acute myeloid leukemia (Buchholz et al., 2000). They targeted *loxP* sites to the mouse homologs of the genes at the breakpoints of this translocation, *Aml* and *Eto*, then crossed the double-*loxP* mice to *Nestin-Cre* mice, which express Cre later in development. While this model circumvents the embryonic lethality of the previously described *Aml/Eto* knock-in (Yergeau et al., 1997) and improves the model by generating both products of the translocation, *Nestin* does not express in hematapoietic lineages, so it was not possible to study leukemia in these mice. A similar system was used to generate the translocation between *Mll* and *Af9*, the mouse genes homologous to the genes found in the human t(9;11) translocations in acute leukemias (Collins et al., 2000). Translocations were detected in ES cells but only in the brain of mice crossed to a *PGK-Cre* line. In both cases, other Cre lines will be necessary to induce the translocation in the appropriate cell type.

Overexpression of Oncogenes by Gene Targeting

As an alternative to expressing oncogenes using transgenic approaches, gene targeting can be used to transplace part of or a whole gene with a mutated copy. Because such constructs are targeted to endogenous loci, they are expressed and regulated normally.

Cdk4: Endocrine Epithelial Tumors. G_1/S cell-cycle checkpoint genes are among the most frequently deregulated targets in human malignancies (reviewed in Ruas and Peters, 1998; Sherr, 2000). D-type cyclins associate with two cyclin-dependent kinases, Cdk4 and Cdk6, to inactivate Rb1. The INK4 family serves as a negative regulator of Cdk4 and Cdk6 by blocking formation of the cyclin-Cdk complex (reviewed in Sherr and Roberts, 1999), and ablation of this negative regulation results in uncontrolled cell growth and neoplasia. Mice that carry a mutation responsible for hereditary melanomas in the INK4-binding domain of Cdk4 (R24C) develop a wide spectrum of tumors including endocrine epithelial, mesenchymatous, and lymphoid tumors (Rane et al., 1999; Sotillo et al., 2001a; Wolfel et al., 1995; Zuo et al., 1996). In contrast to earlier findings that loss of function of a single INK4 family member is not sufficient to induce sporadic tumors (Sherr, 2000), these *Cdk4* knock-in mice showed high tumor susceptibility, illustrating the pivotal role of negative regulation of Cdk4. *Cdk4* knock-in mice were also highly susceptible to melanoma following carcinogenic treatment (Rane et al., 2002; Sotillo et al., 2001b). Melanomas induced in this model have no alterations in the $p19^{ARF}$/p53 pathway, suggesting specific involvement of the $p16^{INK4a}$/Cdk4/Rb1 pathway in melanoma development.

MEN2B: C-cell Thyroid Hyperplasia. Approximately 95% of human multiple endocrine neoplasia type 2B (MEN2B) cases result from a M918T substitution in the RET receptor tyrosine kinase (Carlson et al., 1994; Hofstra et al., 1994). This substitution confers oncogenicity through an alteration of the three-dimensional structure of the tyrosine-binding pocket (reviewed in Ponder, 1995). Homozygous knock-in mice carrying the murine equivalent of the M918T mutation (M919T, ret^{MEN2B}) developed C-cell hyperplasia of the thyroid and pheochromocytoma in the adrenal gland, which resembles human MEN2B (Smith-Hicks et al., 2000). This model also resolved the controversy over whether the M919T substitution induces a gain- or loss-of-function in the RET receptor tyrosine kinase in the mouse, as the kidneys and enteric nervous system of $ret^{MEN2B/MEN2B}$ mice were apparently normal, suggesting that the tumors specific to $ret^{MEN2B/MEN2B}$ homozygotes must be due to a gain-of-function allele.

Inducible Oncogenes

Although conventional transgenics and gene-targeting techniques are powerful tools for gain-of-function studies, they cannot accurately model sporadic human tumors, as uniformly high oncogene expression levels do not accurately model stochastic mutations in isolated single cells surrounded by a field of normal cells. Thus, conditional models have been developed that allow a variety of levels of control over the expression of the mutated allele(s) (Deng et al., 1996; Garcia et al., 1999).

Conditional Models of Small-Cell Lung Cancer. *K-RAS* is a gene mutated in approximately 30% of human non-small-cell lung adenocarcinomas (Minamoto et al., 2000). Chapter 14 describes pharmacological approaches to target Ras-mutated tumors. Four different murine models mimicking the random activation of *K-Ras* in lung cancer have now been generated, with the eventual goal of being able to use this model to test novel therapeutics. All four models mutated the gene at codon 12, showed similar results, and showcase the range of conditional techniques available.

Johnson et al. used a hit-and-run approach (Hasty et al., 1991). Two different "hits" were used, both of which resulted in a duplication of exon 1 and surrounding regions; one carried two mutated (G12D) copies of exon 1, and the second had one mutant and one normal copy. The "run" (removal of one copy by homologous recombination and return to a functional allele) was allowed to occur randomly in the mouse. All mice carrying a mutant-mutant hit developed non-small-cell lung adenomas by 200 days, while all those with a mutant-normal hit showed tumors by 300 days. Some mice also developed thymic lymphomas and skin papillomas. On a *p53* null background, the mice developed a greater number of more aggressive tumors more quickly (Johnson et al., 2001).

A second group (Fisher et al., 2001) placed the mutation under the control of a tet-repressor system, in which the mutant *K-Ras* was under the control of doxcyline (Dox) in type 2 alveolar cells (Gossen and Bujard, 1992). Addition of Dox to the system activated the mutant *K-Ras*, and within 3 days, regions of increased proliferation were seen in the lungs. Within 3 months, the lung tumor burden was so high that the lungs were twice normal size. Amazingly, withdrawal of Dox, even after 2 months, when multiple large adenomas and adenocarcinomas were present in the lungs, resulted in regression of tumors, caused mainly by apoptosis of tumor cells. One month after Dox withdrawal, only small regions of hyperplasia remained, showing that *K-Ras* is not only required for tumorigenesis but also for maintenance of tumors and thereby validating K-Ras as a drug target in established adenocarcinomas. As in the previous study (Johnson et al., 2001), mice on a *p53* null background developed more tumors with a shorter latency. The tet-repressor system used in this study clearly provides good control of mutant *K-Ras* expression, but the model lacks the stochastic features of the others.

Meuwissen et al. used a transgene consisting of the mutant *K-Ras* linked to an IRES-reporter gene cassette, and a strong promoter, with a floxed *green fluorescent protein* (*GFP*) cassette between them. An adenovirus expressing Cre (Anton and Graham, 1995) was introduced intratracheally to delete the floxed cassette and activate the mutant transgene in virally exposed cells. Due to the inefficiency of the adenoviral Cre system, the tumors began as focal lesions surrounded by normal tissues retaining the floxed *GFP* cassette. Within 9–13 weeks, all treated mice had developed multiple adenocarcinomas (Meuwissen et al., 2001).

Jackson et al. produced mice carrying the mutated *K-Ras* gene preceded by a floxed "transcriptional" stop site. The floxed stop site was randomly removed by intranasal administration of adenoviral Cre (Anton and Graham, 1995). Because the major focus of this study was initiation and progression, the viral dose was varied, resulting in a dose-dependent tumor burden. When given a lower viral dose, mice began developing lung hyperplasias within 2 weeks, which progressed to adenocarcinomas by 16 weeks. No tumors were seen in normal mice, or in any area outside of the lungs, indicating that this method allowed for control over both temporal and spatial aspects of tumor induction (Jackson et al., 2001).

These systems primarily demonstrate that activation of this single oncogene may be rate-limiting if not sufficient for lung tumorigenesis in the mouse: Increased prolif-eration was seen very soon after activation of the transgene, tumors developed rapidly, and tumorigenesis could be accelerated by certain mutant backgrounds. Arguably, *K-Ras* is expressed at high levels in two of the models, but given that very similar results were observed in the different studies, mutant *K-Ras* can transform at various levels of expression with potentially a small number of other genetic or epigenetic changes.

Methods of Conditional Activation of a Transgene. The *K-Ras* models illustrate many of the prevailing technologies for conditional activation of a transgene. The tet-repressor system appears to be adequately regulated, as evidenced by the almost complete regression of tumors after removal of Dox in the *K-ras* tet-repressor system (Fisher et al., 2001). The tet-repressor system works through transcriptional regulation and this technology has been developed relatively recently. The first con-ditional system that was successfully used in a cancer model used estrogen receptor fusions, in which gene activity is controlled by a very different mechanism (Eilers et al., 1989). In this system, an oncogene is fused to the hormone-binding domain of the estrogen receptor (ER). The oncogene is activated when ER binds to tamoxifen but is sequestered and inactive in the absence of this antiestrogen. Tamoxifen-treated mice carrying a transgene consisting of the ER fused to an activated form of *c-Myc* in thymocytes showed a 62% tumor incidence (thymic lymphomas) by 300 days if given tamoxifen from birth. If given tamoxifen from 3 weeks of age, 38% had tumors by 300 days. However, 22% of mice not given any tamoxifen at all developed tumors in the same time span (Blyth et al., 2000). This background is consistent with that seen in the original study (Eilers et al., 1989), and although it may be tolerable for some studies, the tet-repressor system appears to exhibit tighter control and circumvents the need to create fusion proteins.

One strength of both the tet-repressor and ER systems lies in their ability to test if an activated oncogene is required for tumor formation and tumor maintenance. In the cases published to date (Chin et al., 1997, 1999; Felsher and Bishop, 1999; Fisher et al., 2001), shutting off the oncogene, even at a point when animals carry a heavy tumor burden, results in remission in a large percentage of animals. Felsher and Bishop used the tet-repressor system to activate *c-MYC* in hematapoetic cells upon withdrawal of Dox. In the absence of Dox, all 20 mice tested died of T-cell-derived tumors within 5 months. However, of 20 mice with a fairly heavy tumor burden, 90% showed regression of tumors, and 80% exhibited remission for up to 30 weeks after readdition of Dox to the diet. This suggests that if the proper drugs and drug targets are identified, regression even of later-stage tumors may be possible (Felsher and Bishop, 1999).

TUMOR SUPPRESSOR MUTATIONS

The availability of TSG knockout mice has greatly facilitated our understanding of the mechanisms involved in tumor development and progression in humans. These mice have been used to model many tumor suppressor–related cancer syndromes. Knock-out models include representatives from caretakers involved in DNA damage repair (Table 11-2A), gatekeepers involved in cell cycle control and apoptosis (Table 11-2B), as well as genes involved in cell signaling and differentiation (Table 11-2C). The complex interactions between TSGs are highlighted by mouse mutants with loss of two TSGs (double knockouts; Table 11-3). In addition, many of these TSG knockouts show enhanced sensitivity (elevated tumorigenesis) to radiation and chemical carcinogens (Table 11-4).

Homozygous null mutants of many tumor suppressor genes are embryonic lethals. Therefore, conditional knockout alleles have been generated. Conditional mutations enable the loss of the second allele (the second hit; Knudson, 1971) to be regulated. Since recombinases are rarely 100% efficient, the random nature of mutagenesis in human cancers and the interaction of mutant and normal cells in the microenvironment is more accurately modeled in these mutants. By controlling the temporal and spatial generation of cells with the desired genotype, researchers are in effect establishing an experimental paradigm where the rate of LOH is artificially increased.

Null Mutations of DNA Repair Genes

Mismatch Repair Genes Msh3 and Msh6. DNA mismatch repair (MMR) is critical for the maintenance of genomic stability and functions by recognizing replication-generated mismatches and mismatches in heteroduplex recombination inter-mediates, as well as playing a role in responses to DNA damage. In *Escherichia coli*, MMR is effected by a heterodimer of a MutS and a MutL protein; however, all eukaryotic organisms possess multiple MutS homologs (MSH proteins) and MutL homologs (MLH proteins). In mammalian cells, four MutL homologs (PMS1, PMS2, MLH1, MLH3) and five MutS homologs (MSH2–6) have been identified.

Germ-line mutations in human MMR genes are directly responsible for most cases of hereditary nonpolyposis colorectal cancer (HNPCC), characterized mainly by early-onset carcinomas of the colon (Fishel et al., 1993; Leach et al., 1993; Watson and Lynch, 1993; Bronner et al., 1994; Nicolaides et al., 1994; Papadopoulos et al., 1994). Somatic mutations in MMR genes underlie some sporadic cancers (Wheeler et al., 2000); however, many mouse MMR mutants are not accurate models of human HNPCC. For example, $Pms2^{-/-}$ mice develop lymphomas and sarcomas but not intestinal adenomas or adenocarcinomas (Prolla et al., 1998). $Msh2^{-/-}$ mice primarily develop lymphomas (in at least 80% of the cases) but do not develop late-onset intestinal adenocarcinoma associated with Apc inactivation. In both cases, the heterozygotes are normal and healthy (de Wind et al., 1998; Kohonen-Corish et al., 2002; Reitmair et al., 1996; Whiteside et al., 2002). Similarly, $Mlh1^{-/-}$ mice develop lymphomas, intestinal adenomas, and adenocarcinomas by 1 year of age (Baker et al., 1996; Prolla et al., 1998), and $Msh6^{-/-}$ mice show a reduced life span, developing a spectrum of mostly gastrointestinal tract (GIT) tumors and lymphomas (Edelmann et al., 1997). $Msh3^{-/-}$, $Msh6^{-/-}$ mice show increased and earlier tumorigenicity (predominantly GIT or lymphoid in origin) compared with $Msh3^{-/-}$ or $Msh6^{-/-}$

TABLE 11-2A. Mouse Knockouts of Tumor Suppressor Genes Involved in DNA Damage Repair

Gene	Function	Mutations in the Gene in Humans	Heterozygous Mouse Phenotype	Homozygous Mouse Phenotype	References
Ataxia telangiectasia mutated (*Atm*)	ATM is a kinase involved in repairing DNA damage, responding to DSBs.	ATM mutations are responsible for the rare genetic disorder ataxia telangiectasia (AT), characterized by immunodeficiency, progressive cellular ataxia, radiosensitivity, defects in cell cycle checkpoints, and a predisposition to leukemia/lymphoma.	Healthy, although exhibit radiosensitivity.	Growth retardation. Neurologic dysfunction. Defective T-lymphocyte maturation. Radiosensitivity. Predisposition to cancer (thyroid lymphomas).	Barlow et al., 1996; Elson et al., 1996; Xu et al., 1996
ATM and Rad3 related (*Atr*)	ATR is a kinase involved in repairing DNA damage, responding to DSBs, UV-induced damage, and replication arrest.	No cancer has yet been associated with an ATR mutation in humans.	Aged mice show increased tumor incidence.	Die before ε8.5.	Brown and Baltimore, 2000; de Klein et al., 2000
Brca1	BRCA1 expression increased in the S phase of the cell cycle and is phosphorylated in a cell cycle–dependent manner in response to DNA damage.	*BRCA1* mutations account for at least 80% of families with both breast and ovarian cancer.	Hypomorphic *Brca1* mutations with a partial loss of Brca1 function die at ε10–13[d] (with spina bifida, anencephaly, and increased neuroepithelial apoptosis).	Die at ε10–13[d] (due to neural tube abnormalities).	Brodie and Deng, 2001; Gowen et al., 1996; Hakem et al., 1996; Liu et al., 1996; Ludwig et al., 1997

Brca2	Putative role as a caretaker involved in DNA damage repair and maintenance of genomic integrity.	BRCA2 mutations are responsible for 32% of hereditary breast cancers (in females).	Some hypomorphic Brca2 mutants survive to adulthood (but show abnormal tissue differentiation, a lack of germ cells, and develop thymic lymphomas by 12–14 weeks). Mammary gland tumors have not been observed.	Die at ε7.5–9.5[d] (due to underdevelopment).	Connor et al., 1997; Friedman et al., 1998; Ludwig et al., 1997; Sharan et al., 1997; Suzuki et al., 1997
Nijmegen breakage syndrome gene, NBS1	NBS1, the product of the gene underlying the disease, forms a multimeric complex with hMRE11/hRAD50 nuclease and recruits them to the sites of DNA damage.	NBS is an autosomal-recessive disease characterized by elevated sensitivity to ionizing radiation that induces double-strand breaks and a high frequency of malignancies.	Viable and healthy, and did not develop cancer spontaneously (within the 14-month study). Tumors were not apparent after being irradiated.	Embryonic lethality at the blastocyst stage (due to growth retardation and increased apoptosis). $Nbs1^{m/m}$ mutant mice (in which the N-terminal exons of Nbs1 have been disrupted) are viable, growth retarded, hypersensitive to ionizing radiation, exhibit multiple lymphoid developmental defects, and rapidly develop thymic lymphoma.	

(continued)

T A B L E 11-2A (*continued*)

Gene	Function	Mutations in the Gene in Humans	Heterozygous Mouse Phenotype	Homozygous Mouse Phenotype	References
				Female $Nbs1^{m/m}$ mice are sterile due to oogenesis failure. Most systematic and cellular defects identified in $Nbs1^{m/m}$ mice recapitulate those in NBS patients and are essentially identical to those observed in $Atm^{-/-}$ mice. $Nbs1^{\Delta B/\Delta B}$ hypomorphic mutant mice (in which the BRCT domain has been deleted) are viable.	Kang et al., 2002; Williams et al., 2002; Zhu et al., 2001
$Msh2^a$	A DNA MMR gene. MSH2–MSH3 and MSH2–MSH6 protein complexes are responsible for recognition of mispaired bases during MMR.	Mutations in the human MMR genes *MSH2*, *MLH1*, *PMS1*, and *PMS2* are responsible for most cases of hereditary HNPCC (characterized by early-onset carcinomas of the colon, as well as cancers of the endometrium, stomach, upper urinary tract, small intestine, and ovary). Mutations in *MSH2* and *MLH1* account for the majority of HNPCC families with germ-line mutations,			

		PMS1 and *PMS2* account for ≤10% of such families.	Mice do not develop spontaneous intestinal or colon tumors.	Succumb to disease within the first year, with lymphomas observed in ≥80% of cases. Develop late-onset intestinal adenocarcinoma (associated with APC inactivation). Predisposed to tumors triggered by chronic inflammation.	de Wind et al., 1998; Kohonen-Corish et al, 2002; Reitmair et al., 1996; Whiteside et al., 2002
Msh6 (aka *GTBP* and *p160*)	See *Msh2.*		A slightly reduced life span compared to wild-type mice. 28% develop tumors (most frequently non-Hodgkin's lymphoma followed by GIT tumors).	Reduced life span. Develop a spectrum of tumors (mostly GIT tumors and B- and T-cell lymphomas).	Edelmann et al., 1997
Mlh1	Involved in the MMR pathway and meiotic crossing over.	See *Msh2.*	Healthy.	Similar phenotype to *Msh2*−/− mice. Develop adenocarcinomas, intestinal adenomas, and lymphomas (plus skin tumors and sarcomas to a lesser extent) by 1 year of age. Sterile.	Baker et al., 1996; Prolla et al., 1998

(continued)

T A B L E 11-2A (continued)

Gene	Function	Mutations in the Gene in Humans	Heterozygous Mouse Phenotype	Homozygous Mouse Phenotype	References
Pms2	Involved in the MMR pathway and meiotic crossing over.	See Msh2.	Healthy.	Develop lymphomas and sarcomas but not intestinal adenocarcinomas/adenomas (by the age of 17 months).[b] Males are infertile.	Prolla et al., 1998
Blm	A RecQ DNA helicase involved in transcription, DNA repair, and replication.	Mutations in BLM result in Bloom's syndrome (a condition characterized by predisposition to a wide variety of malignancies).	Healthy.	Prone to developing a broad spectrum of cancers (29% developed tumors by 20 months of age) due to increased rate of somatic LOH.	Luo et al., 2000
Xeroderma pigmentosum group A gene (Xpa)	Involved in repairing DNA damage via the NER pathway.	Mutations in XPA cause the rare AR disease, xeroderma pigmentosum (XP). XP patients show an impaired ability to repair UV-induced DNA damage, and as a result have >1000-fold increased risk of developing UV-induced skin cancer.	Healthy.	Complete deficiency in NER. >1000-fold higher risk of developing UV-induced skin cancer.[c]	van Steeg et al., 2000

[a] Msh3$^{-/-}$ and Msh3$^{+/+}$ mice developed tumors late in life with a similar incidence (although some Msh3$^{-/-}$ mice developed GI tumors similar to those seen in Msh2$^{-/-}$, Mlh1$^{-/-}$, and Msh6$^{-/-}$ mice). However, the small number of tumors detected in these mice questions the role of Msh3 as a tumor suppressor (Edelmann et al., 2000). The DNA mismatch repair genes Msh3 and Msh6 cooperate in intestinal tumor suppression.

[b] Pms1$^{+/-}$ and Pms1$^{-/-}$ mice do not develop tumors (Prolla et al., 1998).

[c] Another member of the NER DNA repair family is XPC. However, while Xpc$^{-/-}$ mice show elevated mutation rates, this does not lead to an increased tumor incidence or premature aging as seen with Xpa$^{-/-}$ mice (Sands et al., 1995; Wijnhoven et al., 2000).

[d] ε = embryonic day.

TABLE 11-2B. Mouse Knockouts of Tumor Suppressor Genes Involved in Regulating the Cell Cycle and Apoptosis

Gene	Function	Mutations in the Gene in Humans	Heterozygous Mouse Phenotype	Homozygous Mouse Phenotype	References
Retinoblastoma gene (*Rb1*)	Plays an important role during the G1 phase of the cell cycle, as well as apoptosis, and is phosphorylated by cyclin-cyclin-dependent kinases (CDKs). Rb1 represses the transcription of genes required for DNA replication and cell division.	Mutations in one allele of *Rb1* have been found in both inherited and sporadic cases of retinoblastoma, as well as cases of osteosarcoma, prostate cancer, and breast cancer.	*Rb1*[+/−] mice develop pituitary gland tumors from 6 to 8 months on.	Die at ε12–15 (embryos show severe defects in central neurogenesis, fetal liver erythropoiesis, myogenesis, and lens development).	Clarke et al., 1992; Jacks et al., 1992; Lee et al., 1996
p53	A nuclear phosphoprotein that functions as a tumor suppressor by binding to DNA at specific sites (p53 activity is regulated by interactions with the E3 ligase, MDM2). p53 controls the G1 checkpoint of the cell cycle by inducing the transcription of the cyclin/CDK inhibitor, *p21*, and can induce apoptosis of a cell if its damaged DNA cannot be repaired.	*p53* is the most commonly mutated tumor suppressor gene in human cancers. Inherited p53 mutations are associated with Li-Fraumeni syndrome, characterized by an increased risk (50% chance by age 30) for breast and lung carcinomas, soft tissue sarcomas, brain tumors, osteosarcoma, and leukemia).	*p53*[+/−] mice are predisposed to tumorigenesis (tumor-free for the first 9 months, with 50% developing lymphomas, osteosarcomas, and soft tissue sarcomas by 18 months of age); comparable with that observed for Li-Fraumeni syndrome patients.	Viable (although a subset of p53-deficient embryos die in utero due to exencephaly). Show enhanced susceptibility to cancer, usually developing tumors before 6 months of age (mostly lymphomas, although sarcomas and testicular teratomas also develop), and die before 10 months of age.	Armstrong et al., 1995; Donehower et al., 1992; Jacks et al., 1994a; Liu et al., 2000; Purdie et al., 1994
Pten (aka *Mmac1* and *Tep1*)	A phosphatase and tensin homolog that functions by maintaining a low threshold of cellular PIP₃, antagonizing PI₃K signaling and	*PTEN* is commonly mutated in human cancers. Germ-line mutations cause the AD hamartoma disorders: Cowden disease,	Exhibit hallmark features of PTEN-associated human hamartoma syndromes: Young mice develop	Die at ε6.5–9.5 (embryos show poorly organized ectodermal and mesodermal layers, and overgrowth in the cephalic and caudal regions).	Di Cristofano et al., 1998, 2001; Stambolic et al., 2000; Suzuki et al., 1998, 2001

(continued)

T A B L E 11-2B (*continued*)

Gene	Function	Mutations in the Gene in Humans	Heterozygous Mouse Phenotype	Homozygous Mouse Phenotype	References
	activating the protein kinase, PKB/Akt.	Lhermitte-Duclos disease, Bannayan-Zonana syndrome (all show multiple benign tumors and increased susceptibility to breast, thyroid, and brain cancers).	thymic and peripheral lymphomas. Females develop mammary and endometrial neoplasias. Aged mice develop GIT hamartomas, prostate hyperplasias, adrenal gland neoplasias, and skin and colon hyperplasias and dysplasias.		
$p19^{ARF}$ (*ARF*)	The *INK4a* locus in mice encodes two independent but overlapping genes[a] $p16^{INK4a}$ and $p19^{ARF}$: $p16^{INK4a}$ is a CKI regulating the ability of Rb1 to control G_1 exit. $p19^{ARF}$ negatively regulates Mdm2 function and activates p53 in response to particular signals (induces apoptosis or cell cycle arrest).	The *Ink4a* locus is frequently mutated in human cancers. Germ-line mutations predispose individuals to familial melanomas, and sporadic mutations increase the chance of sporadic pancreatic and brain malignancies.	Develop lymphomas, sarcomas, and hemangiomas (although after a longer latency compared to $ARF^{-/-}$ mice).	Highly prone to tumor development (fibrosarcomas, lymphomas, and other rare tumors). 80% develop tumors and die within 1 year of age.	Kamijo et al., 1997, 1999
Lats1	A mammalian homolog of the *Drosophila* large tumor suppressor (LATS) gene, and is a serine-threonine kinase capable of modulating CDC2 activity.	No cancer has yet been associated with a *LATS1* mutation in humans.	Healthy.	Viable but underdeveloped. Develop ovarian tumors and soft tissue sarcomas.	St. John et al., 1999

p27^{Kip1}	A cyclin-CKI controlling cell cycle progression (blocks G$_1$ progression and S-phase entry).	Low expression is generally associated with increased tumor size and poor prognosis in cancer patients.	Healthy	Display a syndrome of multiorgan hyperplasia, including gigantism, female sterility, and tumorigenesis of the pituitary pars intermedia.	Fero et al., 1996
Fhit	A diadenosine polyphosphate hydrolase whose reintroduction causes programmed cell death and suppresses tumor formation in *fhit*-cells.	*Fhit* is inactivated early in epithelial tumor development, particularly in lung and other tissues in which tumors follow exposure to environmental carcinogens.	Increased cancer incidence. Increased susceptibility to carcinogen-induced sebaceous and gastric carcinomas. Oral gene transfer of viral vectors expressing the human *FHIT* gene into *Fhit*$^{+/-}$ mice inhibited tumor development.	Same as the heterozygotes.	Croce et al., 1999; Dumon et al., 2001; Fong et al., 2000; Ishii et al., 2001

^{a}Each gene has its own promoter followed by 3 exons; exon 1 is specific to each gene, whereas exons 2 and 3 are shared (although they are read in different frames).

TABLE 11-2C. Mouse Knockouts of Tumor Suppressor Genes Involved in Cell Signaling and Differentiation

Gene	Function	Mutations in the Gene in Humans	Heterozygous Mouse Phenotype	Homozygous Mouse Phenotype	References
Patched gene (ptc)	The human homolog of the Drosophila segment polarity gene, patched, PTC, controls cell growth and specification in the developing and postnatal tissues. PTC is a Sonic hedgehog (Shh) receptor.	PTC is mutated in individuals with Gorlin syndrome (or nevoid basal cell carcinoma). PTC+/− individuals show developmental and skeletal anomalies, and develop a variety of tumors including basal cell carcinoma and medulloblastoma. They also show radiation sensitivity.	Development of spontaneous cerebellar brain tumors, with 14% of CNS tumors in the posterior fossa by 10 months of age. Develop many of the features characteristic of Gorlin syndrome and exhibit a high incidence of rhabdomyosarcomas. Show increased incidence of radiation-induced teratogenesis.	Die at ε9.5–10.5 (show open and overgrown neural tubes).	Aszterbaum et al., 1999; Goodrich et al., 1997; Hahn et al., 1998; Wetmore et al., 2000
Nf1	Neurofibromin (the protein encoded by Nf1) is highly homologous to mammalian p120Ras GTPase-activating protein (GAP), known to regulate the GTP status of the protooncogene p21-Ras.	Germ-line mutations in Nf1 result in neurofibromatosis type 1 (NF1)—a common autosomal-dominant condition associated with benign peripheral nerve sheath tumors (neurofibromas) and predisposition to optic gliomas, astrocytomas, glioblastomas, pheochromocytomas, and myeloid leukemia.	Increased predisposition to pheochromocytoma and myeloid leukemia at 1 year of age. No development of the human hallmarks of neurofibromas.	Die at ε11–13.5 (due to heart defects and enlarged superior ganglia).	Branman et al., 1994; Jacks et al., 1994b
Nf2	Merlin (the protein encoded by Nf2) is a member of the 4.1 family of	Neurofibromatosis type 2 (NF2) is a rare, severe, inherited condition of humans, resulting in the	Develop a variety of highly metastatic tumors at 10–30 months of age	Die at ε6.5–7 (due to a failure to initiate gastrulation).	McClatchey et al., 1997, 1998

Gene				References
	cytoskeleton-associated proteins.	development of spinal tumors, meningioma, and vestibular schwannoma.	(including osteosarcoma, lymphoma, lung adenocarcinoma, hepatocellular carcinoma, and fibrosarcoma). This contrasts to narrow spectrum of benign tumors observed in human NF2 patients.	Takaku et al., 1998, 1999
Smad4	SMAD4 belongs to the SMAD gene family, which has key roles in regulating gene expression in the TGF-β1 signaling pathways. Activation of Smads causes their translocation from the cytoplasm to the nucleus, where they function as transcription factors.	Mutations in the SMAD4 (DPC4) gene are associated with pancreatic and colorectal cancer, as well as familial juvenile polyposis (an autosomal-dominant disease in which individuals are predisposed to inflammatory polyps and gastrointestinal cancer).	Fertile and appeared normal $\geq$ 1 year, although they had developed multiple gastric and duodenal polyps by 1.5–2 years of age. Although epithelium lining the polyp glands was mostly hyperplastic, showing little cellular atypia, foci with obvious dysplastic signs were also observed. Histopathology of the gastric and duodenal polyps in the Smad4$^{+/-}$ mice resembles human juvenile polyps.	Embryonic lethal.
Vhl	The VHL gene product (pVHL) forms multimeric protein	Germ-line mutations in the VHL gene in humans cause von Hippel–Lindau	Vhl$^{+/-}$ mice develop cavernous hemangiomas of the	Die at ε10.5–12.5 (due to a lack of placental vasculogenesis).	Gnarra et al., 1997; Haase et al., 2001

(continued)

T A B L E 11-2C (continued)

Gene	Function	Mutations in the Gene in Humans	Heterozygous Mouse Phenotype	Homozygous Mouse Phenotype	References
	complexes with Cullin-2, Rbx1, and elongins B and C, and has been shown to negatively regulate hypoxia response genes through ubiquitination of the α-subunit of hypoxia-inducible factor.	(VHL) syndrome, characterized by a dominantly inherited predisposition to develop highly angiogenic tumors.	liver (a rare manifestation of the human disease).		
Adenomatous polyposis coli gene (Apc)	The APC gene plays a major regulatory role in the Wnt signaling pathway by destabilizing β-catenin, thereby suppressing cell growth.	The majority of hereditary (such as adenomatous polyposis coli) and sporadic colorectal tumors show a loss of APC function.	Develop multiple intestinal neoplasia. Min (multiple intestinal neoplasia) is a mutant allele of the murine Apc locus (induced by ENU treatment), encoding a nonsense mutation at codon 850, and $Apc^{Min/+}$ mice are predisposed to intestinal and mammary tumors.	Die before $\varepsilon 8.0$.	Fodde et al., 1994; Moser et al., 1990, 1995; Oshima et al., 1995; Su et al., 1992
p110γ	The catalytic subunit of PI$_3$Kγ–a PI$_3$K, that regulates an array of fundamental cellular responses, such as proliferation, transformation, differentiation, and protection from apoptosis. PI$_3$K-mediated activation of the cell survival kinase PKB/Akt and negative regulation of PI$_3$K signaling by the PTEN TSG are key regulatory	In humans, p110γ protein expression is lost in primary colorectal adenocarcinomas from patients and in colon cancer cell lines.	Healthy.	Shorter life span than heterozygote mice. Older mice show increased incidence of premature death associated with progressive weight loss and the development of spontaneous, malignant epithelial tumors in the colorectum.	Sasaki et al., 2000

c-ski	An oncogene that affects cell growth and is involved in the regulation of muscle differentiation. c-Ski acts as a corepressor and binds to other corepressors (N-CoR/SMRT and mSin3A), which complex with HDAC.	No cancer has yet been associated with a c-SKI mutation in humans.	Increased susceptibility to tumorigenesis.	Decreased myofiber development in addition to abnormalities in pattern formation (such as defects in neuronal and craniofacial patterning).	Berk et al., 1997
CCAAT/enhancer-binding protein epsilon (C/EBPε)	A transcription factor preferentially expressed in granulocytes and lymphoid cells, and thought to play a role in myeloid development.	No cancer has yet been associated with an ATR mutation in humans.	Healthy.	Develop normally but fail to generate functional neutrophils and eosinophils. Die by 3–5 months of age due to opportunistic infections and tissue destruction. End-stage mice also show myelodysplasia.	Yamanaka et al., 1997
α-Inhibin	Important in the regulation of cell proliferation and differentiation in a variety of tissues. Inhibins are composed of two subunits derived from genes of the TGFβ superfamily.	Inhibin synthesis and secretion are prominent features of many ovarian tumors, particularly granulosa cell tumors and mucinous cystadenocarcinomas.	Healthy.	Infertile. Develop gonadal tumors (mixed or incompletely differentiated gonadal stromal tumors) within 4 weeks of age.	Matzuk et al., 1992
Cdx2	The human homolog of the Drosophila homeobox gene, caudal, which functions as a transcription factor.	CDX2 is expressed in intestinal epithelium and is markedly downregulated in colon tumors. While few CDX2 mutations predisposing to	Variable phenotype including tail abnormalities, stunted growth, and a homeotic shift of vertebrae.	Die between ε3.5 and 5.5.	Chawengsaksophak et al., 1997

(continued)

225

TABLE 11-2C (continued)

Gene	Function	Mutations in the Gene in Humans	Heterozygous Mouse Phenotype	Homozygous Mouse Phenotype	References
		sporadic colorectal cancer have been identified, it is agreed that loss of CDX2 contributes to the progression of some sporadic colorectal tumors.	Develop multiple intestinal tumors (most notably in the proximal colon) within 3 months of age.		
Lkb1 (Stk11)	A serine/threonine kinase.	Germ-line mutations of the LKB1 gene are associated with Peutz-Jeghers syndrome (PJS), characterized by mucocutaneous pigmentation and gastrointestinal hamartoma with an increased risk of cancer development.	Develop intestinal polyps identical to those seen in individuals affected with PJS. Develop hepatocellular carcinomas (with a sex difference in the susceptibility).	Die between ε8.5 and 9.5.	Bardeesy et al., 2002; Jishage et al., 2002; Miyoshi et al., 2002; Nakau et al., 2002

ε = embryonic day.

TABLE 11-3. Double Mutants: Mouse Knockouts of Two or More Tumor Suppressor Genes

Genes	Phenotype	References
Apc^{Min} and Blm	$Apc^{Min}/-$, $Blm^{-/-}$ mice develop significantly increased numbers of intestinal polyps compared to $Apc^{Min}/-$, $Blm^{+/-}$ mice (increased tumor formation in the absence of Blm is presumably due to the increased rate of somatic LOH).	Luo et al., 2000
Apc and $Msh6 \pm Msh3$	$Apc^{+/-}$, $Msh6^{-/-}$ mice show reduced survival and a 6–7-fold increase in intestinal tumor development. In contrast, $Apc^{+/-}$, $Msh3^{-/-}$ mice show no difference in survival and intestinal tumor development from $Apc^{+/-}$ mice. However, $Apc^{+/-}$, $Msh6^{-/-}$, $Msh3^{-/-}$ mice show a further decreased survival rate compared to $Apc^{+/-}$, $Msh6^{-/-}$ mice, due to an increased development of intestinal tumors at a younger age.	Kuraguchi et al., 2001
Apc and $Mlh1$	$Apc^{+/-}$, $Mlh1^{-/-}$ mice show a 40–100-fold increase in GIT tumor incidence compared to $Mlh1^{-/-}$.	Edelmann et al., 1999
Apc and $Pms2$	Whereas $Pms2^{-/-}$ mice do not develop intestinal tumors, $Apc^{+/-}$, $Pms2^{-/-}$ mice develop three times the number of small intestinal adenomas and four times the number of colon adenomas relative to $Apc^{+/-}$ and $Apc^{+/-}$, $Pms2^{+/-}$ mice.	Baker et al., 1998
Apc and $Smad4$	Mice heterozygous for $Smad4$ and Apc ($Apc^{+/-}$, $Smad4^{+/-}$) develop a greater number of intestinal polyps than $Apc^{+/-}$ mice.	Takaku et al., 1998; Taketo and Takaku, 2000
Apc and $Cox-2$	In the absence of cyclooxygenase 2, $Apc^{+/-}$ mice ($Apc^{+/-}$, $Cox-2^{-/-}$) develop intestinal polyps that are significantly smaller in size and fewer in number.	Oshima et al., 1996
$Rb1$ and $p107$	$Rb1^{+/-}$, $p107^{-/-}$ mice do not show any altered tumor predisposition when compared with $Rb1^{+/-}$ mice but develop multiple dysplastic lesions of the retina that are absent in $Rb1^{+/-}$ and $p107^{-/-}$ mice. $Rb1^{-/-}$, $p107^{-/-}$ mice develop retinoblastomas.	Lee et al., 1996; Robanus-Maandag et al., 1998
$Rb1$ and $p53$	$Rb1^{+/-}$, $p53^{-/-}$ mice show reduced viability and exhibit novel pathology including pinealoblastomas, islet cell tumors, bronchial epithelial hyperplasia, and retinal dysplasia.	Williams et al., 1994
$Rb1$ and $E2f1$	$Rb1^{+/-}$, $E2f1^{-/-}$ mice show a reduced frequency of pituitary and thyroid tumors compared to $Rb1^{+/-}$ mice, as well as a greatly lengthened life span. $Rb1^{-/-}$, $E2f1^{-/-}$ mice die at $\epsilon17$ (with anemia and defective skeletal muscle and lung development).	Tsai et al., 1998; Yamasaki et al., 1998
Atm and $Rag2$	$Atm^{-/-}$, $Rag2^{-/-}$ mice develop thymomas (although at a lower frequency than $Atm^{-/-}$ mice), as well as other nonthymic malignancies (in contrast to $Atm^{-/-}$ mice).	Petiniot et al., 2000
Atm and $p53$	$Atm^{-/-}$, $p53^{-/-}$ mice exhibit accelerated tumor formation compared to $Atm^{-/-}$ or $p53^{-/-}$ mice.	Westphal et al., 1997
$p53$ and Ptc	$Ptc^{+/-}$, $p53^{-/-}$ mice show a dramatic increase in the incidence and accelerated development (prior to 12 weeks of age) of medulloblastoma. No change in tumor incidence was observed in $Ptc^{+/-}$, $Apc^{Min}/-$ or in $Ptc^{+/-}$, $p19ARF^{-/-}$ mice.	Wetmore et al., 2001

(continued)

TABLE 11-3 (continued)

Genes	Phenotype	References
p53 and c-Myc	$p53^{-/-}$ mice expressing a transgene for human c-Myc (CD2-myc), $p53^{-/-}$/CD2-Myc were viable but developed thymic lymphomas with dramatically increased frequency and reduced latency compared to both parental groups. In contrast, no significant increase in tumor incidence was seen in $p53^{+/-}$/CD2-Myc mice compared to $p53^{+/+}$/CD2-Myc mice.	Blyth et al., 1995
p53 and Nf1	$Nf1^{+/-}, p53^{+/-}$ mice show a reduced life span and develop a range of astrocytoma stages, from low-grade astrocytoma to glioblastoma multiforme. This model mimics human secondary glioblastoma involving p53 loss.	Reilly et al., 2000
p53 and Terc	Telomere attrition in aging telomerase-deficient p53 mutant ($Terc^{-/-}, p53^{-/-}$) mice promotes the development of epithelial cancers (by fusion-bridge breakage, leading to the formation of complex nonreciprocal translocations).	Artandi et al., 2000
$p16^{INK4a}$ and $p19^{ARF}$ (Ink4a locus)	$INK4a^{-/-}, ARF^{+/-}$ mice (in which both $p16^{INK4a}$ and $p19^{ARF}$ are deficient due to deletion of their common exons) show a moderate increase in fibrosarcomas, lymphomas, squamous cell carcinomas, and angiosarcomas. $INK4a^{-/-}, ARF^{-/-}$ mice show an increased susceptibility to cancer, with most developing sarcomas and lymphomas by 7 months of age. However, these mice do not develop melanomas (as seen in humans with mutations in the Ink4a locus).	Orlow et al., 1999
$p16^{INK4a}, p19^{ARF},$ and H-Ras	$INK4a/AFRF^{-/-}$ mice overexpressing an activated human Ras ($H-Ras^{G12V}$) gene in melanocytes develop cutaneous melanomas with high penetrance by 5.5 months of age (not seen in $INK4a/AFRF^{ex2-3-/-}$ mice).	Chin et al., 1997
$p16^{INK4a}, p19^{ARF},$ and Pten	Compared with $Pten^{+/-}$ mice, $Ink4a/Arf^{+/-}, Pten^{+/-}$ and $Ink4a/Arf^{-/-}, Pten^{+/-}$ mice presented with a much earlier onset of endometrial atypical hyperplasia, a condition considered to be a precursor of endometrial carcinoma.	You et al., 2002
Msh3 and Msh6	$Msh3^{-/-}, Msh6^{-/-}$ mice showed tumor development at a much younger age, as well as increased tumor development (predominantly gastrointestinal or lymphoid [non-Hodgkin's] in origin), compared to $Msh3^{-/-}$ or $Msh6^{-/-}$ mice.	de Wind et al., 1999; Edelmann et al., 2000
Pten and Cdkn1b	$Pten^{+/-}, Cdkn1b^{-/-}$ accelerates spontaneous neoplastic transformation and the incidence of tumors of various histological origins. More specifically, these mice develop prostate carcinoma at complete penetrance by 3 months of age (which mimics the time course and pathological features of human prostate cancer).	Di Cristofano et al., 2001

TABLE 11-4. Tumor Suppressor Gene Mouse Knockouts Showing Increased Sensitivity (Tumor Incidence) to Carcinogens

Gene	Carcinogen	Resulting Phenotype	References
Fhit	Chemical	$Fhit^{+/-}$ and $Fhit^{-/-}$ mice are highly susceptible to tumor induction by N–nitrosomethylbenzylamine (78–89% exhibited forestomach and squamocolumnar junction tumors, versus 7% of $Fhit^{+/+}$ controls).	Fong et al., 2000; Zanesi et al., 2001
Msh2	Chemical	$Msh2^{-/-}$ mice succumb to lymphomas at an early age; however, lymphomagenesis can be synergistically enhanced by exposure to ENU.	de Wind et al., 1998
Xpa	Chemical and radiation	$Xpa^{-/-}$ mice develop intestinal tumors when they are exposed to UV-B, benzo[a]pyrene or 2-aceto-amino-fluorene.	van Steeg et al., 2000
Atm	Radiation	$Atm^{+/-}$ and $Atm^{-/-}$ mice show increased sensitivity to sublethal doses of γ-irradiation (displaying decreased survival and premature hair graying, similar to AT patient radiosensitivity).	Barlow et al., 1996
Nbs	Radiation	$Nbs1^{m/m}$ mice die within 10 days after irradiation, whereas most $Nbs1^{+/+}$ mice are viable for at least 2 months after irradiation.	Kang et al., 2002
p53	Chemical and radiation	$p53^{-/-}$ mice are also extremely susceptible to ionizing radiation or chemical carcinogen (dimethylnitrosamine)-induced tumorigenesis.	Harvey et al., 1993; Kemp et al., 1994 Qin et al., 1999, 2000
Pms2	Chemical	$Pms2^{-/-}$ mice show increased susceptibility to ENU-induced thymic lymphomas. $Pms2^{+/-}$ mice show increased susceptibility to ENU-induced intestinal tumors.	
p27	Chemical and radiation	$p27^{+/-}$ and $p27^{-/-}$ mice are predisposed to tumors in multiple tissues when treated with γ-irradiation or a chemical carcinogen (whereas untreated mice only develop tumors of pituitary origin).	Fero et al., 1998
INK4a/ARF	Chemical and radiation	$INK4a/ARF^{ex2-3+/-}$ mice treated with DMBA or UV-B show an earlier onset of cancer susceptibility (mostly sarcomas and lymphomas) compared to untreated $INK4a/ARF^{ex2-3+/-}$ mice.	Orlow et al., 1999

229

single-knockout mice (de Wind et al., 1999; Edelmann et al., 2000). Table 11-3 includes more examples of MMR double-knockout mice.

Brca2 and Breast Cancer. As discussed in Chapter 6, germ-line alterations of the breast cancer susceptibility genes *BRCA1* or *BRCA2* result in susceptibility to breast and ovarian cancer, and account for about 10% of familial breast cancer cases and about 1.5–2.0% of all breast cancer cases (Venkitaraman, 2002). The cellular function of BRCA2 is not fully resolved, but there is evidence to support roles in transcriptional transactivation and DNA repair (Milner et al., 1997; Sharan et al., 1997). Contrary to expectation, $Brca2^{+/-}$ mice do not show a tumor predisposition (Ludwig et al., 1997; Sharan et al., 1997; Suzuki et al., 1997). Although most homozygous mutations in the *Brca2* gene are embryonic lethal (Friedman et al., 1998; Ludwig et al., 1997; Sharan et al., 1997; Suzuki et al., 1997), some $Brca2^{-/-}$ mutants survive to adulthood (Connor et al., 1997; Friedman et al., 1998). These mice show a range of defects, depending on the allele, including abnormal tissue differentiation, a lack of germ cells, development of lethal thymic lymphomas, significantly increased overall tumor incidence, and decreased survival compared with their heterozygous littermates (Connor et al., 1997; McAllister et al., 2002). However, mammary gland tumors have not been observed in *Brca2* knockout mice, in direct contrast to the human pathology.

Brca2 conditional knockout mice carrying a Cre transgene driven by the *whey acidic protein* promoter (*WAP-Cre*) are tumor prone. The tumors arising in these mice appear to have lost both *Brca2* alleles, exhibit aneuploidy and structural chromosomal aberrations, and carry mutations in *p53* (Ludwig et al., 2001). An elegant co-conditional model using both *Brca2* ($Brca2^{F11}$) and *p53* ($p53^{F2-10}$) conditional alleles has been described by Jonkers et al. Conditional *p53* should accelerate tumorigenesis while circumventing the nonepithelial tumor burden that *p53* null mice develop at an early age. An epithelial-specific *K14* promoter was used to drive Cre expression, to inactivate both conditional alleles in normal and mammary gland epithelia. Skin and breast tumors developed in these mice. The absence of tumors in other tissues where *K14-Cre* is expressed (thymus, esophagus, etc.) suggested that the effects of *p53* and *Brca2* were most important in skin and mammary gland epithelium. The study was one of the first to use a model carrying two conditional knockouts and showed that mutations in mouse *Brca2* can induce a human tumor spectrum but that inactivation of *p53* is necessary for *Brca2*-related tumorigenesis (Jonkers et al., 2001).

Cell Cycle and Apoptosis Genes

Rb1: Models of Familial Retinoblastoma. RB1 is phosphorylated by cyclin-dependent kinases (CDKs) and plays important roles during the G_1 phase of the cell cycle and in apoptosis by repressing transcription of genes required for DNA replication and cell division. Mutations in *RB1* have been found in both inherited and sporadic cases of retinoblastoma (a childhood malignancy of the retina), as well as in osteosarcomas, prostate, and breast cancers (reviewed in Zheng and Lee, 2001). Mice carrying mutant *Rb1* alleles are cancer prone, but they do not accurately mimic the human phenotype: $Rb1^{+/-}$ mice develop pituitary gland tumors from 6 to 8 months of age, and $Rb1^{-/-}$ mice die between embryonic days 13.5 and 15.5, although the developing retina appears normal (Clarke et al., 1992; Jacks et al., 1992; Lee et al., 1992). As other members of the Rb family can compensate for the loss of Rb1 in the murine eye, mice have been generated with various combinations of inactivated genes, such as $p107$ (an Rb-related nuclear phosphoprotein) and $p53$. $Rb1^{+/-}$, $p107^{-/-}$ mice do not show any altered tumor predisposition when compared with $Rb1^{+/-}$ mice but develop multiple dysplastic lesions of the retina that are not found in $Rb1^{+/-}$ or $p107^{-/-}$ mice (Lee et al., 1996). $Rb^{-/-}$, $p107^{-/-}$ chimeric mice develop retinoblastoma (Robanus-Maandag et al., 1998), while $Rb1^{+/-}$, $p53^{-/-}$ mice show reduced viability and exhibit pinealoblastomas, islet cell tumors, bronchial epithelial hyperplasia, and retinal dysplasia (Williams et al., 1994).

Two groups have constructed conditional alleles of $Rb1$ to circumvent $Rb1^{-/-}$ embryonic lethality. Vooijs et al. chose to use the Flp/frt recombinase system and a $POMC$-Flp (pituitary-specific promoter) mouse line. $Rb1^{frt/frt}$, $POMC$-Cre mice died rapidly from pituitary tumors, depending on the Flp line used. $Rb1^{frt/+}$, $POMC$-Cre mice had an average tumor latency of 9 months, this being comparable to that of $Rb1$ heterozygotes (Jacks et al., 1992). $Rb1$ inactivation appeared to be an early causative event in tumor formation, as it was inactivated in early hyperplastic areas. Thus, the Flp/frt system can be as effective and efficient as Cre/$loxP$ in generating conditional knockouts (Vooijs et al., 1998).

A co-conditional $p53$/$Rb1$ model was generated by a group interested in looking at glial differentiation and transformation. Conditional $loxP$ alleles were deleted using $GFAP$-Cre, which was believed to be primarily restricted to astroglia but was also active in extra granular layers (EGL) in the cerebellum. Glial tumors were not observed, but all of the $GFAP$-Cre, $Rb1^{loxP/loxP}$, $p53^{loxP/loxP}$ mutant mice developed medulloblastomas (highly aggressive tumors of the embryoid cerebellum) and died by 3–4 months of age. By 16 months of age, 75% of the $GFAP$-Cre, $Rb1^{loxP/+}$, $p53^{loxP/loxP}$ mice had also died of medulloblastomas. All tumors analyzed clearly showed EGL derivation and had undergone recombination of the conditional $Rb1$ and lost the wild-type $Rb1$ allele (Marino et al., 2000). Thus, the combination of Cre lines with conditional tumor suppressor alleles is facilitating the development of new and better tumor models.

p53: The Most Commonly Mutated TSG.   p53, the most commonly mutated TSG in human cancers, is a nuclear phosphoprotein that functions by binding DNA at specific sites and is regulated by interactions with MDM2, an E3 ubiquitin ligase (reviewed in Guimaraes and Hainaut, 2002). p53 controls the G_1 checkpoint of the cell cycle by inducing the transcription of the cyclin/CDK inhibitor $p21$ and can induce apoptosis of a cell if its damaged DNA cannot be repaired. Mice bearing null mutations of $p53$ are viable (Donehower et al., 1992), although a subset of $p53$-deficient embryos die _in utero_ due to exencephaly (Armstrong et al., 1995; Sah et al., 1995), with 75% developing tumors before 6 months of age and 100% dying before 10 months of age. A $p53^{-/-}$ background can dramatically affect the tumor frequency and latency in TSG mutant mice. In addition to the $Brca2^{+/-}$ example we discussed, this background has been shown to accelerate tumor formation in $Atm^{-/-}$ mice (Westphal et al., 1997), $ptc^{+/-}$ mice (Wetmore et al., 2001), aging telomerase-deficient mice ($Terc^{-/-}$; Artandi et al., 2000), and mice expressing a transgene for human c-MYC ($CD2$-MYC; Blyth et al., 1995). More information can be found in Table 11-3. $p53^{-/-}$ mice are also extremely susceptible to ionizing radiation- or chemical carcinogen- induced tumorigenesis (see Table 11-4).

In humans, inherited $p53$ mutations are associated with Li-Fraumeni syndrome, characterized by an increased risk of breast and lung carcinomas, soft tissue sarcomas, brain tumors, osteosarcoma, and leukemia (reviewed in Malkin, 1994). The spectrum and time line for development of tumors in $p53^{+/-}$ mice is generally similar to that seen in Li-Fraumeni syndrome patients: Mice are tumor-free for the first 9 months, but 50% develop osteosarcomas, soft tissue sarcomas, and lymphomas by 18 months of age (Donehower et al., 1992; Jacks et al., 1994a; Purdie et al., 1994). Different genetic backgrounds affect tumorigenesis differently—for example, testicular tumors are elevated on the 129 background (Donehower et al., 1992), and mammary tumors are seen in 50% of the females on the BALB/c background (Kuperwasser et al., 2000). Similar strain-dependent phenotypes occur in mice lacking *Rb1*-related genes. Myeloid hyperplasia, growth deficiency, and accelerated cell cycle are seen in $p107^{-/-}$ mice on a BALB/cJ background, while $p107^{-/-}$ mice on the C57BL/6J background are normal (LeCouter et al., 1998). For more information on the genetics and genomics of modifier genes, see Chapter 12.

RNAi—in which a small double-stranded RNA carrying homology to an endogenous gene induces silencing of the endogenous gene—has been used to mimic loss of p53 function in vivo without complete loss of the *p53* gene (see Shi, 2003, for a review of RNAi in mammalian systems). Three short hairpin RNAs (shRNAs) targeted against *p53* were introduced into retroviral vectors (Hemann et al., 2003). Infection of cultured cells with these constructs resulted in suppression of *p53* expression to varying degrees. The constructs were tested in vivo using a $E\mu$-*myc* transgenic mouse line; mice carrying this oncogene develop B-cell lymphomas by 6 months of age (Adams et al., 1985). $E\mu$-*myc* transgenic mice on a $p53^{+/-}$ background have accelerated tumorigenesis, and resultant tumors always lose the wild-type copy of *p53* (Schmitt et al., 1999). The retroviral shRNA vectors were used to infect $p53^{+/-}$, $E\mu$-*myc* hematapoetic stem cells (HSCs). Infected HSCs were injected into lethally irradiated recipient mice, and tumorigenic latency was assessed.

Analysis indicated that the greater the suppression of *p53* by the shRNA, the shorter the tumor latency in mice carrying that construct. The inclusion of a *GFP* gene in the retroviral vectors meant tumor progression could be followed in vivo as discussed later in this chapter. Interestingly, many of the shRNA tumors were still $p53^{+/-}$, indicating that suppression of *p53* expression by RNAi is sufficient to mimic LOH of *p53*. However, while these $p53^{+/-}$ tumors were deficient in apoptosis, they did not show other phenotypes, such as aneuploidy, common to $p53^{-/-}$ tumors. An earlier study, in which *Bcl* or a dominant-negative *caspase 9* (apoptosis-related genes downstream of *p53*) were introduced into $p53^{+/-}$, $E\mu$-*myc* HSCs by retroviral infection, produced similar results and also utilized GFP for bioimaging of resultant tumors (Schmitt et al., 2002).

TSGs Involved in Signaling and Differentiation

APC: Models of Colorectal Cancer. The human *APC* gene product plays a major regulatory role in the Wnt signaling pathway. *APC* can facilitate the destabilization of ß-catenin, a protein involved in cell adhesion and signal transduction (Polakis, 1997; Willert and Nusse, 1998). Germ-line losses in *APC* lead to familial adenomatous polyposis (FAP), an autosomal dominant syndrome that imparts a predisposition to colorectal cancer (Groden et al., 1991), and somatic mutations have been found in sporadic cases of colorectal cancers (Powell et al., 1992) and a subset of

HNPCC-derived tumors (Huang et al., 1996; Konishi et al., 1996). Several mouse *Apc* models have been established, the first of which was the Min (multiple intestinal neoplasia) mouse, which carries an ENU-derived nonsense mutation at codon 850. $Apc^{Min/+}$ mice are predisposed to intestinal and mammary tumors (Moser et al., 1990; Su et al., 1992). Polyp multiplicity in Min mice is greatly influenced by genetic background and the *Mom1* (*Modifier of Min 1*) modifier locus on mouse chromosome 4 (Dietrich et al., 1993; Moser et al., 1992)—a semidominant modifier of polyp size and multiplicity (Gould and Dove, 1997) that encodes the *secretory type II phospholipase A₂* (*Pla2g2a*) gene (MacPhee et al., 1995). A second modifier locus, *Modifier of Min 2* (*Mom2*), has been identified on mouse chromosome 18 (Silverman et al., 2002). *Mom2* acts in a dominant fashion and has stronger effects on reducing polyp multiplicity than the *Mom1* gene product. Chapter 12 covers modifier screens on the *Min* mouse.

Gene targeting techniques have also been used to generate $Apc^{+/-}$ mice, which develop multiple intestinal neoplasias. $Apc^{-/-}$ mice die early in embryogenesis (Fodde et al., 1994; Moser et al., 1995; Oshima et al., 1995). A hypomorphic mutation of the *Apc* allele in which only the N-terminal 1638 amino acids are expressed (Apc^{1638T}) results in mice that are growth retarded but do not have an increased incidence of tumors ($Apc^{1638T/1638T}$; Smits et al., 1999). The tumorigenesis of *Apc*-heterozygous mice can be modified by mutations in MMR genes, including *Msh6, Mlh1, Pms2*, and the colorectal TSG, *Smad4*. For example, $Apc^{+/-}$, $Msh6^{-/-}$ mice show reduced survival and a six- to seven-fold increase in intestinal tumor development, while $Apc^{+/-}$, $Msh6^{-/-}$, $Msh3^{-/-}$ mice show a further decreased survival rate compared to $Apc^{+/-}$, $Msh6^{-/-}$ mice, due to an increased development of intestinal tumors at a younger age (Kuraguchi et al., 2001). Further examples are detailed in Table 11-3.

Although most of the *Apc* alleles have provided excellent models for intestinal adenomas, these mice succumb at a young age to a large tumor burden in the small intestine, precluding the study of colon tumorigenesis, which is more common in human FAP (Moser et al., 1990; Su et al., 1992). Shibata et al. have generated an *Apc* conditional mutant mouse to study early events in colonic adenoma formation. Mice carrying a floxed allele were treated with adenoviral Cre introduced by colonic injection. At 3 months of age, 80% of the $Apc^{c/c}$ mice had many colonic adenomas, and, as expected, all tumors exhibited two recombined alleles of *Apc* (Shibata et al., 1997).

Nf2: A Model of Familial Neurofibromatosis. Neurofibromatosis type 2 (NF2) is a familial dominant disorder characterized in humans by schwannomas and meningiomas caused by a germ-line mutation in one copy of *NF2*. *NF2* mutations are also found in sporadic schwannomas. While $Nf2^{+/-}$ mice are cancer prone, they exhibit osteosarcomas and hepatocellular carcinomas at an advanced age, and null mutants die in early embryogenesis. These mice were useful in proving that *Nf2* acts as a typical tumor suppressor, but they do not accurately model the human condition (McClatchey et al., 1997, 1998); thus, a conditional mutant allele and a recombinase line in which Cre is driven by the Schwann cell–specific rat *P0* promoter were generated (Giovannini et al., 2000). This was used in conjunction with two mutant alleles mimicking common mutations in human NF2 families. $Nf2^{c/-}$, *P0*-Cre mice died before weaning due to craniofacial abnormalities, lack of molar eruption, and severe otitis media. $Nf2^{c/c}$, *P0-Cre* mice developed schwannomas after 10 months of age. All tumors that were checked had lost both copies of the floxed region.

ANALYSIS OF MOUSE CANCER MODELS

DNA Copy Number Changes and Rearrangements

Genetic changes in tumors have been examined with ever finer resolution as molecular information about the genome has grown increasingly dense. At a primary level, tumors have been examined for cytogenetically visible changes, but this is not an ideal method for mouse chromosomes, which are quite similar in size and banding patterns. Basic cytogenetic profiles have been improved upon with the development of spectral karyotyping (SKY). In this technique, each chromosome is "painted" with a differently colored tag. This enables the detection of chromosome translocations, deletions, and duplications associated with the development of tumors in mice (Liyanage et al., 1996; Schrock et al., 1996). For example, multiple chromosome aberrations, including a constant rearrangement on chromosome 14 at the T-cell receptor α/δ locus, were revealed in thymic lymphomas from $Atm^{-/-}$ mice (Liyanage et al., 2000). In addition, tumors from c-Myc transgenic mice analyzed using SKY demonstrated chromosomal alterations (McCormack et al., 1998; Weaver et al., 1999), and a chromosome 2 deletion was predominant in APL transgenic mice (Zimonjic et al., 2000). While SKY analysis is useful for screening chromosomal rearrangements, the requirement for metaphase chromosome preparations from tumor tissue makes it unsuitable for general application, and the genetic resolution still remains at the cytogenetic level.

In human malignancies, a change in gene dosage caused by deletions and amplifications contributes to the process of tumorigenesis by inactivating TSGs or activating protooncogenes. The technique of comparative genomic hybridization (CGH) was developed to circumvent the problem of obtaining metaphase spreads from solid tumors (Kallioniemi et al., 1992) and is discussed extensively in Chapter 3. In this method, genomic DNA from tumor and normal tissues are labeled with different fluorochromes and cohybridized to normal metaphase chromosomes. Changes in the ratio of the fluorescent signals reflect changes in DNA copy number. The CGH approach has been used to screen changes in DNA copy number in several transgenic mouse models (Shi et al., 1997; Wu et al., 2002). CGH on metaphase chromosomes, however, has only cytogenetic resolution, which cannot detect small changes. Hybridization of genomic DNA isolated from a tumor to an array of mapped genomic DNA, spotted onto glass slides, greatly improves the mapping resolution (Cai et al., 2002; Hodgson et al., 2001; Pinkel et al., 1998; Pollack et al., 1999; Schrock et al., 1996; Solinas-Toldo et al., 1997).

Loss of heterozygosity can also be detected using simple sequence-length polymorphism (SSLP) markers, though this is not as high-throughput as CGH analysis. Genome-wide screening of changes in DNA copy number using SSLP markers has thus not been widely reported but has been used for fine physical mapping of LOH in tumors in certain mouse models (Luo et al., 2000), or used in conjunction with other genome-wide tools (Cai et al., 2002; Hodgson et al., 2001).

Differences in Gene Expression

Expression profiles are molecular signatures that are unique to each tumor (see Chapters 5 and 6 and Resor et al., 2001 for a specific discussion of arrays in murine cancer). Using microarrays, the intensity ratio of fluorescent signals—and thus the corresponding levels of gene expression—from tumor and normal cDNA can be simultaneously defined for thousands of genes. This technique has been applied to identify genetic markers that might predict prognosis or responsiveness of a tumor to chemotherapeutic agents in mice and humans. For example, metastasis- or invasion-associated differences in gene expression profiles have been assessed in osteosarcoma, squamous carcinoma, and lung cancer tumor models (Chen et al., 2001; Dong et al., 2001; Khanna et al., 2001). Genes related to cell growth, apoptosis, angiogenesis, cell adherence, the cytoskeleton, and signal transduction pathways have been shown to be expressed differentially in metastatic or invasive tumor tissues.

Microarray technology has also been used to profile gene expression changes following treatment with antineoplastic drugs or hormonal therapy in mice with tumor cell xenografts (Amler et al., 2000; Zembutsu et al., 2002). Although the technology is very powerful, microarray profiles reveal many changes between tumors and normal tissues—or even between different stages of tumor development—and many of these differences will reflect secondary or tertiary changes that are often quite different from one tumor to the next. It should be stressed that while most of the differentially expressed genes are not primarily causal in transformation, they can be excellent markers. Transgenic and knockout models provide a consistent genetic background with which to perform transcriptional profiling because tumors can be carefully staged and the primary genetic lesions are known.

Bioimaging

Although sensitive and reliable in vitro genome-wide screening tools have been developed, in vitro analysis has some limitations. Since only a selected part of the whole tumor is evaluated, it gives temporal but not real-time information. In addition, tissue sampling is usually invasive, and analysis procedures take time. Imaging the dynamic real-time process of tumor development in living mice is a sensitive and noninvasive way to study the mechanisms of tumor development. Several bioimaging strategies have been developed. These include nuclear imaging methods such as computerized tomography (CT), nuclear magnetic resonance imaging (MRI), positron emission tomography (PET), single-photon emission computed tomography (SPECT), bioluminescent imaging, and near-infrared fluorescence probe imaging (reviewed in Weissleder, 2002; Weissleder et al., 1999).

Although nuclear imaging yields high-resolution tumor images, the application of this approach requires expensive equipment and an experienced operator. Bioluminescent imaging has attracted attention as a sensitive, inexpensive, and rapid imaging method for evaluating tumors. Expression of a bioluminescent substrate such as firefly luciferase or *GFP* as a reporter in growing transformed cells reveals dynamic features of neoplasias in vivo (Contag et al., 2000; Edinger et al., 1999). The luciferase strategy has been applied in real-time whole-body tumor imaging because an external light source is not required for emission of a signal from the luciferase-expressing tumor cells, and some of the emitted light can be detected through body tissues. Efficient assessment of the response to anticancer chemotherapy using bioluminescent imaging has been applied to orthotopic tumor models (Rehemtulla et al., 2000;

Sweeney et al., 1999). Luciferase-expressing sporadic tumors from conditional *Rb1* knockout mice were monitored by bioluminescent imaging (Vooijs et al., 2002). This study showed that efficient monitoring of chemoresponsiveness is possible. This strategy was reported to be sensitive enough to detect even a small number of early-stage marrow micrometastases (Wetterwald et al., 2002).

Photon signal penetration from luciferase-expressing cells makes this approach possible for whole-body imaging. However, luciferase activity requires the exogenous delivery of the substrate luciferin. An alternative method for real-time optical imaging is to express *GFP* in tumors and to monitor the fluorescence externally using a fluorescent stereomicroscope or a fluorescence light box (Hoffman, 2001). The sensitivity of this technique allows for single-cell resolution of tumor tissue. Quantification of metastases in prostate, lung, and pancreatic carcinomas has revealed extensive metastasis in liver, skeleton, lung, and the gastrointestinal tract (Bouvet et al., 2002; Maeda et al., 2000; Yang et al., 1998, 1999, 2000, 2002). These bioimaging studies have contributed to the understanding of the dynamic physiology of tumor cell growth and metastasis and allow for early detection of microinvasions in vivo. Bioimaging in mouse models is a powerful tool for the quantitative real-time monitoring of the response to chemotherapeutics.

CONCLUSION AND PERSPECTIVES

Since the 1980s, there has been an enormous change in the development of mouse models of cancer. Hundreds of different models have been developed by numerous laboratories. Most of these models are designed to replicate the molecular lesions in genes that are mutated or aberrantly expressed in human tumors. These models have gradually increased in their sophistication. In their earliest form, massive overexpression of potent oncogenes was used, but gradually these models have evolved to recapitulate the process of neoplastic transformation more realistically. Mutant oncogene(s) can be turned on and tumor suppressor gene(s) can be turned off in just a few cells in specific tissues, generating premalignant cells in a normal tissue environment and thereby replicating early stages of the genetic cascades that are responsible for cancer.

Although in their earliest form these models were crude representations of cancer as a disease, analysis of the molecular changes in the tumors that arise in these strains has begun to reveal some of the underlying mechanisms as well as collaborations between genes that drive tumorigenesis. Moreover, mouse models have begun to reveal mechanistic insights into many genes involved in human cancers that were not apparent when the genes were first identified. These insights have often come from analysis of developmental defects in knockouts as well as studies on cell lines isolated from these strains.

The ability to regulate timing and tissue specificity of specific genetic events in inbred mice is yielding uniform, controllable, and physiologically appropriate tumor development. In turn, these tumors are providing fertile ground for further genetic analyses facilitated by our increasingly detailed knowledge of the mouse and human genomes. Thus, models are no longer just models but research systems that provide foundations for discovery of novel genes and mechanisms. These discoveries can be tested and modeled in next-generation mice, completing a virtuous cycle of discovery that will drive oncogenomics for many years.

ACKNOWLEDGMENTS

Work in the Bradley laboratory is supported by The Wellcome Trust. D. M. Thompson was a Howard Hughes Medical Institute Predoctoral Fellow. L. van der Weyden was a C. J. Martin/R. G. Menzies Fellow of the Australian Medical Research Council.

REFERENCES

Adams, J. M., Harris, A. W., Pinkert, C. A., Corcoran, L. M., Alexander, W. S., Cory, S., Palmiter, R. D., and Brinster, R. L. (1985). The c-myc oncogene driven by immunoglobulin enhancers induces lymphoid malignancy in transgenic mice. *Nature 318*, 533–538.

Amler, L. C., Agus, D. B., LeDuc, C., Sapinoso, M. L., Fox, W. D., Kern, S., Lee, D., Wang, V., Leysens, M., Higgins, B., et al. (2000). Dysregulated expression of androgen-responsive and nonresponsive genes in the androgen-independent prostate cancer xenograft model CWR22-R1. *Cancer Res 60*, 6134–6141.

Andrechek, E. R., Hardy, W. R., Siegel, P. M., Rudnicki, M. A., Cardiff, R. D., and Muller, W. J. (2000). Amplification of the neu/erbB-2 oncogene in a mouse model of mammary tumorigenesis. *Proc Natl Acad Sci USA 97*, 3444–3449.

Anton, M., and Graham, F. L. (1995). Site-specific recombination mediated by an adenovirus vector expressing the Cre recombinase protein: A molecular switch for control of gene expression. *J Virol 69*, 4600–4606.

Arbeit, J. M., Munger, K., Howley, P. M., and Hanahan, D. (1993). Neuroepithelial carcinomas in mice transgenic with human papillomavirus type 16 E6/E7 ORFs. *Am J Pathol 142*, 1187–1197.

Arbeit, J. M., Munger, K., Howley, P. M., and Hanahan, D. (1994). Progressive squamous epithelial neoplasia in K14-human papillomavirus type 16 transgenic mice. *J Virol 68*, 4358–4368.

Arbeit, J. M., Howley, P. M., and Hanahan, D. (1996). Chronic estrogen-induced cervical and vaginal squamous carcinogenesis in human papillomavirus type 16 transgenic mice. *Proc Natl Acad Sci USA 93*, 2930–2935.

Armstrong, J. F., Kaufman, M. H., Harrison, D. J., and Clarke, A. R. (1995). High-frequency developmental abnormalities in p53-deficient mice. *Curr Biol 5*, 931–936.

Artandi, S. E., Chang, S., Lee, S. L., Alson, S., Gottlieb, G. J., Chin, L., and DePinho, R. A. (2000). Telomere dysfunction promotes non-reciprocal translocations and epithelial cancers in mice. *Nature 406*, 641–645.

Aszterbaum, M., Epstein, J., Oro, A., Douglas, V., LeBoit, P. E., Scott, M. P., and Epstein, E. H., Jr. (1999). Ultraviolet and ionizing radiation enhance the growth of BCCs and trichoblastomas in patched heterozygous knockout mice. *Nat Med 5*, 1285–1291.

Baker, S. M., Plug, A. W., Prolla, T. A., Bronner, C. E., Harris, A. C., Yao, X., Christie, D. M., Monell, C., Arnheim, N., Bradley, A., et al. (1996). Involvement of mouse Mlh1 in DNA mismatch repair and meiotic crossing over. *Nat Genet 13*, 336–342.

Baker, S. M., Harris, A. C., Tsao, J. L., Flath, T. J., Bronner, C. E., Gordon, M., Shibata, D., and Liskay, R. M. (1998). Enhanced intestinal adenomatous polyp formation in Pms2−/−; Min mice. *Cancer Res 58*, 1087–1089.

Bardeesy, N., Sinha, M., Hezel, A. F., Signoretti, S., Hathaway, N. A., Sharpless, N. E., Loda, M., Carrasco, D. R., and DePinho, R. A. (2002). Loss of the Lkb1 tumour suppressor provokes intestinal polyposis but resistance to transformation. *Nature 419*, 162–167.

Bargmann, C. I., and Weinberg, R. A. (1988). Increased tyrosine kinase activity associated with the protein encoded by the activated neu oncogene. *Proc Natl Acad Sci USA 85*, 5394–5398.

Barlow, C., Hirotsune, S., Paylor, R., Liyanage, M., Eckhaus, M., Collins, F., Shiloh, Y., Crawley, J. N., Ried, T., Tagle, D., and Wynshaw-Boris, A. (1996). Atm-deficient mice: A paradigm of ataxia telangiectasia. *Cell 86*, 159–171.

Baron, U., and Bujard, H. (2000). Tet repressor–based system for regulated gene expression in eukaryotic cells: Principles and advances. *Methods Enzymol 327*, 401–421.

Berk, M., Desai, S. Y., Heyman, H. C., and Colmenares, C. (1997). Mice lacking the ski protooncogene have defects in neurulation, craniofacial, patterning, and skeletal muscle development. *Genes Dev 11*, 2029–2039.

Blyth, K., Terry, A., O'Hara, M., Baxter, E. W., Campbell, M., Stewart, M., Donehower, L. A., Onions, D. E., Neil, J. C., and Cameron, E. R. (1995). Synergy between a human c-myc transgene and p53 null genotype in murine thymic lymphomas: Contrasting effects of homozygous and heterozygous p53 loss. *Oncogene 10*, 1717–1723.

Blyth, K., Stewart, M., Bell, M., James, C., Evan, G., Neil, J. C., and Cameron, E. R. (2000). Sensitivity to myc-induced apoptosis is retained in spontaneous and transplanted lymphomas of CD2-mycER mice. *Oncogene 19*, 773–782.

Bouchard, L., Lamarre, L., Tremblay, P. J., and Jolicoeur, P. (1989). Stochastic appearance of mammary tumors in transgenic mice carrying the MMTV/c-neu oncogene. *Cell 57*, 931–936.

Bouvet, M., Wang, J., Nardin, S. R., Nassirpour, R., Yang, M., Baranov, E., Jiang, P., Moossa, A. R., and Hoffman, R. M. (2002). Real-time optical imaging of primary tumor growth and multiple metastatic events in a pancreatic cancer orthotopic model. *Cancer Res 62*, 1534–1540.

Brannan, C. I., Perkins, A. S., Vogel, K. S., Ratner, N., Nordlund, M. L., Reid, S. W., Buchberg, A. M., Jenkins, N. A., Parada, L. F., and Copeland, N. G. (1994). Targeted disruption of the neurofibromatosis type-1 gene leads to developmental abnormalities in heart and various neural crest–derived tissues. *Genes Dev 8*, 1019–1029.

Brodie, S. G., and Deng, C. X. (2001). BRCA1-associated tumorigenesis: What have we learned from knockout mice? *Trends Genet 17*, S18–22.

Bronner, C. E., Baker, S. M., Morrison, P. T., Warren, G., Smith, L. G., Lescoe, M. K., Kane, M., Earabino, C., Lipford, J., Lindblom, A., et al. (1994). Mutation in the DNA mismatch repair gene homologue hMLH1 is associated with hereditary non-polyposis colon cancer. *Nature 368*, 258–261.

Brown, E. J., and Baltimore, D. (2000). ATR disruption leads to chromosomal fragmentation and early embryonic lethality. *Genes Dev 14*, 397–402.

Buchholz, F., Refaeli, Y., Trumpp, A., and Bishop, J. M. (2000). Inducible chromosomal translocation of AML1 and ETO genes through Cre/loxP-mediated recombination in the mouse. *EMBO Rep 1*, 133–139.

Butel, J. S., Sepulveda, A. R., Finegold, M. J., and Woo, S. L. (1990). SV40 large T antigen directed by regulatory elements of the human alpha-1-antitrypsin gene. A transgenic mouse system that exhibits stages in liver carcinogenesis. *Intervirology 31*, 85–100.

Cai, W. W., Mao, J. H., Chow, C. W., Damani, S., Balmain, A., and Bradley, A. (2002). Genome-wide detection of chromosomal imbalances in tumors using BAC microarrays. *Nat Biotechnol 20*, 393–396.

Carlson, K. M., Dou, S., Chi, D., Scavarda, N., Toshima, K., Jackson, C. E., Wells, S. A., Jr., Goodfellow, P. J., and Donis-Keller, H. (1994). Single missense mutation in the tyrosine kinase catalytic domain of the RET protooncogene is associated with multiple endocrine neoplasia type 2B. *Proc Natl Acad Sci USA 91*, 1579–1583.

Chawengsaksophak, K., James, R., Hammond, V. E., Kontgen, F., and Beck, F. (1997). Homeosis and intestinal tumours in Cdx2 mutant mice. *Nature 386*, 84–87.

Chen, J. J., Peck, K., Hong, T. M., Yang, S. C., Sher, Y. P., Shih, J. Y., Wu, R., Cheng, J. L., Roffler, S. R., Wu, C. W., and Yang, P. C. (2001). Global analysis of gene expression in invasion by a lung cancer model. *Cancer Res 61*, 5223–5230.

Chin, L., Pomerantz, J., Polsky, D., Jacobson, M., Cohen, C., Cordon-Cardo, C., Horner, J. W., II, and DePinho, R. A. (1997). Cooperative effects of INK4a and ras in melanoma susceptibility in vivo. *Genes Dev 11*, 2822–2834.

Chin, L., Tam, A., Pomerantz, J., Wong, M., Holash, J., Bardeesy, N., Shen, Q., O'Hagan, R., Pantginis, J., Zhou, H., et al. (1999). Essential role for oncogenic Ras in tumour maintenance. *Nature 400*, 468–472.

Chiu, I. M., Touhalisky, K., and Baran, C. (2001). Multiple controlling mechanisms of FGF1 gene expression through multiple tissue-specific promoters. *Prog Nucleic Acid Res Mol Biol 70*, 155–174.

Cho, J. Y., Sagartz, J. E., Capen, C. C., Mazzaferri, E. L., and Jhiang, S. M. (1999). Early cellular abnormalities induced by RET/PTC1 oncogene in thyroid-targeted transgenic mice. *Oncogene 18*, 3659–3665.

Christofori, G., Naik, P., and Hanahan, D. (1994). A second signal supplied by insulin-like growth factor II in oncogene-induced tumorigenesis. *Nature 369*, 414–418.

Clarke, A. R., Maandag, E. R., van Roon, M., van der Lugt, N. M., van der Valk, M., Hooper, M. L., Berns, A., and te Riele, H. (1992). Requirement for a functional Rb-1 gene in murine development. *Nature 359*, 328–330.

Collins, E. C., Pannell, R., Simpson, E. M., Forster, A., and Rabbitts, T. H. (2000). Interchromosomal recombination of Mll and Af9 genes mediated by cre-loxP in mouse development. *EMBO Rep 1*, 127–132.

Connor, F., Bertwistle, D., Mee, P. J., Ross, G. M., Swift, S., Grigorieva, E., Tybulewicz, V. L., and Ashworth, A. (1997). Tumorigenesis and a DNA repair defect in mice with a truncating Brca2 mutation. *Nat Genet 17*, 423–430.

Contag, C. H., Jenkins, D., Contag, P. R., and Negrin, R. S. (2000). Use of reporter genes for optical measurements of neoplastic disease in vivo. *Neoplasia 2*, 41–52.

Croce, C. M., Sozzi, G., and Huebner, K. (1999). Role of FHIT in human cancer. *J Clin Oncol 17*, 1618–1624.

DeCaprio, J. A., Ludlow, J. W., Figge, J., Shew, J. Y., Huang, C. M., Lee, W. H., Marsilio, E., Paucha, E., and Livingston, D. M. (1988). SV40 large tumor antigen forms a specific complex with the product of the retinoblastoma susceptibility gene. *Cell 54*, 275–283.

de Klein, A., Muijtjens, M., van Os, R., Verhoeven, Y., Smit, B., Carr, A. M., Lehmann, A. R., and Hoeijmakers, J. H. (2000). Targeted disruption of the cell-cycle checkpoint gene ATR leads to early embryonic lethality in mice. *Curr Biol 10*, 479–482.

Deng, G., Lu, Y., Zlotnikov, G., Thor, A. D., and Smith, H. S. (1996). Loss of heterozygosity in normal tissue adjacent to breast carcinomas. *Science 274*, 2057–2059.

de Wind, N., Dekker, M., van Rossum, A., van der Valk, M., and te Riele, H. (1998). Mouse models for hereditary nonpolyposis colorectal cancer. *Cancer Res 58*, 248–255.

de Wind, N., Dekker, M., Claij, N., Jansen, L., van Klink, Y., Radman, M., Riggins, G., van der Valk, M., van't Wout, K., and te Riele, H. (1999). HNPCC-like cancer predisposition in mice through simultaneous loss of Msh3 and Msh6 mismatch-repair protein functions. *Nat Genet 23*, 359–362.

Di Cristofano, A., Pesce, B., Cordon-Cardo, C., and Pandolfi, P. P. (1998). Pten is essential for embryonic development and tumour suppression. *Nat Genet 19*, 348–355.

Di Cristofano, A., De Acetis, M., Koff, A., Cordon-Cardo, C., and Pandolfi, P. P. (2001). Pten and p27KIP1 cooperate in prostate cancer tumor suppression in the mouse. *Nat Genet 27*, 222–224.

Dietrich, W. F., Lander, E. S., Smith, J. S., Moser, A. R., Gould, K. A., Luongo, C., Borenstein, N., and Dove, W. (1993). Genetic identification of Mom-1, a major modifier locus affecting Min-induced intestinal neoplasia in the mouse. *Cell 75*, 631–639.

Dietrich, W. F., Radany, E. H., Smith, J. S., Bishop, J. M., Hanahan, D., and Lander, E. S. (1994). Genome-wide search for loss of heterozygosity in transgenic mouse tumors reveals candidate tumor suppressor genes on chromosomes 9 and 16. *Proc Natl Acad Sci USA 91*, 9451–9455.

Donehower, L. A., Harvey, M., Slagle, B. L., McArthur, M. J., Montgomery, C. A., Jr., Butel, J. S., and Bradley, A. (1992). Mice deficient for p53 are developmentally normal but susceptible to spontaneous tumours. *Nature 356*, 215–221.

Dong, G., Loukinova, E., Chen, Z., Gangi, L., Chanturita, T. I., Liu, E. T., and Van Waes, C. (2001). Molecular profiling of transformed and metastatic murine squamous carcinoma cells by differential display and cDNA microarray reveals altered expression of multiple genes related to growth, apoptosis, angiogenesis, and the NF-kappaB signal pathway. *Cancer Res 61*, 4797–4808.

Dumon, K. R., Ishii, H., Fong, L. Y., Zanesi, N., Fidanza, V., Mancini, R., Vecchione, A., Baffa, R., Trapasso, F., During, M. J., et al. (2001). FHIT gene therapy prevents tumor development in Fhit-deficient mice. *Proc Natl Acad Sci USA 98*, 3346–3351.

Edelmann, W., Yang, K., Umar, A., Heyer, J., Lau, K., Fan, K., Liedtke, W., Cohen, P. E., Kane, M. F., Lipford, J. R., et al. (1997). Mutation in the mismatch repair gene Msh6 causes cancer susceptibility. *Cell 91*, 467–477.

Edelmann, W., Yang, K., Kuraguchi, M., Heyer, J., Lia, M., Kneitz, B., Fan, K., Brown, A. M., Lipkin, M., and Kucherlapati, R. (1999). Tumorigenesis in Mlh1 and Mlh1/Apc1638N mutant mice. *Cancer Res 59*, 1301–1307.

Edelmann, W., Umar, A., Yang, K., Heyer, J., Kucherlapati, M., Lia, M., Kneitz, B., Avdievich, E., Fan, K., Wong, E., et al. (2000). The DNA mismatch repair genes Msh3 and Msh6 cooperate in intestinal tumor suppression. *Cancer Res 60*, 803–807.

Edinger, M., Sweeney, T. J., Tucker, A. A., Olomu, A. B., Negrin, R. S., and Contag, C. H. (1999). Noninvasive assessment of tumor cell proliferation in animal models. *Neoplasia 1*, 303–310.

Eilers, M., Picard, D., Yamamoto, K. R., and Bishop, J. M. (1989). Chimaeras of myc oncoprotein and steroid receptors cause hormone-dependent transformation of cells. *Nature 340*, 66–68.

Elson, A., Wang, Y., Daugherty, C. J., Morton, C. C., Zhou, F., Campos-Torres, J., and Leder, P. (1996). Pleiotropic defects in ataxia-telangiectasia protein-deficient mice. *Proc Natl Acad Sci USA 93*, 13084–13089.

Evans, M. J., and Kaufman, M. H. (1981). Establishment in culture of pluripotential cells from mouse embryos. *Nature 292*, 154–156.

Ewald, D., Li, M., Efrat, S., Auer, G., Wall, R. J., Furth, P. A., and Hennighausen, L. (1996). Time-sensitive reversal of hyperplasia in transgenic mice expressing SV40 T antigen. *Science 273*, 1384–1386.

Felsher, D. W., and Bishop, J. M. (1999). Reversible tumorigenesis by MYC in hematopoietic lineages. *Mol Cell 4*, 199–207.

Fero, M. L., Rivkin, M., Tasch, M., Porter, P., Carow, C. E., Firpo, E., Polyak, K., Tsai, L. H., Broudy, V., Perlmutter, R. M., et al. (1996). A syndrome of multiorgan hyperplasia with features of gigantism, tumorigenesis, and female sterility in p27(Kip1)-deficient mice. *Cell 85*, 733–744.

Fero, M. L., Randel, E., Gurley, K. E., Roberts, J. M., and Kemp, C. J. (1998). The murine gene p27Kip1 is haplo-insufficient for tumour suppression. *Nature 396*, 177–180.

Fishel, R., Lescoe, M. K., Rao, M. R., Copeland, N. G., Jenkins, N. A., Garber, J., Kane, M., and Kolodner, R. (1993). The human mutator gene homolog MSH2 and its association with hereditary nonpolyposis colon cancer. *Cell 75*, 1027–1038.

Fisher, G. H., Wellen, S. L., Klimstra, D., Lenczowski, J. M., Tichelaar, J. W., Lizak, M. J., Whitsett, J. A., Koretsky, A., and Varmus, H. E. (2001). Induction and apoptotic regression of lung adenocarcinomas by regulation of a K-Ras transgene in the presence and absence of tumor suppressor genes. *Genes Dev 15*, 3249–3262.

Fodde, R., Edelmann, W., Yang, K., van Leeuwen, C., Carlson, C., Renault, B., Breukel, C., Alt, E., Lipkin, M., Khan, P. M., et al. (1994). A targeted chain-termination mutation in the mouse Apc gene results in multiple intestinal tumors. *Proc Natl Acad Sci USA 91*, 8969–8973.

Folkman, J., Watson, K., Ingber, D., and Hanahan, D. (1989). Induction of angiogenesis during the transition from hyperplasia to neoplasia. *Nature 339*, 58–61.

Fong, L. Y., Fidanza, V., Zanesi, N., Lock, L. F., Siracusa, L. D., Mancini, R., Siprashvili, Z., Ottey, M., Martin, S. E., Druck, T., et al. (2000). Muir-Torre-like syndrome in Fhit-deficient mice. *Proc Natl Acad Sci USA 97*, 4742–4747.

Friedman, L. S., Thistlethwaite, F. C., Patel, K. J., Yu, V. P., Lee, H., Venkitaraman, A. R., Abel, K. J., Carlton, M. B., Hunter, S. M., Colledge, W. H., et al. (1998). Thymic lymphomas in mice with a truncating mutation in Brca2. *Cancer Res 58*, 1338–1343.

Furth, P. A., Li, M., and Hennighausen, L. (1998). Studying development of disease through temporally controlled gene expression in the salivary gland. *Ann NY Acad Sci 842*, 181–187.

Garcia, S. B., Park, H. S., Novelli, M., and Wright, N. A. (1999). Field cancerization, clonality, and epithelial stem cells: The spread of mutated clones in epithelial sheets. *J Pathol 187*, 61–81.

Giovannini, M., Robanus-Maandag, E., van der Valk, M., Niwa-Kawakita, M., Abramowski, V., Goutebroze, L., Woodruff, J. M., Berns, A., and Thomas, G. (2000). Conditional biallelic Nf2 mutation in the mouse promotes manifestations of human neurofibromatosis type 2. *Genes Dev 14*, 1617–1630.

Gnarra, J. R., Ward, J. M., Porter, F. D., Wagner, J. R., Devor, D. E., Grinberg, A., Emmert-Buck, M. R., Westphal, H., Klausner, R. D., and Linehan, W. M. (1997). Defective placental vasculogenesis causes embryonic lethality in VHL-deficient mice. *Proc Natl Acad Sci USA 94*, 9102–9107.

Goodrich, L. V., Milenkovic, L., Higgins, K. M., and Scott, M. P. (1997). Altered neural cell fates and medulloblastoma in mouse patched mutants. *Science 277*, 1109–1113.

Gordon, J. W., and Ruddle, F. H. (1981). Integration and stable germ line transmission of genes injected into mouse pronuclei. *Science 214*, 1244–1246.

Gossen, M., and Bujard, H. (1992). Tight control of gene expression in mammalian cells by tetracycline-responsive promoters. *Proc Natl Acad Sci USA 89*, 5547–5551.

Gould, K. A., and Dove, W. F. (1997). Localized gene action controlling intestinal neoplasia in mice. *Proc Natl Acad Sci USA 94*, 5848–5853.

Gowen, L. C., Johnson, B. L., Latour, A. M., Sulik, K. K., and Koller, B. H. (1996). Brca1 deficiency results in early embryonic lethality characterized by neuroepithelial abnormalities. *Nat Genet 12*, 191–194.

Greenberg, N. M., DeMayo, F., Finegold, M. J., Medina, D., Tilley, W. D., Aspinall, J. O., Cunha, G. R., Donjacour, A. A., Matusik, R. J., and Rosen, J. M. (1995). Prostate cancer in a transgenic mouse. *Proc Natl Acad Sci USA 92*, 3439–3443.

Groden, J., Thliveris, A., Samowitz, W., Carlson, M., Gelbert, L., Albertsen, H., Joslyn, G., Stevens, J., Spirio, L., Robertson, M., et al. (1991). Identification and characterization of the familial adenomatous polyposis coli gene. *Cell 66*, 589–600.

Guimaraes, D. P., and Hainaut, P. (2002). TP53: A key gene in human cancer. *Biochimie 84*, 83–93.

Gupta, S., Ahmad, N., Marengo, S. R., MacLennan, G. T., Greenberg, N. M., and Mukhtar, H. (2000). Chemoprevention of prostate carcinogenesis by alpha-difluoromethylornithine in TRAMP mice. *Cancer Res 60*, 5125–5133.

Gupta, S., Hastak, K., Ahmad, N., Lewin, J. S., and Mukhtar, H. (2001). Inhibition of prostate carcinogenesis in TRAMP mice by oral infusion of green tea polyphenols. *Proc Natl Acad Sci USA 98*, 10350–10355.

Guy, C. T., Webster, M. A., Schaller, M., Parsons, T. J., Cardiff, R. D., and Muller, W. J. (1992). Expression of the neu protooncogene in the mammary epithelium of transgenic mice induces metastatic disease. *Proc Natl Acad Sci USA 89*, 10578–10582.

Haase, V. H., Glickman, J. N., Socolovsky, M., and Jaenisch, R. (2001). Vascular tumors in livers with targeted inactivation of the von Hippel–Lindau tumor suppressor. *Proc Natl Acad Sci USA 98*, 1583–1588.

Hahn, H., Wojnowski, L., Zimmer, A. M., Hall, J., Miller, G., and Zimmer, A. (1998). Rhabdomyosarcomas and radiation hypersensitivity in a mouse model of Gorlin syndrome. *Nat Med 4*, 619–622.

Hakem, R., de la Pompa, J. L., Sirard, C., Mo, R., Woo, M., Hakem, A., Wakeham, A., Potter, J., Reitmair, A., Billia, F., et al. (1996). The tumor suppressor gene Brca1 is required for embryonic cellular proliferation in the mouse. *Cell 85*, 1009–1023.

Hanahan, D. (1985). Heritable formation of pancreatic beta-cell tumours in transgenic mice expressing recombinant insulin/simian virus 40 oncogenes. *Nature 315*, 115–122.

Hann, B., and Balmain, A. (2001). Building "validated" mouse models of human cancer. *Curr Opin Cell Biol 13*, 778–784.

Harris, H., Miller, O. J., Klein, G., Worst, P., and Tachibana, T. (1969). Suppression of malignancy by cell fusion. *Nature 223*, 363–368.

Harvey, M., McArthur, M. J., Montgomery, C. A., Jr., Butel, J. S., Bradley, A., and Donehower, L. A. (1993). Spontaneous and carcinogen-induced tumorigenesis in p53-deficient mice. *Nat Genet 5*, 225–229.

Hasty, P., Ramirez-Solis, R., Krumlauf, R., and Bradley, A. (1991). Introduction of a subtle mutation into the Hox-2.6 locus in embryonic stem cells. *Nature 350*, 243–246.

Hasty, P., Abuin, A., and Bradley, A. (2000). Gene targeting, principles, and practice in mammalian cells. In *Gene Targeting*, A. L. Joyner (ed.). Oxford University Press, Oxford, England, pp. 1–35.

He, L. Z., Tribioli, C., Rivi, R., Peruzzi, D., Pelicci, P. G., Soares, V., Cattoretti, G., and Pandolfi, P. P. (1997). Acute leukemia with promyelocytic features in PML/RARalpha transgenic mice. *Proc Natl Acad Sci USA 94*, 5302–5307.

He, L. Z., Guidez, F., Tribioli, C., Peruzzi, D., Ruthardt, M., Zelent, A., and Pandolfi, P. P. (1998). Distinct interactions of PML-RARalpha and PLZF-RARalpha with co-repressors determine differential responses to RA in APL. *Nat Genet 18*, 126–135.

He, L. Z., Bhaumik, M., Tribioli, C., Rego, E. M., Ivins, S., Zelent, A., and Pandolfi, P. P. (2000). Two critical hits for promyelocytic leukemia. *Mol Cell 6*, 1131–1141.

Hemann, M. T., Fridman, J. S., Zilfou, J. T., Hernando, E., Paddison, P. J., Cordon-Cardo, C., Hannon, G. J., and Lowe, S. W. (2003). An epi-allelic series of p53 hypomorphs created by stable RNAi produces distinct tumor phenotypes in vivo. *Nat Genet 33*, 396–400.

Hodgson, G., Hager, J. H., Volik, S., Hariono, S., Wernick, M., Moore, D., Nowak, N., Albertson, D. G., Pinkel, D., Collins, C., et al. (2001). Genome scanning with array CGH delineates regional alterations in mouse islet carcinomas. *Nat Genet 29*, 459–464.

Hoffman, R. M. (2001). Visualization of GFP-expressing tumors and metastasis in vivo. *Biotechniques 30*, 1016–1022, 1024–1026.

Hofstra, R. M., Landsvater, R. M., Ceccherini, I., Stulp, R. P., Stelwagen, T., Luo, Y., Pasini, B., Hoppener, J. W., van Amstel, H. K., Romeo, G., et al. (1994). A mutation in the RET proto-oncogene associated with multiple endocrine neoplasia type 2B and sporadic medullary thyroid carcinoma. *Nature 367*, 375–376.

Huang, J., Papadopoulos, N., McKinley, A. J., Farrington, S. M., Curtis, L. J., Wyllie, A. H., Zheng, S., Willson, J. K., Markowitz, S. D., Morin, P., et al. (1996). APC mutations in colorectal tumors with mismatch repair deficiency. *Proc Natl Acad Sci USA 93*, 9049–9054.

Huettner, C. S., Zhang, P., Van Etten, R. A., and Tenen, D. G. (2000). Reversibility of acute B-cell leukaemia induced by BCR-ABL1. *Nat Genet 24*, 57–60.

Ishii, H., Dumon, K. R., Vecchione, A., Trapasso, F., Mimori, K., Alder, H., Mori, M., Sozzi, G., Baffa, R., Huebner, K., and Croce, C. M. (2001). Effect of adenoviral transduction of the fragile histidine triad gene into esophageal cancer cells. *Cancer Res 61*, 1578–1584.

Jacks, T. (1996). Tumor suppressor gene mutations in mice. *Annu Rev Genet 30*, 603–636.

Jacks, T., Fazeli, A., Schmitt, E. M., Bronson, R. T., Goodell, M. A., and Weinberg, R. A. (1992). Effects of an Rb mutation in the mouse. *Nature 359*, 295–300.

Jacks, T., Remington, L., Williams, B. O., Schmitt, E. M., Halachmi, S., Bronson, R. T., and Weinberg, R. A. (1994a). Tumor spectrum analysis in p53-mutant mice. *Curr Biol 4*, 1–7.

Jacks, T., Shih, T. S., Schmitt, E. M., Bronson, R. T., Bernards, A., and Weinberg, R. A. (1994b). Tumour predisposition in mice heterozygous for a targeted mutation in Nf1. *Nat Genet 7*, 353–361.

Jackson, E. L., Willis, N., Mercer, K., Bronson, R. T., Crowley, D., Montoya, R., Jacks, T., and Tuveson, D. A. (2001). Analysis of lung tumor initiation and progression using conditional expression of oncogenic K-ras. *Genes Dev 15*, 3243–3248.

Jishage, K., Nezu, J., Kawase, Y., Iwata, T., Watanabe, M., Miyoshi, A., Ose, A., Habu, K., Kake, T., Kamada, N., et al. (2002). Role of Lkb1, the causative gene of Peutz-Jeghers syndrome, in embryogenesis and polyposis. *Proc Natl Acad Sci USA 99*, 8903–8908.

Johnson, L., Mercer, K., Greenbaum, D., Bronson, R. T., Crowley, D., Tuveson, D. A., and Jacks, T. (2001). Somatic activation of the K-ras oncogene causes early onset lung cancer in mice. *Nature 410*, 1111–1116.

Jonkers, J., Meuwissen, R., van der Gulden, H., Peterse, H., van der Valk, M., and Berns, A. (2001). Synergistic tumor suppressor activity of BRCA2 and p53 in a conditional mouse model for breast cancer. *Nat Genet 29*, 418–425.

Kallioniemi, A., Kallioniemi, O. P., Sudar, D., Rutovitz, D., Gray, J. W., Waldman, F., and Pinkel, D. (1992). Comparative genomic hybridization for molecular cytogenetic analysis of solid tumors. *Science 258*, 818–821.

Kamijo, T., Zindy, F., Roussel, M. F., Quelle, D. E., Downing, J. R., Ashmun, R. A., Grosveld, G., and Sherr, C. J. (1997). Tumor suppression at the mouse INK4a locus mediated by the alternative reading frame product p19ARF. *Cell 91*, 649–659.

Kamijo, T., Bodner, S., van de Kamp, E., Randle, D. H., and Sherr, C. J. (1999). Tumor spectrum in ARF-deficient mice. *Cancer Res 59*, 2217–2222.

Kang, J., Bronson, R. T., and Xu, Y. (2002). Targeted disruption of NBS1 reveals its roles in mouse development and DNA repair. *EMBO J 21*, 1447–1455.

Kemp, C. J., Wheldon, T., and Balmain, A. (1994). p53-deficient mice are extremely susceptible to radiation-induced tumorigenesis. *Nat Genet 8*, 66–69.

Khanna, C., Khan, J., Nguyen, P., Prehn, J., Caylor, J., Yeung, C., Trepel, J., Meltzer, P., and Helman, L. (2001). Metastasis-associated differences in gene expression in a murine model of osteosarcoma. *Cancer Res 61*, 3750–3759.

Kinzler, K. W., and Vogelstein, B. (1997). Cancer-susceptibility genes. Gatekeepers and caretakers. *Nature 386*, 761, 763.

Kitagawa, T., Hino, O., Lee, G. H., Li, H., Liu, J., Nomura, K., Ohtake, K., Furuta, Y., and Aizawa, S. (1991). Multistep hepatocarcinogenesis in transgenic mice harboring SV40 T-antigen gene. *Princess Takamatsu Symp 22*, 349–360.

Knudson, A. G. (2000). Chasing the cancer demon. *Annu Rev Genet 34*, 1–19.

Knudson, A. G., Jr. (1971). Mutation and cancer: Statistical study of retinoblastoma. *Proc Natl Acad Sci USA 68*, 820–823.

Kohonen-Corish, M. R., Daniel, J. J., te Riele, H., Buffinton, G. D., and Dahlstrom, J. E. (2002). Susceptibility of Msh2-deficient mice to inflammation-associated colorectal tumors. *Cancer Res 62*, 2092–2097.

Konishi, M., Kikuchi-Yanoshita, R., Tanaka, K., Muraoka, M., Onda, A., Okumura, Y., Kishi, N., Iwama, T., Mori, T., Koike, M., et al. (1996). Molecular nature of colon tumors in hereditary nonpolyposis colon cancer, familial polyposis, and sporadic colon cancer. *Gastroenterology 111*, 307–317.

Kovalchuk, A. L., Qi, C. F., Torrey, T. A., Taddesse-Heath, L., Feigenbaum, L., Park, S. S., Gerbitz, A., Klobeck, G., Hoertnagel, K., Polack, A., et al. (2000). Burkitt lymphoma in the mouse. *J Exp Med 192*, 1183–1190.

Kuperwasser, C., Hurlbut, G. D., Kittrell, F. S., Dickinson, E. S., Laucirica, R., Medina, D., Naber, S. P., and Jerry, D. J. (2000). Development of spontaneous mammary tumors in BALB/c p53 heterozygous mice. A model for Li-Fraumeni syndrome. *Am J Pathol 157*, 2151–2159.

Kuraguchi, M., Yang, K., Wong, E., Avdievich, E., Fan, K., Kolodner, R. D., Lipkin, M., Brown, A. M., Kucherlapati, R., and Edelmann, W. (2001). The distinct spectra of tumor-associated Apc mutations in mismatch repair-deficient Apc1638N mice define the roles of MSH3 and MSH6 in DNA repair and intestinal tumorigenesis. *Cancer Res 61*, 7934–7942.

Lane, D. P., and Crawford, L. V. (1979). T antigen is bound to a host protein in SV40-transformed cells. *Nature 278*, 261–263.

Leach, F. S., Nicolaides, N. C., Papadopoulos, N., Liu, B., Jen, J., Parsons, R., Peltomaki, P., Sistonen, P., Aaltonen, L. A., Nystrom-Lahti, M., et al. (1993). Mutations of a mutS homolog in hereditary nonpolyposis colorectal cancer. *Cell 75*, 1215–1225.

LeCouter, J. E., Kablar, B., Hardy, W. R., Ying, C., Megeney, L. A., May, L. L., and Rudnicki, M. A. (1998). Strain-dependent myeloid hyperplasia, growth deficiency, and accelerated cell cycle in mice lacking the Rb-related p107 gene. *Mol Cell Biol 18*, 7455–7465.

Leder, A., Pattengale, P. K., Kuo, A., Stewart, T. A., and Leder, P. (1986). Consequences of widespread deregulation of the c-myc gene in transgenic mice: Multiple neoplasms and normal development. *Cell 45*, 485–495.

Lee, E. Y., Chang, C. Y., Hu, N., Wang, Y. C., Lai, C. C., Herrup, K., Lee, W. H., and Bradley, A. (1992). Mice deficient for Rb are nonviable and show defects in neurogenesis and haematopoiesis. *Nature 359*, 288–294.

Lee, M. H., Williams, B. O., Mulligan, G., Mukai, S., Bronson, R. T., Dyson, N., Harlow, E., and Jacks, T. (1996). Targeted disruption of p107: Functional overlap between p107 and Rb. *Genes Dev 10*, 1621–1632.

Li, B., Rosen, J. M., McMenamin-Balano, J., Muller, W. J., and Perkins, A. S. (1997). neu/ERBB2 cooperates with p53-172H during mammary tumorigenesis in transgenic mice. *Mol Cell Biol 17*, 3155–3163.

Liu, C. Y., Flesken-Nikitin, A., Li, S., Zeng, Y., and Lee, W. H. (1996). Inactivation of the mouse Brca1 gene leads to failure in the morphogenesis of the egg cylinder in early postimplantation development. *Genes Dev 10*, 1835–1843.

Liu, G., McDonnell, T. J., Montes de Oca Luna, R., Kapoor, M., Mims, B., El-Naggar, A. K., and Lozano, G. (2000). High metastatic potential in mice inheriting a targeted p53 missense mutation. *Proc Natl Acad Sci USA 97*, 4174–4179.

Liyanage, M., Coleman, A., du Manoir, S., Veldman, T., McCormack, S., Dickson, R. B., Barlow, C., Wynshaw-Boris, A., Janz, S., Wienberg, J., et al. (1996). Multicolour spectral karyotyping of mouse chromosomes. *Nat Genet 14*, 312–315.

Liyanage, M., Weaver, Z., Barlow, C., Coleman, A., Pankratz, D. G., Anderson, S., Wynshaw-Boris, A., and Ried, T. (2000). Abnormal rearrangement within the alpha/delta T-cell receptor locus in lymphomas from Atm-deficient mice. *Blood 96*, 1940–1946.

Ludwig, T., Chapman, D. L., Papaioannou, V. E., and Efstratiadis, A. (1997). Targeted mutations of breast cancer susceptibility gene homologs in mice: Lethal phenotypes of Brca1, Brca2, Brca1/Brca2, Brca1/p53, and Brca2/p53 nullizygous embryos. *Genes Dev 11*, 1226–1241.

Ludwig, T., Fisher, P., Murty, V., and Efstratiadis, A. (2001). Development of mammary adenocarcinomas by tissue-specific knockout of Brca2 in mice. *Oncogene 20*, 3937–3948.

Luo, G., Santoro, I. M., McDaniel, L. D., Nishijima, I., Mills, M., Youssoufian, H., Vogel, H., Schultz, R. A., and Bradley, A. (2000). Cancer predisposition caused by elevated mitotic recombination in Bloom mice. *Nat Genet 26*, 424–429.

MacPhee, M., Chepenik, K. P., Liddell, R. A., Nelson, K. K., Siracusa, L. D., and Buchberg, A. M. (1995). The secretory phospholipase A2 gene is a candidate for the Mom1 locus, a major modifier of ApcMin-induced intestinal neoplasia. *Cell 81*, 957–966.

Maeda, H., Segawa, T., Kamoto, T., Yoshida, H., Kakizuka, A., Ogawa, O., and Kakehi, Y. (2000). Rapid detection of candidate metastatic foci in the orthotopic inoculation model of androgen-sensitive prostate cancer cells introduced with green fluorescent protein. *Prostate 45*, 335–340.

Malkin, D. (1994). p53 and the Li-Fraumeni syndrome. *Biochim Biophys Acta 1198*, 197–213.

Marino, S., Vooijs, M., van Der Gulden, H., Jonkers, J., and Berns, A. (2000). Induction of medulloblastomas in p53-null mutant mice by somatic inactivation of Rb in the external granular layer cells of the cerebellum. *Genes Dev 14*, 994–1004.

Maroulakou, I. G., Anver, M., Garrett, L., and Green, J. E. (1994). Prostate and mammary adenocarcinoma in transgenic mice carrying a rat C3(1) simian virus 40 large tumor antigen fusion gene. *Proc Natl Acad Sci USA 91*, 11236–11240.

Matzuk, M. M., Finegold, M. J., Su, J. G., Hsueh, A. J., and Bradley, A. (1992). Alpha-inhibin is a tumour-suppressor gene with gonadal specificity in mice. *Nature 360*, 313–319.

McAllister, K. A., Bennett, L. M., Houle, C. D., Ward, T., Malphurs, J., Collins, N. K., Cachafeiro, C., Haseman, J., Goulding, E. H., Bunch, D., et al. (2002). Cancer susceptibility of mice with a homozygous deletion in the COOH-terminal domain of the Brca2 gene. *Cancer Res 62*, 990–994.

McClatchey, A. I., Saotome, I., Ramesh, V., Gusella, J. F., and Jacks, T. (1997). The Nf2 tumor suppressor gene product is essential for extraembryonic development immediately prior to gastrulation. *Genes Dev 11*, 1253–1265.

McClatchey, A. I., Saotome, I., Mercer, K., Crowley, D., Gusella, J. F., Bronson, R. T., and Jacks, T. (1998). Mice heterozygous for a mutation at the Nf2 tumor suppressor locus develop a range of highly metastatic tumors. *Genes Dev 12*, 1121–1133.

McCormack, S. J., Weaver, Z., Deming, S., Natarajan, G., Torri, J., Johnson, M. D., Liyanage, M., Ried, T., and Dickson, R. B. (1998). Myc/p53 interactions in transgenic mouse mammary development, tumorigenesis and chromosomal instability. *Oncogene 16*, 2755–2766.

Mellon, P. L., Wetsel, W. C., Windle, J. J., Valenca, M. M., Goldsmith, P. C., Whyte, D. B., Eraly, S. A., Negro-Vilar, A., and Weiner, R. I. (1992). Immortalized hypothalamic gonadotropin-releasing hormone neurons. *Ciba Found Symp 168*, 104–117; discussion 117–126.

Mentor-Marcel, R., Lamartiniere, C. A., Eltoum, I. E., Greenberg, N. M., and Elgavish, A. (2001). Genistein in the diet reduces the incidence of poorly differentiated prostatic adenocarcinoma in transgenic mice (TRAMP). *Cancer Res 61*, 6777–6782.

Meuwissen, R., Linn, S. C., van der Valk, M., Mooi, W. J., and Berns, A. (2001). Mouse model for lung tumorigenesis through Cre/lox controlled sporadic activation of the K-Ras oncogene. *Oncogene 20*, 6551–6558.

Milner, J., Ponder, B., Hughes-Davies, L., Seltmann, M., and Kouzarides, T. (1997). Transcriptional activation functions in BRCA2. *Nature 386*, 772–773.

Minamoto, T., Mai, M., and Ronai, Z. (2000). K-ras mutation: Early detection in molecular diagnosis and risk assessment of colorectal, pancreas, and lung cancers—a review. *Cancer Detect Prev 24*, 1–12.

Mitelman, F., Johansson, B., Mandahl, N., and Mertens, F. (1997). Clinical significance of cytogenetic findings in solid tumors. *Cancer Genet Cytogenet 95*, 1–8.

Miyoshi, H., Nakau, M., Ishikawa, T. O., Seldin, M. F., Oshima, M., and Taketo, M. M. (2002). Gastrointestinal hamartomatous polyposis in Lkb1 heterozygous knockout mice. *Cancer Res 62*, 2261–2266.

Moser, A. R., Pitot, H. C., and Dove, W. F. (1990). A dominant mutation that predisposes to multiple intestinal neoplasia in the mouse. *Science 247*, 322–324.

Moser, A. R., Dove, W. F., Roth, K. A., and Gordon, J. I. (1992). The Min (multiple intestinal neoplasia) mutation: Its effect on gut epithelial cell differentiation and interaction with a modifier system. *J Cell Biol 116*, 1517–1526.

Moser, A. R., Shoemaker, A. R., Connelly, C. S., Clipson, L., Gould, K. A., Luongo, C., Dove, W. F., Siggers, P. H., and Gardner, R. L. (1995). Homozygosity for the Min allele of Apc results in disruption of mouse development prior to gastrulation. *Dev Dyn 203*, 422–433.

Muller, W. J., Sinn, E., Pattengale, P. K., Wallace, R., and Leder, P. (1988). Single-step induction of mammary adenocarcinoma in transgenic mice bearing the activated c-neu oncogene. *Cell 54*, 105–115.

Muthuswamy, S. K., Siegel, P. M., Dankort, D. L., Webster, M. A., and Muller, W. J. (1994). Mammary tumors expressing the neu proto-oncogene possess elevated c-Src tyrosine kinase activity. *Mol Cell Biol 14*, 735–743.

Nakau, M., Miyoshi, H., Seldin, M. F., Imamura, M., Oshima, M., and Taketo, M. M. (2002). Hepatocellular carcinoma caused by loss of heterozygosity in Lkb1 gene knockout mice. *Cancer Res 62*, 4549–4553.

Nicolaides, N. C., Papadopoulos, N., Liu, B., Wei, Y. F., Carter, K. C., Ruben, S. M., Rosen, C. A., Haseltine, W. A., Fleischmann, R. D., Fraser, C. M., et al. (1994). Mutations of two PMS homologues in hereditary nonpolyposis colon cancer. *Nature 371*, 75–80.

Nusse, R., van Ooyen, A., Cox, D., Fung, Y. K., and Varmus, H. (1984). Mode of proviral activation of a putative mammary oncogene (int-1) on mouse chromosome 15. *Nature 307*, 131–136.

Nusse, R., Brown, A., Papkoff, J., Scambler, P., Shackleford, G., McMahon, A., Moon, R., and Varmus, H. (1991). A new nomenclature for int-1 and related genes: The Wnt gene family. *Cell 64*, 231.

Olson, D. C., Deng, C., and Hanahan, D. (1998). Fibroblast growth factor receptor 4, implicated in progression of islet cell carcinogenesis by its expression profile, does not contribute functionally. *Cell Growth Differ 9*, 557–564.

Orlow, I., Rabbani, F., Chin, L., Pomerantz, J., Ligeois, N., Dudas, M., Depinho, R., and Cordon-Cardo, C. (1999). Involvement of the Ink4a gene (p16 and p19arf) in murine tumorigenesis. *Int J Oncol 15*, 17–24.

Oshima, M., Oshima, H., Kitagawa, K., Kobayashi, M., Itakura, C., and Taketo, M. (1995). Loss of Apc heterozygosity and abnormal tissue building in nascent intestinal polyps in mice carrying a truncated Apc gene. *Proc Natl Acad Sci USA 92*, 4482–4486.

Oshima, M., Dinchuk, J. E., Kargman, S. L., Oshima, H., Hancock, B., Kwong, E., Trzaskos, J. M., Evans, J. F., and Taketo, M. M. (1996). Suppression of intestinal polyposis in Apc delta716 knockout mice by inhibition of cyclooxygenase 2 (COX-2). *Cell 87*, 803–809.

Pandolfi, P. P. (2001). in vivo analysis of the molecular genetics of acute promyelocytic leukemia. *Oncogene 20*, 5726–5735.

Papadopoulos, N., Nicolaides, N. C., Wei, Y. F., Ruben, S. M., Carter, K. C., Rosen, C. A., Haseltine, W. A., Fleischmann, R. D., Fraser, C. M., Adams, M. D., et al. (1994). Mutation of a mutL homolog in hereditary colon cancer. *Science 263*, 1625–1629.

Petiniot, L. K., Weaver, Z., Barlow, C., Shen, R., Eckhaus, M., Steinberg, S. M., Ried, T., Wynshaw-Boris, A., and Hodes, R. J. (2000). Recombinase-activating gene (RAG) 2-mediated V(D)J recombination is not essential for tumorigenesis in Atm-deficient mice. *Proc Natl Acad Sci USA 97*, 6664–6669.

Pinkel, D., Segraves, R., Sudar, D., Clark, S., Poole, I., Kowbel, D., Collins, C., Kuo, W. L., Chen, C., Zhai, Y., et al. (1998). High resolution analysis of DNA copy number variation using comparative genomic hybridization to microarrays. *Nat Genet 20*, 207–211.

Polakis, P. (1997). The adenomatous polyposis coli (APC) tumor suppressor. *Biochim Biophys Acta 1332*, F127–147.

Pollack, J. R., Perou, C. M., Alizadeh, A. A., Eisen, M. B., Pergamenschikov, A., Williams, C. F., Jeffrey, S. S., Botstein, D., and Brown, P. O. (1999). Genome-wide analysis of DNA copy-number changes using cDNA microarrays. *Nat Genet 23*, 41–46.

Ponder, B. A. (1995). Mutations of the RET proto-oncogene in multiple endocrine neoplasia type 2. *Cancer Surv 25*, 195–205.

Powell, S. M., Zilz, N., Beazer-Barclay, Y., Bryan, T. M., Hamilton, S. R., Thibodeau, S. N., Vogelstein, B., and Kinzler, K. W. (1992). APC mutations occur early during colorectal tumorigenesis. *Nature 359*, 235–237.

Prolla, T. A., Baker, S. M., Harris, A. C., Tsao, J. L., Yao, X., Bronner, C. E., Zheng, B., Gordon, M., Reneker, J., Arnheim, N., et al. (1998). Tumour susceptibility and spontaneous mutation in mice deficient in Mlh1, Pms1 and Pms2 DNA mismatch repair. *Nat Genet 18*, 276–279.

Purdie, C. A., Harrison, D. J., Peter, A., Dobbie, L., White, S., Howie, S. E., Salter, D. M., Bird, C. C., Wyllie, A. H., Hooper, M. L., et al. (1994). Tumour incidence, spectrum and ploidy in mice with a large deletion in the p53 gene. *Oncogene 9*, 603–609.

Qian, F., Hanahan, D., and Weissman, I. L. (2001). L-selectin can facilitate metastasis to lymph nodes in a transgenic mouse model of carcinogenesis. *Proc Natl Acad Sci USA 98*, 3976–3981.

Qin, X., Liu, L., and Gerson, S. L. (1999). Mice defective in the DNA mismatch gene PMS2 are hypersensitive to MNU induced thymic lymphoma and are partially protected by transgenic expression of human MGMT. *Oncogene 18*, 4394–4400.

Qin, X., Shibata, D., and Gerson, S. L. (2000). Heterozygous DNA mismatch repair gene PMS2-knockout mice are susceptible to intestinal tumor induction with N-methyl-N-nitrosourea. *Carcinogenesis 21*, 833–838.

Rabbitts, T. H. (1994). Chromosomal translocations in human cancer. *Nature 372*, 143–149.

Raghow, S., Kuliyev, E., Steakley, M., Greenberg, N., and Steiner, M. S. (2000). Efficacious chemoprevention of primary prostate cancer by flutamide in an autochthonous transgenic model. *Cancer Res 60*, 4093–4097.

Raghow, S., Hooshdaran, M. Z., Katiyar, S., and Steiner, M. S. (2002). Toremifene prevents prostate cancer in the transgenic adenocarcinoma of mouse prostate model. *Cancer Res 62*, 1370–1376.

Rane, S. G., Dubus, P., Mettus, R. V., Galbreath, E. J., Boden, G., Reddy, E. P., and Barbacid, M. (1999). Loss of Cdk4 expression causes insulin-deficient diabetes and Cdk4 activation results in beta-islet cell hyperplasia. *Nat Genet 22*, 44–52.

Rane, S. G., Cosenza, S. C., Mettus, R. V., and Reddy, E. P. (2002). Germ line transmission of the Cdk4(R24C) mutation facilitates tumorigenesis and escape from cellular senescence. *Mol Cell Biol 22*, 644–656.

Rehemtulla, A., Stegman, L. D., Cardozo, S. J., Gupta, S., Hall, D. E., Contag, C. H., and Ross, B. D. (2000). Rapid and quantitative assessment of cancer treatment response using in vivo bioluminescence imaging. *Neoplasia 2*, 491–495.

Reilly, K. M., Loisel, D. A., Bronson, R. T., McLaughlin, M. E., and Jacks, T. (2000). Nf1;Trp53 mutant mice develop glioblastoma with evidence of strain-specific effects. *Nat Genet 26*, 109–113.

Reitmair, A. H., Redston, M., Cai, J. C., Chuang, T. C., Bjerknes, M., Cheng, H., Hay, K., Gallinger, S., Bapat, B., and Mak, T. W. (1996). Spontaneous intestinal carcinomas and skin neoplasms in Msh2-deficient mice. *Cancer Res 56*, 3842–3849.

Resor, L., Bowen, T. J., and Wynshaw-Boris, A. (2001). Unraveling human cancer in the mouse: Recent refinements to modeling and analysis. *Hum Mol Genet 10*, 669–675.

Robanus-Maandag, E., Dekker, M., van der Valk, M., Carrozza, M. L., Jeanny, J. C., Dannenberg, J. H., Berns, A., and te Riele, H. (1998). p107 is a suppressor of retinoblastoma development in pRb-deficient mice. *Genes Dev 12*, 1599–1609.

Rous, P. (1983). Landmark article (*JAMA* 1911;56:198). Transmission of a malignant new growth by means of a cell-free filtrate. By Peyton Rous. *JAMA 250*, 1445–1449.

Rowley, J. D. (1998). The critical role of chromosome translocations in human leukemias. *Ann Rev Genet 32*, 495–519.

Ruas, M., and Peters, G. (1998). The p16INK4a/CDKN2A tumor suppressor and its relatives. *Biochim Biophys Acta 1378*, F115–177.

Sah, V. P., Attardi, L. D., Mulligan, G. J., Williams, B. O., Bronson, R. T., and Jacks, T. (1995). A subset of p53-deficient embryos exhibit exencephaly. *Nat Genet 10*, 175–180.

Sands, A. T., Abuin, A., Sanchez, A., Conti, C. J., and Bradley, A. (1995). High susceptibility to ultraviolet-induced carcinogenesis in mice lacking XPC. *Nature 377*, 162–165.

Sasaki, T., Irie-Sasaki, J., Horie, Y., Bachmaier, K., Fata, J. E., Li, M., Suzuki, A., Bouchard, D., Ho, A., Redston, M., et al. (2000). Colorectal carcinomas in mice lacking the catalytic subunit of PI(3)Kgamma. *Nature 406*, 897–902.

Scheffner, M., Werness, B. A., Huibregtse, J. M., Levine, A. J., and Howley, P. M. (1990). The E6 oncoprotein encoded by human papillomavirus types 16 and 18 promotes the degradation of p53. *Cell 63*, 1129–1136.

Schmidt, E. E., Taylor, D. S., Prigge, J. R., Barnett, S., and Capecchi, M. R. (2000). Illegitimate Cre-dependent chromosome rearrangements in transgenic mouse spermatids. *Proc Natl Acad Sci USA 97*, 13702–13707.

Schmitt, C. A., McCurrach, M. E., de Stanchina, E., Wallace-Brodeur, R. R., and Lowe, S. W. (1999). INK4a/ARF mutations accelerate lymphomagenesis and promote chemoresistance by disabling p53. *Genes Dev 13*, 2670–2677.

Schmitt, C. A., Fridman, J. S., Yang, M., Baranov, E., Hoffman, R. M., and Lowe, S. W. (2002). Dissecting p53 tumor suppressor functions in vivo. *Cancer Cell 1*, 289–298.

Schoenenberger, C. A., Andres, A. C., Groner, B., van der Valk, M., LeMeur, M., and Gerlinger, P. (1988). Targeted c-myc gene expression in mammary glands of transgenic mice induces mammary tumours with constitutive milk protein gene transcription. *EMBO J 7*, 169–175.

Schrock, E., du Manoir, S., Veldman, T., Schoell, B., Wienberg, J., Ferguson-Smith, M. A., Ning, Y., Ledbetter, D. H., Bar-Am, I., Soenksen, D., et al. (1996). Multicolor spectral karyotyping of human chromosomes. *Science 273*, 494–497.

Sharan, S. K., Morimatsu, M., Albrecht, U., Lim, D. S., Regel, E., Dinh, C., Sands, A., Eichele, G., Hasty, P., and Bradley, A. (1997). Embryonic lethality and radiation hypersensitivity mediated by Rad51 in mice lacking Brca2. *Nature 386*, 804–810.

Sherr, C. J. (2000). The Pezcoller lecture: Cancer cell cycles revisited. *Cancer Res 60*, 3689–3695.

Sherr, C. J., and Roberts, J. M. (1999). CDK inhibitors: Positive and negative regulators of G1-phase progression. *Genes Dev 13*, 1501–1512.

Shi, Y. (2003). Mammalian RNAi for the masses. *Trends Genet 19*, 9–12.

Shi, Y. P., Naik, P., Dietrich, W. F., Gray, J. W., Hanahan, D., and Pinkel, D. (1997). DNA copy number changes associated with characteristic LOH in islet cell carcinomas of transgenic mice. *Genes Chromosomes Cancer 19*, 104–111.

Shibata, H., Toyama, K., Shioya, H., Ito, M., Hirota, M., Hasegawa, S., Matsumoto, H., Takano, H., Akiyama, T., Toyoshima, K., et al. (1997). Rapid colorectal adenoma formation initiated by conditional targeting of the Apc gene. *Science 278*, 120–123.

Siegel, P. M., Dankort, D. L., Hardy, W. R., and Muller, W. J. (1994). Novel activating mutations in the neu proto-oncogene involved in induction of mammary tumors. *Mol Cell Biol 14*, 7068–7077.

Silverman, K. A., Koratkar, R., Siracusa, L. D., and Buchberg, A. M. (2002). Identification of the modifier of Min 2 (Mom2) locus, a new mutation that influences Apc-induced intestinal neoplasia. *Genome Res 12*, 88–97.

Slamon, D. J., Clark, G. M., Wong, S. G., Levin, W. J., Ullrich, A., and McGuire, W. L. (1987). Human breast cancer: Correlation of relapse and survival with amplification of the HER-2/neu oncogene. *Science 235*, 177–182.

Slamon, D. J., Godolphin, W., Jones, L. A., Holt, J. A., Wong, S. G., Keith, D. E., Levin, W. J., Stuart, S. G., Udove, J., Ullrich, A., et al. (1989). Studies of the HER-2/neu protooncogene in human breast and ovarian cancer. *Science 244*, 707–712.

Smith-Hicks, C. L., Sizer, K. C., Powers, J. F., Tischler, A. S., and Costantini, F. (2000). C-cell hyperplasia, pheochromocytoma and sympathoadrenal malformation in a mouse model of multiple endocrine neoplasia type 2B. *EMBO J 19*, 612–622.

Smits, R., Kielman, M. F., Breukel, C., Zurcher, C., Neufeld, K., Jagmohan-Changur, S., Hofland, N., van Dijk, J., White, R., Edelmann, W., et al. (1999). Apc1638T: A mouse model delineating critical domains of the adenomatous polyposis coli protein involved in tumorigenesis and development. *Genes Dev 13*, 1309–1321.

Solinas-Toldo, S., Lampel, S., Stilgenbauer, S., Nickolenko, J., Benner, A., Dohner, H., Cremer, T., and Lichter, P. (1997). Matrix-based comparative genomic hybridization: Biochips to screen for genomic imbalances. *Genes Chromosomes Cancer 20*, 399–407.

Sotillo, R., Dubus, P., Martin, J., de la Cueva, E., Ortega, S., Malumbres, M., and Barbacid, M. (2001a). Wide spectrum of tumors in knock-in mice carrying a Cdk4 protein insensitive to INK4 inhibitors. *EMBO J 20*, 6637–6647.

Sotillo, R., Garcia, J. F., Ortega, S., Martin, J., Dubus, P., Barbacid, M., and Malumbres, M. (2001b). Invasive melanoma in Cdk4-targeted mice. *Proc Natl Acad Sci USA 98*, 13312–13317.

Stambolic, V., Tsao, M. S., Macpherson, D., Suzuki, A., Chapman, W. B., and Mak, T. W. (2000). High incidence of breast and endometrial neoplasia resembling human Cowden syndrome in pten+/− mice. *Cancer Res 60*, 3605–3611.

Stehelin, D., Varmus, H. E., Bishop, J. M., and Vogt, P. K. (1976). DNA related to the transforming gene(s) of avian sarcoma viruses is present in normal avian DNA. *Nature 260*, 170–173.

Stevens, L. C. (1970). Experimental production of testicular teratomas in mice of strains 129, A/He, and their F1 hybrids. *J Natl Cancer Inst 44*, 923–929.

Stewart, T. A., Pattengale, P. K., and Leder, P. (1984). Spontaneous mammary adenocarcinomas in transgenic mice that carry and express MTV/myc fusion genes. *Cell 38*, 627–637.

St. John, M. A., Tao, W., Fei, X., Fukumoto, R., Carcangiu, M. L., Brownstein, D. G., Parlow, A. F., McGrath, J., and Xu, T. (1999). Mice deficient of Lats1 develop soft-tissue sarcomas, ovarian tumours and pituitary dysfunction. *Nat Genet 21*, 182–186.

Su, L. K., Kinzler, K. W., Vogelstein, B., Preisinger, A. C., Moser, A. R., Luongo, C., Gould, K. A., and Dove, W. F. (1992). Multiple intestinal neoplasia caused by a mutation in the murine homolog of the APC gene. *Science 256*, 668–670.

Suzuki, A., de la Pompa, J. L., Hakem, R., Elia, A., Yoshida, R., Mo, R., Nishina, H., Chuang, T., Wakeham, A., Itie, A., et al. (1997). Brca2 is required for embryonic cellular proliferation in the mouse. *Genes Dev 11*, 1242–1252.

Suzuki, A., de la Pompa, J. L., Stambolic, V., Elia, A. J., Sasaki, T., del Barco Barrantes, I., Ho, A., Wakeham, A., Itie, A., Khoo, W., et al. (1998). High cancer susceptibility and embryonic lethality associated with mutation of the PTEN tumor suppressor gene in mice. *Curr Biol 8*, 1169–1178.

Suzuki, A., Yamaguchi, M. T., Ohteki, T., Sasaki, T., Kaisho, T., Kimura, Y., Yoshida, R., Wakeham, A., Higuchi, T., Fukumoto, M., et al. (2001). T cell-specific loss of Pten leads to defects in central and peripheral tolerance. *Immunity 14*, 523–534.

Sweeney, T. J., Mailander, V., Tucker, A. A., Olomu, A. B., Zhang, W., Cao, Y., Negrin, R. S., and Contag, C. H. (1999). Visualizing the kinetics of tumor-cell clearance in living animals. *Proc Natl Acad Sci USA 96*, 12044–12049.

Takaku, K., Oshima, M., Miyoshi, H., Matsui, M., Seldin, M. F., and Taketo, M. M. (1998). Intestinal tumorigenesis in compound mutant mice of both Dpc4 (Smad4) and Apc genes. *Cell 92*, 645–656.

Takaku, K., Miyoshi, H., Matsunaga, A., Oshima, M., Sasaki, N., and Taketo, M. M. (1999). Gastric and duodenal polyps in Smad4 (Dpc4) knockout mice. *Cancer Res 59*, 6113–6117.

Taketo, M. M., and Takaku, K. (2000). Gastrointestinal tumorigenesis in Smad4 (Dpc4) mutant mice. *Hum Cell 13*, 85–95.

Thomas, K. R., and Capecchi, M. R. (1987). Site-directed mutagenesis by gene targeting in mouse embryo-derived stem cells. *Cell 51*, 503–512.

Tsai, K. Y., Hu, Y., Macleod, K. F., Crowley, D., Yamasaki, L., and Jacks, T. (1998). Mutation of E2f-1 suppresses apoptosis and inappropriate S phase entry and extends survival of Rb-deficient mouse embryos. *Mol Cell 2*, 293–304.

Tsukamoto, A. S., Grosschedl, R., Guzman, R. C., Parslow, T., and Varmus, H. E. (1988). Expression of the int-1 gene in transgenic mice is associated with mammary gland hyperplasia and adenocarcinomas in male and female mice. *Cell 55*, 619–625.

van Steeg, H., Mullenders, L. H., and Vijg, J. (2000). Mutagenesis and carcinogenesis in nucleotide excision repair-deficient XPA knock out mice. *Mutat Res 450*, 167–180.

Venkitaraman, A. R. (2002). Cancer susceptibility and the functions of BRCA1 and BRCA2. *Cell 108*, 171–182.

Vooijs, M., van der Valk, M., te Riele, H., and Berns, A. (1998). Flp-mediated tissue-specific inactivation of the retinoblastoma tumor suppressor gene in the mouse. *Oncogene 17*, 1–12.

Vooijs, M., Jonkers, J., Lyons, S., and Berns, A. (2002). Noninvasive imaging of spontaneous retinoblastoma pathway-dependent tumors in mice. *Cancer Res 62*, 1862–1867.

Wang, T. C., Cardiff, R. D., Zukerberg, L., Lees, E., Arnold, A., and Schmidt, E. V. (1994). Mammary hyperplasia and carcinoma in MMTV-cyclin D1 transgenic mice. *Nature 369*, 669–671.

Watson, P., and Lynch, H. T. (1993). Extracolonic cancer in hereditary nonpolyposis colorectal cancer. *Cancer 71*, 677–685.

Weaver, Z. A., McCormack, S. J., Liyanage, M., du Manoir, S., Coleman, A., Schrock, E., Dickson, R. B., and Ried, T. (1999). A recurring pattern of chromosomal aberrations in mammary gland tumors of MMTV-cmyc transgenic mice. *Genes Chromosomes Cancer 25*, 251–260.

Wechter, W. J., Leipold, D. D., Murray, E. D., Jr., Quiggle, D., McCracken, J. D., Barrios, R. S., and Greenberg, N. M. (2000). E-7869 (R-flurbiprofen) inhibits progression of prostate cancer in the TRAMP mouse. *Cancer Res 60*, 2203–2208.

Weissleder, R. (2002). Scaling down imaging: Molecular mapping of cancer in mice. *Nature Rev Cancer 2*, 11–18.

Weissleder, R., Tung, C. H., Mahmood, U., and Bogdanov, A., Jr. (1999). In vivo imaging of tumors with protease-activated near-infrared fluorescent probes. *Nat Biotechnol 17*, 375–378.

Westphal, C. H., Rowan, S., Schmaltz, C., Elson, A., Fisher, D. E., and Leder, P. (1997). atm and p53 cooperate in apoptosis and suppression of tumorigenesis, but not in resistance to acute radiation toxicity. *Nat Genet 16*, 397–401.

Wetmore, C., Eberhart, D. E., and Curran, T. (2000). The normal patched allele is expressed in medulloblastomas from mice with heterozygous germ-line mutation of patched. *Cancer Res 60*, 2239–2246.

Wetmore, C., Eberhart, D. E., and Curran, T. (2001). Loss of p53 but not ARF accelerates medulloblastoma in mice heterozygous for patched. *Cancer Res 61*, 513–516.

Wetterwald, A., van der Pluijm, G., Que, I., Sijmons, B., Buijs, J., Karperien, M., Lowik, C. W., Gautschi, E., Thalmann, G. N., and Cecchini, M. G. (2002). Optical imaging of cancer metastasis to bone marrow: A mouse model of minimal residual disease. *Am J Pathol 160*, 1143–1153.

Wheeler, J. M., Bodmer, W. F., and Mortensen, N. J. (2000). DNA mismatch repair genes and colorectal cancer. *Gut 47*, 148–153.

Whiteside, D., McLeod, R., Graham, G., Steckley, J. L., Booth, K., Somerville, M. J., and Andrew, S. E. (2002). A homozygous germ-line mutation in the human MSH2 gene predisposes to hematological malignancy and multiple cafe-au-lait spots. *Cancer Res 62*, 359–362.

Wijnhoven, S. W., Kool, H. J., Mullenders, L. H., van Zeeland, A. A., Friedberg, E. C., van der Horst, G. T., van Steeg, H., and Vrieling, H. (2000). Age-dependent spontaneous mutagenesis in Xpc mice defective in nucleotide excision repair. *Oncogene 19*, 5034–5037.

Willert, K., and Nusse, R. (1998). Beta-catenin: A key mediator of Wnt signaling. *Curr Opin Genet Dev 8*, 95–102.

Williams, B. O., Remington, L., Albert, D. M., Mukai, S., Bronson, R. T., and Jacks, T. (1994). Cooperative tumorigenic effects of germline mutations in Rb and p53. *Nat Genet 7*, 480–484.

Williams, B. R., Mirzoeva, O. K., Morgan, W. F., Lin, J., Dunnick, W., and Petrini, J. H. (2002). A murine model of Nijmegen breakage syndrome. *Curr Biol 12*, 648–653.

Wolfel, T., Hauer, M., Schneider, J., Serrano, M., Wolfel, C., Klehmann-Hieb, E., De Plaen, E., Hankeln, T., Meyer zum Buschenfelde, K. H., and Beach, D. (1995). A p16INK4a-insensitive CDK4 mutant targeted by cytolytic T lymphocytes in a human melanoma. *Science 269*, 1281–1284.

Wong, S., and Witte, O. N. (2001). Modeling Philadelphia chromosome positive leukemias. *Oncogene 20*, 5644–5659.

Wu, Y., Renard, C. A., Apiou, F., Huerre, M., Tiollais, P., Dutrillaux, B., and Buendia, M. A. (2002). Recurrent allelic deletions at mouse chromosomes 4 and 14 in Myc-induced liver tumors. *Oncogene 21*, 1518–1526.

Xu, Y., Ashley, T., Brainerd, E. E., Bronson, R. T., Meyn, M. S., and Baltimore, D. (1996). Targeted disruption of ATM leads to growth retardation, chromosomal fragmentation during meiosis, immune defects, and thymic lymphoma. *Genes Dev 10*, 2411–2422.

Yamanaka, R., Barlow, C., Lekstrom-Himes, J., Castilla, L. H., Liu, P. P., Eckhaus, M., Decker, T., Wynshaw-Boris, A., and Xanthopoulos, K. G. (1997). Impaired granulopoiesis, myelodysplasia, and early lethality in CCAAT/enhancer binding protein epsilon-deficient mice. *Proc Natl Acad Sci USA 94*, 13187–13192.

Yamasaki, L., Bronson, R., Williams, B. O., Dyson, N. J., Harlow, E., and Jacks, T. (1998). Loss of E2F-1 reduces tumorigenesis and extends the lifespan of Rb1(+/-)mice. *Nat Genet 18*, 360–364.

Yang, M., Hasegawa, S., Jiang, P., Wang, X., Tan, Y., Chishima, T., Shimada, H., Moossa, A. R., and Hoffman, R. M. (1998). Widespread skeletal metastatic potential of human lung cancer revealed by green fluorescent protein expression. *Cancer Res 58*, 4217–4221.

Yang, M., Jiang, P., Sun, F. X., Hasegawa, S., Baranov, E., Chishima, T., Shimada, H., Moossa, A. R., and Hoffman, R. M. (1999). A fluorescent orthotopic bone metastasis model of human prostate cancer. *Cancer Res 59*, 781–786.

Yang, M., Baranov, E., Jiang, P., Sun, F. X., Li, X. M., Li, L., Hasegawa, S., Bouvet, M., Al-Tuwaijri, M., Chishima, T., et al. (2000). Whole-body optical imaging of green fluorescent protein-expressing tumors and metastases. *Proc Natl Acad Sci USA 97*, 1206–1211.

Yang, M., Baranov, E., Wang, J. W., Jiang, P., Wang, X., Sun, F. X., Bouvet, M., Moossa, A. R., Penman, S., and Hoffman, R. M. (2002). Direct external imaging of nascent cancer, tumor progression, angiogenesis, and metastasis on internal organs in the fluorescent orthotopic model. *Proc Natl Acad Sci USA 99*, 3824–3829.

Yergeau, D. A., Hetherington, C. J., Wang, Q., Zhang, P., Sharpe, A. H., Binder, M., Marin-Padilla, M., Tenen, D. G., Speck, N. A., and Zhang, D. E. (1997). Embryonic lethality and impairment of haematopoiesis in mice heterozygous for an AML1-ETO fusion gene. *Nat Genet 15*, 303–306.

Yew, P. R., Liu, X., and Berk, A. J. (1994). Adenovirus E1B oncoprotein tethers a transcriptional repression domain to p53. *Genes Dev 8*, 190–202.

You, M. J., Castrillon, D. H., Bastian, B. C., O'Hagan, R. C., Bosenberg, M. W., Parsons, R., Chin, L., and DePinho, R. A. (2002). Genetic analysis of Pten and Ink4a/Arf interactions in the suppression of tumorigenesis in mice. *Proc Natl Acad Sci USA 99*, 1455–1460.

Zanesi, N., Fidanza, V., Fong, L. Y., Mancini, R., Druck, T., Valtieri, M., Rudiger, T., McCue, P. A., Croce, C. M., and Huebner, K. (2001). The tumor spectrum in FHIT-deficient mice. *Proc Natl Acad Sci USA 98*, 10250–10255.

Zembutsu, H., Ohnishi, Y., Tsunoda, T., Furukawa, Y., Katagiri, T., Ueyama, Y., Tamaoki, N., Nomura, T., Kitahara, O., Yanagawa, R., et al. (2002). Genome-wide cDNA microarray screening to correlate gene expression profiles with sensitivity of 85 human cancer xenografts to anticancer drugs. *Cancer Res 62*, 518–527.

Zheng, L., and Lee, W. H. (2001). The retinoblastoma gene: A prototypic and multifunctional tumor suppressor. *Exp Cell Res 264*, 2–18.

Zhu, J., Petersen, S., Tessarollo, L., and Nussenzweig, A. (2001). Targeted disruption of the Nijmegen breakage syndrome gene NBS1 leads to early embryonic lethality in mice. *Curr Biol 11*, 105–109.

Zimonjic, D. B., Pollock, J. L., Westervelt, P., Popescu, N. C., and Ley, T. J. (2000). Acquired, nonrandom chromosomal abnormalities associated with the development of acute promyelocytic leukemia in transgenic mice. *Proc Natl Acad Sci USA 97*, 13306–13311.

Zuo, L., Weger, J., Yang, Q., Goldstein, A. M., Tucker, M. A., Walker, G. J., Hayward, N., and Dracopoli, N. C. (1996). Germline mutations in the p16INK4a binding domain of CDK4 in familial melanoma. *Nat Genet 12*, 97–99.

WEB RESOURCES

Organ-Specific Mouse transgenics

Skin cancer: http://dermatology.bwh.harvard.edu/tg_mice.html/

Breast cancer: http://mammary.nih.gov/models/transgenics/index.html/

Mammary Transgene Database: http://mbcr.bcm.tmc.edu/ermb/mtdb/mtdb.html

General Sites

Internet Resources for Transgenic and Targeted Mutation Research (from the Jackson Laboratory): http://tbase.jax.org/docs/databases.html

TBASE (Transgenic/Targeted Mutation Database): http://tbase.jax.org/

Induced Mutant Resource (IMR)—Jackson Laboratory: www.jax.org/resources/documents/imr/

Transgenic Systems for Mutation Analysis—BigBlue and MutaMouse: http://eden.ceh.uvic.ca/bigblue.htm

Andras Nagy maintains a list of Cre-lines (and conditional mutations): www.mshri.on.ca/nagy/default.htm

Jackson Lab (www.informatics.jax.org) also maintains information on Cre lines and conditional mutations.

The National Cancer Institute has an excellent comprehensive web site of information on mouse models of cancer at http://emice.nci.nih.gov/.

12

GENOME-WIDE MODIFIER SCREENS: HOW THE GENETICS OF CANCER PENETRANCE MAY SHAPE THE FUTURE OF PREVENTION AND TREATMENT

Linda D. Siracusa, Karen A. Silverman, Revati Koratkar, Marina Markova, and Arthur M. Buchberg

INTRODUCTION

The search and characterization of genes that modify the initiation, growth, promotion, and/or progression of cancer constitutes a rapidly evolving field. The mouse provides a powerful mammalian model system to characterize genes that influence cancer risk and the penetrance of tumor phenotypes. The literature has many examples of the influence of modifier loci not only on different forms of cancer but also on other types of genetic disorders and susceptibility to infectious diseases. We focus on mice that carry mutations in the *Apc* gene as models of human colorectal cancer. We review the molecular genomic approaches that have been developed to detect modifier genes in this system (Box 12-1). As these genes become genetically and pharmacologically validated in mice, human geneticists will seek corresponding human populations to study cancer

Oncogenomics: Molecular Approaches to Cancer, Edited by Charles Brenner and David Duggan
ISBN 0-471-22592-4 © 2004 John Wiley & Sons, Inc.

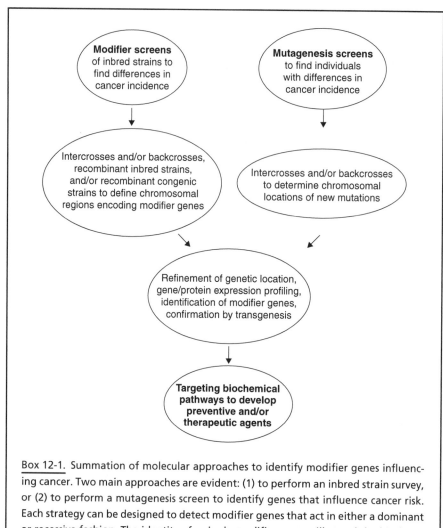

Box 12-1. Summation of molecular approaches to identify modifier genes influencing cancer. Two main approaches are evident: (1) to perform an inbred strain survey, or (2) to perform a mutagenesis screen to identify genes that influence cancer risk. Each strategy can be designed to detect modifier genes that act in either a dominant or recessive fashion. The identity of a single modifier gene will reveal the biochemical pathways it influences. As the number of modifier genes increases for a given phenotype, so too will the number of pathways, thus providing opportunities to target premalignant or malignant cells at multiple stages.

incidence, and novel agents may be tested on patients or at-risk populations. The ultimate goals are to make use of modifier genes for cancer prevention, diagnosis, and treatment.

COLORECTAL CANCER

Colorectal cancer is the second leading cause of cancer morbidity and mortality in the United States and other Western developed countries (Greenlee et al., 2000). Environmental factors have been implicated in the pathogenesis of this disease due to wide variations in colorectal cancer incidence among different populations (Potter, 1995; Rustgi, 1994). Although factors such as diet affect the incidence of disease, genetic factors also play a key role, as indicated by familial clustering of colorectal cancer (Griffioen et al., 1998). Thus, colorectal cancer is the result of interacting genetic and environmental factors, which contribute to tumorigenesis through a complex multistep process (Dunlop, 1997; Ilyas et al., 1999; Rustgi, 1994; Sparks et al., 1998).

FAMILIAL ADENOMATOUS POLYPOSIS AND THE *APC* GENE

Familial adenomatous polyposis (FAP) is a dominantly inherited disorder characterized by the development of hundreds to thousands of benign adenomatous polyps throughout the intestinal tract that have a relatively high probability of progressing to malignant adenocarcinoma (Fearon et al., 1990; Groden et al., 1991). Genetic evidence suggests that the adenomatous polyposis coli (*APC*) gene acts as a classical tumor suppressor gene in both the tumors of FAP patients and in a large proportion of sporadic colorectal tumors, in that both alleles are likely to require inactivation for tumor growth to occur (Miyaki et al., 1994; Miyoshi et al., 1992a; Powell et al., 1992). Individuals with FAP have been shown to inherit one defective *APC* allele, making them unusually susceptible to the development of colorectal adenomas, where the first rate-limiting step appears to be inactivation of the wild-type *APC* allele through somatic mutation and/or loss of heterozygosity (LOH; Groden et al., 1991; Kinzler et al., 1991a; Miyaki et al., 1994; Nishisho et al., 1991; Powell et al., 1992).

In addition to the development of colorectal polyps, FAP patients have an increased predisposition to various benign and malignant extracolonic disease manifestations, such as epidermoid cysts, mandibular osteomas, desmoid tumors, thyroid carcinomas, pancreatic adenocarcinomas, and congenital hypertrophy of the retinal pigment epithelium (CHRPE; Ficari et al., 2000; Lal and Gallinger, 2000; Watson et al., 1995). Duodenal polyps are found in the majority of FAP patients 10–20 years after the development of colorectal polyps; although duodenal polyposis is common, duodenal carcinoma occurs in only 1–5% of FAP patients (Lal and Gallinger, 2000). Desmoid tumors are the second leading cause of death in FAP patients; although benign, these tumors grow and can interfere with organ function. Gardner's syndrome and Turcot's syndrome are variants of FAP (Watson et al., 1995). In Gardner's syndrome, colorectal polyposis is associated with skin fibromas, epidermoid cysts, and benign osteomas of the mandible and long bones (Gardner and Richards, 1953). In Turcot's syndrome, colorectal polyposis is associated with primary central nervous system neoplasia (Hamilton et al., 1995). Mutations in the *APC* gene are also observed in other polyposis syndromes, such as attenuated adenomatous polyposis coli (AAPC) and hereditary flat adenomas syndrome (Nishisho et al., 1991; Spirio et al., 1992).

HEREDITARY NONPOLYPOSIS COLORECTAL CANCER AND THE *APC* GENE

Hereditary nonpolyposis colorectal cancer (HNPCC) is another dominantly inherited form of colorectal cancer. The mechanisms leading to colorectal tumorigenesis have previously been considered as four separate pathways (Ilyas et al., 1999). Two major pathways are the aneuploid pathway and the mismatch repair-defective (MMR) pathway. The aneuploid pathway involves mutations in the *APC, MYC, RAS*, and *TRP53* genes along with LOH of chromosome 18 (Fearon et al., 1990). The MMR pathway involves mutations in genes governing mismatch repair (*MLH1, MSH2, PMS1, PMS2*, and *MSH6*) leading to microsatellite instability (MSI), with subsequent mutations in tumorigenic genes such as *TGFBR2, IGFRII, BAX*, and *CASP5* due to loss of DNA repair functions (Lynch and Lynch, 2000; Markowitz et al., 1995; Ouyang et al., 1997; Rampino et al., 1997; Schwartz et al., 1999; Yamamoto et al., 1997, 1998). In addition, MMR-deficient cells may have reduced apoptotic responses; failure to undergo programmed cell death would facilitate clonal expansion and provide a selective advantage to cells (Fishel, 1998, 1999). However, recent evidence suggests that these pathways may not be mutually exclusive. More than half of HNPCC tumors have either regulatory mutations in the *CTNNB1* gene or mutations in the *APC* gene (Miyaki et al., 1999a), suggesting that the majority of HNPCC carcinomas develop through alteration of the *APC/CTNNB1/TCF* pathway (see below).

SPORADIC COLORECTAL CARCINOMAS HAVE MUTATIONS IN EITHER THE *APC* OR *CTNNB1* GENES

More than 70% of sporadic colorectal tumors have detectable somatic mutations or LOH of *APC* (Miyaki et al., 1994; Miyoshi et al., 1992b; Powell et al., 1992). In addition, 48% of colorectal tumors that did not have mutations in the *APC* gene exhibited mutations in the regulatory domain of the *CTNNB1* gene (Sparks et al., 1998). These findings, coupled with the observation of mutations in *APC* or *CTNNB1* in FAP and HNPCC, highlight the central role of the *APC/CTNNB1/TCF* pathway in colorectal carcinogenesis (Polakis, 1999). Inactivation of APC results in activation of CTNNB1, which in turn interacts with T-cell factor (TCF) transcription factors (Polakis, 1999). Mutations in either *APC* or *CTNNB1* represent an early step in the pathway to carcinoma. Animal models in which the *APC* pathway is perturbed provide important resources for unraveling the molecular mechanisms and gene interactions leading to human colorectal tumorigenesis.

DEVELOPMENTAL EXPRESSION OF THE APC PROTEIN

The APC gene product is expressed in a wide variety of fetal and adult tissues, including the brain, esophagus, eye, liver, and stomach, as well as the intestine and colon (Lal and Gallinger, 2000; Midgley et al., 1997). At the cellular level, APC is found in both the cytoplasm and the nucleus; cytoplasmic APC is often at the leading edges of cells, and nuclear APC has been detected in many tissues, including mammary and colorectal epithelium (Midgley et al., 1997; Nathke et al., 1996; Neufeld and White, 1997). APC protein levels increase at the crypt-villus boundary in the intestines; cells migrate from a position near the base of the crypt to the top of the villus, at which point the cells are sloughed off into the intestinal cavity (van Es et al., 2001). APC is highly expressed in differentiated intestinal epithelial cells, and its levels gradually increase as differentiating cells move up the crypt-villus axis, while levels of β-catenin decline as the cells move up the crypt-villus axis (Fodde and Smits, 2001). In normal human colon, APC expression is limited to cells in the lumenal half of the crypt, which contains nonproliferative, terminally differentiated cells (Midgley et al., 1997; Smith et al., 1993).

STRUCTURE AND FUNCTION OF THE *APC* GENE

APC is located on human chromosome 5q21-q22, is composed of 15 exons with an 8538 bp mRNA, and encodes a 312 kDa protein consisting of 2843 amino acids (Groden et al., 1991; Kinzler et al., 1991b; Nishisho et al., 1991; Fig. 12-1). Exon 15 comprises >75% of the coding sequence of the *APC* gene and is the most common target for both germ-line and somatic mutations (Beroud and Soussi, 1996). The mutation cluster region (MCR) between amino acid 1284 and amino acid 1580 is where ~60% of the APC mutations reside that have been mapped in colorectal tumors (Fig. 12-1; Miyoshi et al., 1992b), while ~34% of the germ-line mutations of APC occur at codons 1061 and 1309 (Fig. 12-1; Beroud and Soussi, 1996).

The *APC* gene encodes a multifunctional protein that controls cell growth and chromosome segregation through several different mechanisms, including regulation of cell adhesion and migration, maintenance of the actin and microtubule components of the cytoskeleton, and processing of multiple cell signaling pathways, including those involved in cell cycle progression and apoptosis (Fig. 12-1; Fearnhead et al., 2001; Fodde et al., 2001b; van Es et al., 2001). Therefore, the loss of *APC* gene function could alter cell cycle parameters, slow intestinal cell migration, alter cell adhesion, and/or prevent programmed cell death.

The *Wnt* signaling pathway plays a key role in development, cellular proliferation, and differentiation, and its dysregulation is involved in the development of various human cancers (Peifer and Polakis, 2000). The APC and β-catenin proteins serve an important role in this signaling pathway, with a critical role of APC in the regulation of cytoplasmic levels of β-catenin. In the absence of Wnt signals, free cytoplasmic β-catenin is phosphorylated through its association with a multiprotein complex containing the scaffolding proteins axin/conductin, glycogen synthase kinase 3b (GSK3B), and APC (Fodde and Smits, 2001; van Es et al., 2001). This complex targets β-catenin for ubiquitination and subsequent proteosomal degradation, preventing it from reaching the nucleus and serving as a transcriptional coactivator.

Activation of the *Wnt* pathway results in the decreased degradation of β-catenin; β-catenin is not targeted for destruction and is free to enter the nucleus (Fodde and Smits, 2001). Once inside the nucleus, β-catenin forms a complex with members of the TCF and lymphoid enhancer factor (LEF) transcription factor families to activate the transcription of several genes such as the oncogene *c-MYC*, and the cell cycle regulatory protein cyclin D1, in addition to other genes (Fearnhead et al., 2001; Fodde and Smits, 2001; van Es et al., 2001). These downstream targets are involved in tumor formation due to their roles in proliferation, apoptosis, and cell cycle progression; thus alteration of normal gene expression may affect cell proliferation rates in normal intestinal epithelial cells, possibly contributing to polyp development.

Mutations in essential components of the *Wnt* signaling pathway, such as APC, β-catenin, or axin/conductin, lead to the inappropriate and continuous activation of target genes, resulting in the development of cancer in a wide variety of tissues (Fodde and Smits, 2001; van Es et al., 2001). Because APC is important in regulating free β-catenin levels, loss of APC function results in increased levels of cytoplasmic β-catenin

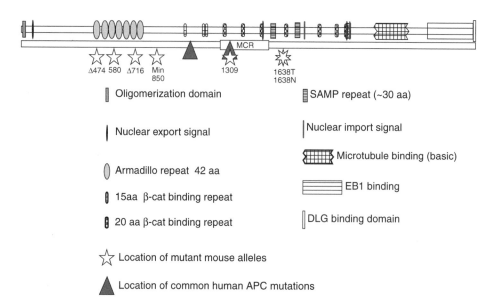

Figure 12-1. Structure of the *APC* gene. The *APC* gene contains several functional domains that mediate protein-protein interactions in cell adhesion, formation of epithelial cell-cell contacts, regulation of β-catenin, and maintenance of cytoskeletal microtubules (Polakis, 1997). The development of cancer is caused by deletion, and thus loss of function, of various domains in the mutant APC protein (van Es et al., 2001). The oligomerization domain at the N-terminus is comprised of heptad repeats that mediate the formation of APC homodimers (Su et al., 1993). The armadillo domain consists of 7 copies of a 42-amino-acid motif that allows APC to bind to protein phosphatase 2A (PP2A) and APC-stimulated guanine nucleotide exchange factor (Asef; Kawasaki et al., 2000; Seeling et al., 1999). The APC-Asef complex is involved in regulation of the actin cytoskeletal network, cell morphology and migration, and neuronal function (Kawasaki et al., 2000). The central portion of APC contains a group of repeats that mediate the binding and downregulation of β-catenin. This group is composed of three 15 amino acid repeats and seven imperfect 20 amino acid repeats (Fodde and Smits, 2001; van Es et al., 2001). The central region is where the majority of protein truncation mutations have been identified in sporadic and inherited mutations of APC. The SAMP repeats, interwoven with the 20 amino acid repeats, bind axin/conductin to form a complex with APC, GSK3B, and β-catenin to regulate the phosphorylation status of β-catenin (Hart et al., 1998; Zeng et al., 1997). The C-terminal region of APC binds the tubulin-binding protein EB1 and the human homolog of the Drosophila disc large tumor suppressor gene (hDLG) involved in maintenance of cell polarity, migration, and blocking of cell proliferation (Matsumine et al., 1996; Su et al., 1995). Nuclear export signals (NES) present at the N-terminus and within the 20 amino acid repeats, and the nuclear import signals present within the 20-amino-acid repeat region are important for the regulated movement of APC and its bound proteins between the nucleus and cytoplasmic compartments (Fearnhead et al., 2001).

The majority of mutations have been identified in APC in sporadic cases of colorectal cancer within the mutation cluster region (MCR; Miyoshi et al., 1992b). The triangles identify the location of the most common germ-line mutations identified in FAP patients; mutations at codons 1061 and 1309 account for ~30% of the known mutations (Nagase and Nakamura, 1993). The stars represent the location of the mouse mutations that have been studied (see Table 12-1).

(Polakis, 1999; Polakis et al., 1999). Accumulation of β-catenin may also be a result of direct activating mutations of the β-catenin gene itself; mutations of β-catenin have been found in a wide variety of tumor types including hepatocellular, colorectal, ovarian, medulloblastoma, prostate, and uterine cancer. Mutations of the β-catenin gene are often identified in colorectal tumors that lack *APC* mutations (Fearnhead et al., 2001; van Es et al., 2001).

β-catenin functions not only as a transducer in the *Wnt* pathway but also as an essential component of adherens junctions, providing the link between E-cadherin and β-catenin, which bind actin and actin-associated proteins (Fodde and Smits, 2001; van Es et al., 2001). The critical interaction between APC and β-catenin provides an indirect link between APC and the regulation of the adherens junction complex. APC may therefore control cell migration and adhesion by regulating the stability and subcellular localization of β-catenin; a defective APC protein may result in an increase in intestinal or colonic cell migration and/or deregulation of cell adhesion, resulting in disorganization of epithelial cells, thus contributing to polyp development (Fodde and Smits, 2001; van Es et al., 2001).

Recent work has provided evidence for a role of APC in chromosome segregation and stability via the interaction of the C-terminal tail of APC and EB1. Embryonic stem cells that are homozygous for either Apc^{Min} or Apc^{1638T} alleles reveal a significantly higher degree of aneuploidy in comparison to wild-type cells (Fodde et al., 2001a; Kaplan et al., 2001). These results highlight the critical role of Apc in the development of colorectal cancer primarily through the chromosomal instability pathway.

MODIFIER GENES CAN INFLUENCE CANCER SUSCEPTIBILITY

Modifier genes or tumor susceptibility genes modify the tumor phenotype through enhancement or suppression of the initiation, growth, promotion, and/or progression to cancer (Balmain, 2002). Modifier genes are responsible for the clinical variation that is observed in many human diseases. The identification and molecular characterization of genetic modifiers of cancer susceptibility may provide novel insights into pathogenesis, leading to a better assessment of cancer risks, and aid in the development of therapeutic agents to decrease cancer susceptibility (Moser et al., 2001; Mott et al., 2000).

FAP is known to have a wide spectrum of phenotypes (Griffioen et al., 1998; Joslyn et al., 1991; Kinzler et al., 1991b; Leppert et al., 1987). Considerable clinical variability exists with respect to the age of disease onset and the number and distribution of colorectal adenomas that develop, as well as the variety of extracolonic manifestations (Nugent et al., 1994). Inter- and intrafamilial variation in phenotype is observed even in FAP patients who inherit the same mutation within the *APC* gene, indicating that other genetic (modifier genes, epigenetic factors) and environmental factors may influence the expression of colorectal disease (Fodde and Khan, 1995; Giardiello et al., 1994; Martin-Denavit et al., 2001; Moser et al., 1995; Paul et al., 1993). The significant clinical variability observed in FAP patients has led to the search for modifier genes that may influence the severity and/or extracolonic manifestations of FAP (Crabtree et al., 2002; Houlston et al., 2001; Sanabria et al., 1996).

QUANTITATIVE TRAIT LOCI IDENTIFICATION IN HUMANS

As was explained in Chapter 4, complex traits are a result of multiple genetic determinants; each individual locus contributes a small effect to the overall phenotype (Darvasi,

1998). Most phenotypic differences between individuals with respect to physiology, disease, growth, and behavior are quantitative in nature (Zwick et al., 2000). These quantitative trait loci (QTLs) may affect quantitative phenotypic trait differences, such as tumor location, size, number, or latency (Balmain, 2002; McPeek, 2000; Mott et al., 2000). QTL analysis is the study of the genetic basis of complex traits with the goal of identifying the genes and pathways that underlie complex diseases (Johnson and Todd, 2000).

Many common diseases, including colorectal cancer, are the result of complex interactions between environmental factors and susceptibility alleles of multiple genes, resulting in clinical heterogeneity (Johnson and Todd, 2000). The clinical variability that is often observed in affected individuals within FAP families that carry the same germ-line *APC* mutation suggests the presence of modifier genes in the human genome. The identification of genetic modifier loci can be extremely difficult due to the variability of environmental factors, as well as the genetic heterogeneity present in the human population (Leppert et al., 1990; Paul et al., 1993; Spirio et al., 1993). Due to the problems confounding the search for human tumor susceptibility alleles, many laboratories have turned to the mouse as a model system (Balmain, 2002). The analysis of mouse strains that are genetically highly susceptible or highly resistant to various cancers allows the identification of the modifier genes that affect cancer phenotypes (Balmain, 2002).

GENETIC RESOURCES FOR QTL ANALYSES IN THE MOUSE

Several chromosomal regions influencing cancer development have already been identified by QTL analysis in the mouse (Balmain and Nagase, 1998; Buchberg and Siracusa, 1995; www.informatics.jax.org). QTL mapping provides the means to identify chromosomal regions that harbor genes whose collective action is responsible for a given complex trait (Balmain and Nagase, 1998; Belknap et al., 2001; Frankel, 1995; Moore and Nagle, 2000; Strachan and Read, 1996; Wakeland et al., 1997). Genetically homozygous inbred strains of mice are a valuable resource for identifying genetic factors influencing these traits (Balmain and Nagase, 1998; Rikke and Johnson, 1998). Each member of an inbred strain is genetically identical; therefore, under controlled environmental conditions, members of a single inbred strain will exhibit characteristic and reproducible phenotypes.

Testing of different inbred strains is the first step to determine which strains are resistant and which strains are susceptible for the desired tumor phenotype. The two strains that exhibit the extremes in phenotype are usually selected for further study. The greater the difference in phenotype, the greater the probability of finding the genetic loci responsible for the phenotypic difference.

Backcrosses or intercrosses between strains that show the extremes in tumor phenotypes, coupled with genotypic and phenotypic analysis of offspring, can reveal the number and sites of chromosomal regions encoding genes responsible for differences in cancer susceptibility (Balmain and Nagase, 1998; Frankel, 1995). The choice of which type of cross to perform is usually based on the phenotype of the F1 hybrid offspring. If the F1 hybrids exhibit an intermediate phenotype, an intercross (F1 × F1) may be chosen; if the F1 hybrids resemble one of the two parental strains, a backcross (F1 × recessive parental strain) may be chosen.

Individual loci may each contribute differently to the total phenotype. As the number of genes responsible for a given trait are increased, phenotype distribution is broadened (Silver, 1995). For example, if a trait is determined by a single locus, the parental phenotypes will be observed in the F2 generation. If two loci are responsible, an intermediate phenotype will be seen in addition to the parental phenotypes. As the number of genes involved increases, the phenotypic distribution of F2 progeny will form a bell-shaped curve (Silver, 1995; Strachan and Read, 1996). Only the phenotypic extremes, which are most likely homozygous for the gene(s) of interest, need to be analyzed to identify modifier loci (Silver, 1995). A genome-wide linkage search can be performed using simple sequence-length polymorphisms (SSLP) or single nucleotide polymorphisms (SNP) distributed at defined intervals throughout the genome (Brookes, 1999; Dietrich et al., 1995). With these methods, genomes of individual mice can be scanned for linkage disequilibrium (LD), where the gene that contributes to a phenotype is linked to the marker being analyzed. Similar SNP-based LD searches are conducted in humans for cancer predisposition traits, as described in Chapter 4. Obviously, human QTL analysis is based on existing families rather than experimental crosses.

An alternative method for identification of chromosomal regions harboring modifier genes is the use of recombinant inbred (RI) and/or recombinant congenic (RC) strains (Taylor, 2000). RI strains are made by intercrossing two already inbred strains followed by sequential brother × sister mating for 20 or more generations (Bailey, 1981). RC strains are made by the same initial intercross followed by backcrosses to one of the parental strains prior to inbreeding (Demant and Hart, 1986). Collections of these strains have already been made by numerous investigators and some sets are commercially available. Once a difference between two inbred strains has been found, the members of the corresponding RI or RC series can be individually tested for the phenotype of interest. The advantages of using RI and/or RC strains is that genotyping has already been performed (Blake et al., 2002) and several members of a single RI/RC line can be tested to ensure the phenotype of each RI/RC line.

Another resource for QTL mapping is the chromosome substitution strains (CSSs), formerly called consomic strains (Nadeau et al., 2000). Each CSS has one of its chromosomes replaced with the homologous chromosome from another strain. A CSS panel is composed of 21 strains, which represent the substitution of autosomes 1 through 19 as well as the X and Y chromosomes. These strains can be individually assessed for cancer susceptibility traits or crossed to *Apc* mutants to establish their tumor profile. As with RI and RC strains, genotypes of the CSSs are already known. A fine structure map of the QTL region can be generated rather quickly by backcrossing a given CSS with the chosen strain and selecting for recombinants that limit the QTL to a small defined interval. Thus, CSSs can enhance the process of positional cloning of a modifier gene (Nadeau et al., 2000).

Regardless of the method chosen, a preliminary chromosomal localization of modifier gene(s) will be obtained; however, the region containing the gene(s) is usually quite large (on the order of 10–20 cM) and may contain several hundred genes. The establishment and testing of congenic strains derived to isolate and narrow the region responsible for tumor suppression on an otherwise susceptible background (or vice versa) has proven critical for refinement of the modifier region. The establishment of the sequence of the mouse genome, with corresponding BAC tiling panels that cover the genome, now allows the identification of candidate genes to be carried out directly and to a high resolution (www.ensembl.org; www.ncbi.nlm.nih.gov). Once the region is narrowed to 1–2 cM, further investigations can proceed by several methods (such as the candidate gene approach, generating transgenic mice with BACs or YACs that cover the region, or deletion testing) to identify the gene(s) responsible for cancer susceptibility. Studies to define qualitative and/or quantitative differences in mRNA transcript and/or protein expression may facilitate the identification of the modifier gene among several candidates in a given region. QTL analysis has already identified numerous loci associated with a host of complex diseases in mammals, and at least four genes mapping to these regions have already been shown to be involved in cancer (Balmain, 2002; Glazier et al., 2002; Korstanje and Paigen, 2002; Nadeau et al., 2000).

MURINE MODELS OF COLORECTAL CANCER

The study of human disease has been greatly facilitated by the use of animal model systems, which provide a means to analyze cellular processes leading to neoplasia (Bedell et al., 1997a, 1997b). As described in Chapter 11, several models for intestinal tumorigenesis have been generated by introducing specific mutations into the murine homolog of the *APC* gene (*Apc*), allowing investigation of its role in polyp initiation through carcinoma progression; these various models are described in Table 12-1.

One model that has been extensively studied is the *Min* mouse, which was discovered through phenotypic screening following ENU mutagenesis (Moser et al., 1990). *Min* mice carry a dominant, fully penetrant mutation in the *Apc* gene, which results in a high spontaneous rate of adenoma development in both the small intestine and colon (Moser et al., 1990; Su et al., 1992). The *Min* mutation, maintained on the C57BL/6 (B6) genetic background, provides an in vivo model for studying interactions of genes in the initiation, growth, and progression of intestinal tumorigenesis. B6 $Apc^{Min/+}$ mice were initially reported to develop an average of 29 tumors throughout their small and large intestines (as counted in one-third of the intestines) and rarely live past 150 days of age (Moser et al., 1990; Su et al., 1992). The premature death of these animals is associated with secondary effects of tumor growth, which include intestinal blockage and bleeding, resulting in severe, chronic anemia.

The *Min* mouse is heterozygous for a nonsense mutation at codon 850 in exon 15 of the *Apc* gene on chromosome 18, which is analogous to mutations frequently found in the *APC* gene in FAP kindreds (Table 12-1; Fig. 12-1; Miyoshi et al., 1992a; Su et al., 1992). In addition to the inherited germ-line Apc^{Min} mutation, all adenomas analyzed from B6 $Apc^{Min/+}$ mice demonstrate loss of the wild-type *Apc* allele, similar to what is seen in the majority of human FAP as well as sporadic colorectal tumors (Levy et al., 1994; Luongo et al., 1994; Miyaki et al., 1994). This finding indicates that in mice, as in humans, an early event in adenoma formation requires the loss of function of both alleles at the *Apc* locus, providing additional evidence for its tumor suppressor function (Luongo et al., 1994; Moser et al., 1992). The reasons for the apparent dominance of loss of function mutations in tumor suppressor genes are discussed in Chapter 1. Genotypic and phenotypic similarities between $Apc^{Min/+}$ mice and FAP patients suggest the $Apc^{Min/+}$ mouse as an important model for this human disease (Klausner, 1999; Moser et al., 1990; Su et al., 1992).

TABLE 12-1. Mutations in the Apc Gene and Their Phenotypic Effects in Mice

Mouse Model	Description of Mutation	Heterozygous Phenotype	Homozygous Phenotype	Size of the Mutant Apc Protein	Apc Functional Domains	References
$Apc^{\Delta 474}$	Targeting vector containing exons 7–10 inserted in exon 9, resulting in frameshift and nonsense codon after exon 10.	Multiple adenomas in the GI tract (>100 small intestinal polyps on B6 background); 19% incidence of mammary tumors.	Not reported.	~55 kDa	Lacks armadillo repeats, all binding regions for β-catenin, axin, tubulin, EB1, and DLG	Sasai et al., 2000
Apc^{580S}	Conditional mutant—loxP sites inserted in introns flanking exon 14.	Normal.	Introduction of Cre-expressing adenovirus leads to colon tumors.	~70 kDa	Lacks armadillo repeats, all binding regions for β-catenin, axin, tubulin, EB1, and DLG	Shibata et al., 1997
$Apc^{\Delta 716}$	Neo cassette inserted in codon 716.	Multiple small intestinal adenomas.	Embryonic lethal.	80 kDa	Lacks all binding regions for β-catenin, axin, tubulin, EB1, and DLG	Oshima et al., 1995
Apc^{Min}	ENU mutagenesis—nonsense mutation in codon 850.	Multiple adenomas, strain dependent.	Embryonic lethal.	95 kDa	Lacks all 20 amino acid repeats for β-catenin regulation	Moser et al., 1990
Apc^{1309}	Not reported	Multiple adenomas in the GI tract (~30).	Not reported	Not reported	Not reported	Quesada et al., 1998
Apc^{1638N}	Neo cassette inserted in the opposite transcriptional orientation as Apc.	3–6 GI adenomas; desmoid tumors, cutaneous cysts, and mammary tumors.	Embryonic lethal.	182 kDa (unstable); low amounts (1–2%)	Lacks all binding regions for tubulin, EB1, and DLG	Fodde et al., 1994; Smits et al. 1998
Apc^{1638T}	Neo cassette inserted in the same transcriptional orientation as Apc.	Normal.	Viable.	182 kDa (stable); normal amounts	Truncation at C-terminus without affecting β-catenin regulatory motifs	Smits et al., 1999

POLYP MULTIPLICITY IN *MIN* MICE IS GREATLY INFLUENCED BY GENETIC BACKGROUND

Hybrid F1 offspring generated from B6 $Apc^{Min}/+$ mice crossed to either AKR/J (AKR), MA/MyJ (MA), or *Mus musculus castaneus* (CAST) mice show a significant decrease in polyp number, as well as an increased life span (Dietrich et al., 1993; Moser et al., 1992). This difference in polyp number suggests that some inbred strains carry modifier genes that reduce polyp multiplicity in $Apc^{Min}/+$ mice. When F1 animals were backcrossed to the parental strains, the phenotype of the offspring resembled each of the parental phenotypes, again providing strong evidence for at least one unlinked dominant gene capable of modifying the $Apc^{Min}/+$ phenotype (Dietrich et al., 1993; Moser et al., 1992).

A modifier locus, called Modifier of *Min 1* (*Mom1*), was subsequently identified and localized to the distal region of mouse chromosome 4 by QTL analysis (Dietrich et al., 1993). The location of the *Mom1* locus was further refined to a 4 cM interval on distal mouse chromosome 4 using congenic strains (Gould et al., 1996b). Analysis of additional inbred mouse strains showed that AKR, MA, CAST, SWR/J, DBA/2J, and BALB/c each carry *Mom1*-resistant (*Mom1^R*) alleles, while B6, BTBR, and 129/SvJ each carry *Mom1*-susceptible (*Mom1^S*) alleles (Dietrich et al., 1993; Gould et al., 1996a). *Mom1* was determined to be a semidominant modifier of intestinal polyp multiplicity and size (Dietrich et al., 1993; Gould et al., 1996a). *Mom1* was estimated to account for ~50% of the genetic variation in polyp number, indicating the presence of other unlinked modifier loci in some highly resistant strain backgrounds (Dietrich et al., 1993; Siracusa and Buchberg, unpublished data).

THE *MOM1* LOCUS AND THE *PLA2G2A* GENE

The candidate gene approach revealed that the gene encoding secretory type II non-pancreatic phospholipase A_2 (*Pla2g2a*) was a strong candidate for the *Mom1* locus (MacPhee et al., 1995). Not only has this gene been shown to map within the same region of chromosome 4 that contains *Mom1* but there is 100% concordance between the *Pla2g2a* genotype and *Mom1* phenotype in the mouse strains studied (Dietrich et al., 1993; Gould and Dove, 1998; MacPhee et al., 1995). High levels of *Pla2g2a* expression were detected in the intestines of mouse strains resistant to polyp formation, such as AKR, MA, and CAST, while extremely low levels were detected in the susceptible B6 strain (MacPhee et al., 1995). A mutation in *Pla2g2a* was subsequently discovered in the susceptible B6 strain, while the resistant AKR, MA, and CAST strains were shown to carry wild-type *Pla2g2a* (MacPhee et al., 1995). Sequence analysis determined that the B6 *Pla2g2a* gene was disrupted by a frameshift mutation in exon 3, resulting in an inactive gene product; strains with a resistant *Mom1^R* allele (AKR, MA, CAST, SWR/J, DBA/2J, and BALB/c) each carried the wild-type *Pla2g2a* allele, while strains with a susceptible *Mom1^S* allele (B6, BTBR, and 129/SvJ) each carried the null *Pla2g2a* allele (Gould et al., 1996a, 1996b; Kennedy et al., 1995; MacPhee et al., 1995).

The current data strongly implicate *Pla2g2a* as a dominant inhibitor of polyp multiplicity in $Apc^{Min}/+$ mice. Previously, a congenic line was created by placing a 35 cM region surrounding *Mom1* from the AKR strain onto a B6 genetic background in order to examine the action of *Mom1* in the absence of additional modifier genes (Gould et al., 1996a, 1996b). A single copy of the $Mom1^R$ AKR allele was able to produce a two-fold reduction in polyp multiplicity and a significant reduction in polyp size (Gould et al., 1996a, 1996b). More recently, one transgenic line was constructed where the $Mom1^R$ AKR allele of *Pla2g2a* was introduced into a susceptible B6 background (Cormier et al., 1997). $Apc^{Min/+}$ offspring overexpressing this *Pla2g2a* cosmid transgene displayed a two-fold reduction in polyp multiplicity and a significant reduction in polyp size, thus providing additional evidence that *Pla2g2a* provides resistance to polyp development and growth (Cormier et al., 1997, 2000). Therefore, one or two wild-type copies of the *Pla2g2a* gene can greatly decrease polyp multiplicity in mice heterozygous for the Apc^{Min} mutation, indicating that the *Pla2g2a* gene encodes the *Mom1* locus and acts as a major modifier of polyp multiplicity in $Apc^{Min/+}$ mice.

THE *PLA2G2A* GENE AND HUMAN COLORECTAL CANCER

The results obtained with $Apc^{Min/+}$ mice have led to the assumption that *PLA2G2A* may also function as a modifier gene in human colorectal tumorigenesis. The homologous human *PLA2G2A* locus has been mapped to human chromosome 1p36-p35 (Praml et al., 1995; Riggins et al., 1995; Tomlinson et al., 1996a). This region is frequently found deleted in various human cancers including colorectal cancer and is thought to contain a modifier of FAP (Dobbie et al., 1997; Haluska et al., 1997; Leister et al., 1990; Tomlinson et al., 1996b). LOH of this region is seen in a significant number of colorectal carcinomas, as well as a large proportion of human sporadic colorectal tumors (Praml et al., 1995). Thus, there is evidence for the existence of a human colorectal tumor suppressor gene in this region that acts to reduce the severity of human FAP. Investigations to determine the role of PLA2G2A in human colorectal cancer are ongoing.

MATING OF *APC* MUTANT MICE TO SELECTED TRANSGENIC AND GENE-TARGETED MUTANTS

Another avenue for detection of modifier genes exists in that we can mate mice carrying a mutation in the *Apc* gene to mice that carry known or introduced mutations in another gene of interest. The choice of which mutant to select involves a number of factors including the likelihood of the gene of interest to be a modifier. Obviously, there is no way to know the outcome in advance, but logical selections can be made based on the temporal and spatial expression pattern of the gene of interest as well as its involvement in defined biochemical and/or physiological pathways.

This approach has already been taken with murine *Apc* mutants. Table 12-2 shows the specific *Apc* mutation and the transgenic or gene-targeted mutation to which mice carrying specific *Apc* mutations were intercrossed. The results to date show that most of the genes selected have a detectable effect on *Apc* phenotypes; only alterations in 2 of 22 genes—namely the *scid* and *Tgfbr2* mutations—did not significantly alter *Apc* phenotypes. Indeed, the results show that absence of particular proteins can increase average polyp numbers, whereas absence of other proteins can decrease average polyp numbers.

The advantages of this approach are that (1) it provides a direct test of a given *Apc* mutation in the presence of a single, defined mutation in a known gene, and

T A B L E 12-2. Cancer Phenotypes of Mutant Apc Mice Mated to Gene-Targeted Mutants

Apc Mutation	Gene	Genotype	Strain Background	Effects on Small Intestinal Polyps	Effects on Colon Polyps	Other Effects	References
Min	Blm	-/-; +/-	C57BL/6J × 129S5 hybrid background	Increase in polyp number in -/- mice	Not Reported	Not reported	Luo et al., 2000; Goss et al., 2002
Δ716	Cox2 (Ptgs2)	-/-; +/-	C57BL/6	Decrease in polyp number and size	Decrease in polyp number and size; no colon polyps in -/-	Decrease in polyp number and size is dosage dependent	Oshima et al., 1996
Min	Cox1 (Ptgs1); Cox2 (Ptgs2)	+/-	B6 × 129/Ola mixed background	Decrease in polyp number	Decrease in polyp size	Not reported	Chulada et al., 2000
Min	Dnmt	S/+	B6 × 129/SvJ mixed background	Decrease in polyp number	Not reported	Not reported	Laird et al., 1995
Min	Dnmt	N/+	B6 × 129/Sv mixed background	Decrease in polyp number and size	Not reported	Not reported	Cormier and Dove, 2000
Min	Dnmt	R/+	B6 × 129/SvJae mixed background	Decrease in polyp number and size	(Colon numbers combined with small intestine numbers)	Not reported	Eads et al., 2002
1638N	Cad1 (Ecad, Um, UVO)	+/-	[C57BL/6JIco × (129/Ola × 129/J mixed background)]F1	Increase in polyp numbers; no change in progression	Not reported	Increase in gastric polyp numbers; no change in progression or desmoid tumor number	Smits et al., 2000a
Min	Egfr	wa2/wa2	B6; B6/Ei; C3H mixed background	Decrease in polyp number	Decrease in polyp number	Not reported	Roberts et al., 2002
Min	Gastrin	-/-	B6 × 129/Sv mixed background	Decrease in polyp number and size	No colon polyps in controls	Increased life expectancy	Koh et al., 2000
Min	Igf2	K10Igf2 transgene expressing excess Igf2	B6 × 129/SvJ hybrid background	No difference in polyp number or size	Increase in polyp number and size	Polyps progress to carcinoma; increase in rectal prolapse	Hassan and Howell, 2000

Model	Gene	Allele	Strain background				Reference
Min	Igf2	+m/−p	B6 × 129/SvJ hybrid background	Decrease in polyp number and size	No difference in polyp number or size	Offspring fostered to wild-type females	Hassan and Howell, 2000
Δ716	Madh4 (Dpc-4, Smad4)	+/− (cis-compound heterozygotes)	B6 × 129/Sv mixed background	Increase in polyp size	Increase in polyp size	Polyps develop into malignant adenocarcinoma; skin epidermoid cysts	Takaku et al., 1998
Min	Mbd4	−/−	C57BL/6	Increase in polyp number	Not reported	Accelerated polyp formation; reduced survival	Millar et al., 2002
Min	Mlh1	−/−; +/−	C57BL/6	Increase in polyp number	Not reported	Increase in cystic intestinal crypt multiplicity; increased desmoid tumorigenesis and epidermoid cyst development	Shoemaker et al., 2000
1638N	Mlh1	−/−	B6 × 129/Ola mixed background	Increase in polyp number	Increase in polyp number	High incidence of carcinoma; shortened life span	Edelmann et al., 1999
Min	Mmp7	−/−	B6 × 129/Sv mixed background	Decrease in polyp number and size	(Colon numbers combined with small intestine numbers)		Wilson et al., 1997
Min	Msh2	−/−	B6 × 129 mixed background	Increase in polyp number	Increase in polyp number	Accelerated polyp phenotype; develop dysplastic colonic aberrant crypt foci (ACF)	Lal et al., 2001
Min	Msh2	−/−	B6 × 129 mixed background	Increase in polyp number	Increase in polyp number; accelerated colonic adenoma growth	Development of aberrant crypt foci (ACF); reduced survival	Reitmair et al., 1996
Min	Msh2	Δ7N/Δ7N	B6 × 129 mixed background	Increase in polyp number	Increase in polyp number	Increase in polyp number	Smits et al., 2000b

(continued)

269

TABLE 12-2 (*continued*)

Apc Mutation	Gene	Genotype	Strain Background	Effects on Small Intestinal Polyps	Effects on Colon Polyps	Other Effects	References
1638N	*Msh2*	Δ7N/Δ7N	B6 × 129 mixed background	Increase in polyp number	Increase in polyp number	Reduced survival	Smits et al., 2000b
1638N	*Msh3*	-/-	C57BL/6	No difference in polyp number		No difference in survival	Kuraguchi et al., 2001
1638N	*Msh6*	-/-	C57BL/6	Increase in polyp number		Reduced survival	Kuraguchi et al., 2001
Min	*MTI/G-Gly* transgene	Overexpression of glycine-extended gastrin in colon	B6 × FVB mixed background	Increase in polyp number and size	No colon polyps in controls		Koh et al., 2000
1638N	*p21*^{waf1}	-/-; +/-	B6, 129/SvEv, black Swiss mixed background	Increase in polyp number and size	No colon polyps in controls	Increase in polyp number and size is dosage dependent; shortened life span	Yang et al., 2001
Min	*Pla2g2a* (*sPla2*)	Wild-type *Pla2g2a* transgene expression on -/- background	C57BL/6	Decrease in polyp number and size	Decrease in polyp number and size	Not reported	Cormier et al., 1997, 2000
Min	*Pla2g4* (*cPla2*)	-/-; +/-	C57BL/6J	Decrease in polyp number and size in -/- mice	No difference in polyp number or size	Not reported	Hong et al., 2001
Min	*Pms2*	-/-; +/-	B6 × 129 mixed background	Increase in polyp number in -/- mice	Increase in polyp number in -/- mice	Early-onset morbidity	Baker et al., 1998
Min	*scid*	-/-	B6 × B6JSz-scid/scid mixed background	No difference in polyp number or progression	No difference in polyp number or progression	Reduced immunoglobulin levels, reduced body weight, increased morbidity	Dudley et al., 1996

				C57BL/6N			
Δ716	Tgfbr2	+/−		No difference in polyp number or size	Not reported		Oshima et al., 1997
Min	Tp53	−/−	C57BL/6, SWR, 129/Ola mixed background	No difference in polyp number or progression	No difference in polyp number or progression	Pancreatic dysplasia, preneoplastic foci, acinar cell adenocarcinoma	Clarke et al., 1995
Min	Tp53	−/−; +/−	B6/129 mixed background	No effect on polyp number, size, or progression	No effect on polyp number, size, or progression	Not reported	Fazeli et al., 1997
Min	Tp53	−/−; +/−	B6/129Sv mixed background	Increase in polyp number; −/− develop invasive tumors	−/− develop invasive tumors	Increase in polyp number is dosage dependent; −/− develop abdominal desmoid fibromas	Halberg et al., 2000

(2) the remainder of the genome is less of an issue. However, one consideration is the background strain that carries each of the mutations. A robust phenotype should be able to be detected regardless of the strain background (mixed or inbred) upon which it is carried, whereas a weak phenotype may be difficult to detect on a single-inbred background and especially difficult to detect (if at all) on a mixed-strain background. This situation may or may not be beneficial, in that the genes that have the best chance of protecting against, or decreasing the incidence of, colorectal cancer are those that exhibit a robust phenotype regardless of the strain background (thus being more akin to the heterogeneity of the human population); molecular therapeutic approaches may not be worth developing for a single gene, which alone may have only a very small effect on colorectal cancer detectable only on a defined homogeneous background. The disadvantages of this approach are that it would be both expensive and time-consuming to individually test each of the ~25,000 protein coding genes in the mammalian genome against a given *Apc* mutation. It is this limitation that leads us to consider mutagenesis studies of the genome as a whole (see below).

MUTAGENESIS APPROACHES TO IDENTIFY MODIFIER LOCI OF INTESTINAL AND COLORECTAL NEOPLASIA

Mutagenesis screens of the mouse genome as a whole (Belknap et al., 2001; Justice et al., 1999; Schimenti and Bucan, 1998) can be useful to identify modifier genes of mutant *Apc* alleles. Modifier genes may affect a variety of biological processes, the final outcome of which is detected as changes in phenotypes such as polyp multiplicity, size, stage, or location within the intestinal tract. Mutagenesis strategies can be designed to detect dominant or recessive mutations that confer resistance to intestinal polyps. In either case, the *Apc^{Min}* mutation enables a sensitized screen to detect such changes in intestinal polyp phenotypes. The design of such screens and the genetic resources necessary to carry them out have been described elsewhere (Justice, 2000; Justice et al., 1999; Schimenti and Bucan, 1998). Mutagenesis screens are powerful because they allow for unbiased discovery of any gene that (for example) increases or decreases tumor number. As described in Chapter 11, technological advances in our ability to image tumors in vivo in mice will also facilitate the identification of modifier loci. The feasibility of success with such screens is demonstrated by the identification of a novel spontaneous mutation that confers resistance to polyps in mutant *Apc* mice (see below).

Dominant suppressors that result from overexpression of a particular gene resulting in suppression of polyps may be useful therapeutic targets, since there is the potential to develop agents to upregulate the expression and/or activity of such genes. Conversely, recessive or haploinsufficient mutations that result in suppression of polyps hold promise as potential drug targets because inhibitors of their function would have a protective effect. From a drug target point of view, recessive mutations that confer resistance would be the best, since they hold the potential of simply developing agents to knock out their function.

In addition to their potential utility in therapy, these modifier genes are of interest at the basic research level; modifier genes are important to understand complex interactions of genes at the cell and/or organ level, and for accurate disease modeling and risk assessment.

IDENTIFICATION OF THE SPONTANEOUS *MOM2* MUTATION

The prospect of performing directed mutagenesis screens to identify modifier loci is realistic in light of the recent finding of a spontaneous mutation that significantly affects the phenotype of Apc^{Min} mice. A new modifier locus, called Modifier of *Min* 2 (*Mom2*), which acts in a dominant fashion to markedly reduce intestinal polyp multiplicity in $Apc^{Min/+}$ mice, was traced to a B6 $Apc^{Min/+}$ male who had been mated with a DBA/2J female (Silverman et al., 2002). This "founder" male lived to be more than 1 year old and had only 33 small intestinal polyps and no large intestinal polyps. In contrast, B6 $Apc^{Min/+}$ males that do not carry the resistant $Mom2^R$ mutation exhibit an average of 90 polyps in the entire small intestine and a 95% incidence of colon polyps by 6 months of age. Polyp numbers along the intestinal tract of offspring from this "exceptional" mating cage resembled a bimodal distribution (Silverman et al., 2002). Further crosses revealed that one resistant *Mom2* allele ($Mom2^R$) can suppress ~90% of polyps in $Apc^{Min/+}$ mice, indicating that *Mom2* acts in a dominant fashion. The effects of the *Mom2* locus on reducing polyp multiplicity in the small and large intestines are stronger than the effects of the *Mom1* locus. The presence of one resistant $Mom2^R$ allele is capable of significantly reducing the penetrance of the Apc^{Min} mutation in the small and large intestines.

Molecular genetic linkage studies of the *Mom2* phenotype showed that the *Mom2* locus most likely resides within a ~10 cM interval bounded by *D18Mit186* and *D18Mit213* (Silverman et al., 2002). The *Mom2* region is syntenic with human chromosome 18q21 and 18q23 (Radice, 2000). Chromosome 18q21 is frequently found to undergo LOH in human colorectal tumors (Takagi et al., 1996; Thiagalingam et al., 1996). At least two genes in this region have been shown to result in intestinal neoplasia when cells undergo LOH, namely *Madh2* and *Madh4* (Koyama et al., 1999; Miyaki et al., 1999b; Tarafa et al., 2000; Xu et al., 2000). In addition, inheritance of an inactivating mutation in *MADH4* is responsible for a subset of the juvenile polyposis disorders (Howe et al., 1998).

Alternatively, other genes within this region of mouse chromosome 18 may have been altered by the *Mom2* mutation. Genes that influence cell division, differentiation, or survival of cells in the intestinal tract may be candidates for the *Mom2* locus. The mechanism by which the resistant $Mom2^R$ allele provides protection from polyp development is under study. It is not yet known whether the protective effects of the $Mom2^R$ mutation are limited to intestinal tissue or whether these effects extend to other *Apc*-induced tumors such as gastric, desmoid, and mammary tumors (Moser et al., 1993; Smits et al., 1998). Refinement of the map position of the *Mom2* locus, cloning of the *Mom2* gene, and characterization of the mutant *Mom2* allele will answer these questions, as well as lead to studies of the effects of the human *MOM2* gene in cancer.

DIETARY MODULATION OF *APC^Min*-INDUCED INTESTINAL NEOPLASIA

Variation in the incidence of colorectal cancer worldwide suggests the influence of diet (www.nih.gov). Diets rich in plant-derived foods, including grains, fruits, and vegetables, reduce the risk for colon cancer. In contrast, a Western-style diet consisting of increased saturated fat and low consumption of fiber, reduced calcium, folic acid, and vitamin D, is associated with an increased risk for colon cancer (Bruce et al., 2000;

Ferguson et al., 2001; Johnson, 2002; Lamprecht and Lipkin, 2001; Riboli and Norat, 2001; Ryan and Weir, 2001; Slattery, 2000).

Mice carrying mutant *Apc* alleles are a powerful system to study the complex genetic and environmental interactions leading to neoplasia, due to their predisposition to develop multiple intestinal adenomas (Fodde and Smits, 2001; Paulsen, 2000). Newmark and colleagues have shown that a rodent diet designed to mimic the human Western diet (increased fat, with reduced calcium, vitamin D, vitamin B12, folic acid, methionine, and choline) could induce colonic tumors in normal B6 mice without carcinogen exposure (Newmark et al., 2001). Another study performed by Kakuni and colleagues indicates that the growth of intestinal polyps in Apc^{Min} mice can be inhibited by food restriction (Kakuni et al., 2002).

Yu and colleagues performed an extensive study of Apc^{Min} mice using nine diets, each differing in fat and fiber content (Yu et al., 2001). Their analyses found that dietary fat predisposes, while fiber protects, animals from the development of small intestinal polyps. Neither high fat nor low fiber significantly altered colonic neoplasia, but diets that produced large amounts of stool resulted in more colon polyps in animals (Yu et al., 2001). Similar studies that increased the fat content more than threefold (from 3% to 10%) and halved the crude fiber content (from 4% to 2%) showed no significant effect on small intestinal polyp numbers but increased colonic polyp numbers by twofold (Wasan et al., 1997). The same study showed that the small intestinal polyp diameter was significantly enlarged in the 10% and 15% fat diet, but no such effect was observed in colon polyp diameter (Wasan et al., 1997).

Another study indicated that consumption of a low-fat diet or vegetable-fruit mix did not decrease the development of polyps compared to a high-fat diet in Apc^{Min} mice (van Kranen et al., 1998). However, a study by a different group found no effect of fat on intestinal polyp formation in Apc^{Min} mice but found that rye decreased small intestinal polyp formation, whereas a beef diet promoted polyp formation (Mutanen et al., 2000). These observed variations in results could be due to differences in the protocols between laboratories (e.g., the age of the mice at the start of the experiment, the duration of feeding time, and/or the source of fat or protein in the diets).

The effects of different dietary supplements have also been tested on Apc^{Min} mice. The addition of indigestible carbohydrates to food, such as short-chain fructo-oligosaccharides, prevented colon polyps in Apc^{Min} mice, compared to other resistant starch (modified) or starch-free wheat-bran diets that had no effect on polyp formation (Pierre et al., 1997). When soy protein was substituted as a protein source in the Western-type high-risk diet, there was no difference in incidence, multiplicity, size, and distribution of intestinal tumors in Apc^{Min} mice (Sorensen et al., 1998).

Studies analyzing the effects of dietary constituents on intestinal tumorigenesis in the Apc^{Min} model have yielded some important observations. Soybean-derived Bowman-Birk inhibitor significantly suppressed polyp development in both the small intestine and colon of Apc^{Min} mice (Kennedy et al., 1996). Mice fed ceramide, sphingomyelin, glucosylceramide, lactosylceramide, and galioside Gd13 (a composition similar in amount and type to that of dairy products) reduced polyps in all sections of the small intestine by normalizing β-catenin localization (Schmelz et al., 2001). There was partial suppression of jejunum polyp multiplicity when Apc^{Min} mice were given bovine lactoferrin (Ushida et al., 1998). Dietary supplementation of a synthetic organoselenium compound (1,4-phenylene *bis*(methylene) selenocyanate) via its action on β-catenin expression and COX2 activity significantly reduced small intestinal and colon polyps in Apc^{Min} mice (Rao et al., 2000). However, dietary folate/choline did not produce consistent effects, suggesting effective folate intervention is more sensitive to temporal and dosage variations (Sibani et al., 2002; Song et al., 2000). Dietary L-methionine supplementation stimulated growth of adenomas in the small intestine of Apc^{Min} mice, with no effects in the colon (Paulsen and Alexander, 2001).

Studies with vitamin D and its noncalcemic synthetic analogue were effective in decreasing polyp size in Apc^{Min} mice (Huerta et al., 2002). The effects of polyunsaturated fatty acids (such as $n-3$ PUFA) on intestinal tumorigenesis were shown to be more effective in the suppression and formation of small intestinal polyps than colon polyps, and suppression of intestinal polyps was inversely correlated to the production of prostaglandins (Paulsen et al., 1997; Petrik et al., 2000). Resveratrol, a natural constituent of grapes, reduced the formation of small intestinal polyps in $Apc^{Min/+}$ mice. The effects of resveratrol are mediated by downregulation of genes that are directly involved in cell cycle progression and tumor growth, and upregulation of genes that are involved in recruitment and activation of immune cells (Schneider et al., 2001). Some studies have reported that diets rich in fruits and vegetables reduce the risk of cancer because of the antioxidant and antiinflammatory properties of fruit/plant-derived phenolic compounds (Churchill et al., 2000). The flavanoid (+)-catechin that is abundant in certain fruits decreased intestinal polyp multiplicity (Weyant et al., 2001), while caffeic acid phenethyl ester and curcumin plant-derived phenolic compounds were effective in suppressing Apc^{Min}-induced intestinal tumorigenesis (Mahmoud et al., 2000; Perkins et al., 2002).

Studies in mice that carry other mutations in the Apc gene have also shown a positive correlation in the incidence of colon cancer with an increased intake of dietary fat and a decreased intake of fiber, calcium, and vitamin D (Hioki et al., 1997; Lipkin, 1997). Studies providing a Western-style diet to $Apc^{1638+/-}$, $p21^{+/-}$ animals resulted in more and larger polyps, with decreased survival of these mice (Yang et al., 2001).

These studies highlight the complexities of various diets and dietary components, and the importance of regulating the dose and length of administration of each dietary supplement for effective chemoprevention. Ultimately, such studies will help to elucidate the interactions between genetics and environment in intestinal tumorigenesis and will help in cancer chemoprevention and treatment (Glinghammar and Rafter, 1999).

EFFICACY OF THERAPEUTIC TARGETS USED IN THE TREATMENT OF *APC*-INDUCED INTESTINAL NEOPLASIA

Numerous studies have tested the effects of different therapeutic agents on intestinal tumorigenesis in mutant Apc mice. Treatment with nonsteroidal antiinflammatory drugs (NSAIDs) is known to reduce the risk of colorectal cancer. Although the precise mechanism of NSAID action remains unclear, suppression of the COX2 enzyme is thought to be of pivotal importance, in part via interference with PGE2 biosynthesis and intracellular calcium levels (Hansen-Petrik et al., 2002). Nonselective inhibitors (piroxicam, sulindac) and selective inhibitors of COX2 (nimesulide, celecoxib) have been effective in reducing polyp multiplicity and size (Beazer-Barclay et al., 1996; Boolbol et al., 1996; Chiu et al., 1997; Jacoby et al., 1996; Lipkin, 1997; Nakatsugi et al., 1997; Ritland et al., 1999). The sulfide metabolite of sulindac is responsible for its antitumor effect by decreasing PGE2 levels in the intestine and restoring mucosal apoptosis levels to normal (Mahmoud et al., 1998a).

Extensive studies by Jacoby and co-workers have shown that the chemopreventive actions of piroxicam and celecoxib are not mediated through thromboxane B2 levels. Though piroxicam decreased thromboxane B2 levels and celecoxib did not, both drugs were effective in reducing polyp number and size despite starting treatment at 55 days of age in Apc^{Min} mice (Jacoby et al., 2000b).

A study by Ritland and Gendler described the duration, kinetics, and timing of piroxicam-induced intestinal polyp suppression in Apc^{Min} mice. Their study showed that treatment for 6 days with piroxicam was effective in reducing polyp numbers. They further showed that intermittent treatment with piroxicam conferred long-term benefits against both nascent and established polyps (Ritland and Gendler, 1999). Furthermore, piroxicam was shown to be effective against polyps arising in the jejunum and ileum region, rather than in the duodenum and colon (Jacoby et al., 2000a; Ritland and Gendler, 1999). Ritland and Gendler's study also demonstrated that the effectiveness of piroxicam and sulindac treatment was strain dependent; polyps arising from B6FVBF1 $Apc^{Min/+}$ mice were significantly more resistant to piroxicam than polyps arising from either B6 $Apc^{Min/+}$ or B6129F1 $Apc^{Min/+}$ mice, suggesting that chemosensitivity may be dependent on strain background (Ritland and Gendler, 1999).

While some studies showed aspirin treatment to be effective in suppression of Apc^{Min}-induced intestinal polyps (Barnes and Lee, 1998; Mahmoud et al., 1998b; Sansom et al., 2001), others could not find a beneficial effect with aspirin treatment alone (Chiu et al., 2000; Reuter et al., 2002). Chiu's study showed that although both aspirin and indomethacin reduce PGE2 levels, only indomethacin was effective in reducing polyp numbers; aspirin was not (Chiu et al., 2000). Another form of salicylate (5-aminosalicylic acid) used in inflammatory bowel disease was not effective in suppressing intestinal polyps induced by the Apc^{Min} mutation (Ritland et al., 1999). These findings suggest that different NSAIDs may have varying impacts on Apc^{Min}-induced tumorigenesis. Another NSAID, R-flurbiprofen, dramatically reduced polyp number and size and consequently increased the survival rate of Apc^{Min} mice; however, some treated mice developed ulcers (Wechter et al., 1997, 2000). Similarly, studies in Apc knockout models ($Apc^{\Delta474}$, $Apc^{\Delta716}$, and Apc^{1309}) with inhibitors of COX1 (Mofezolac) or COX2 (nimesulide, rofecoxib, sulindac, and JTE-522) have shown suppression of intestinal polyps (Kitamura et al., 2002; Oshima et al., 2001; Sasai et al., 2000).

Although highly effective in reducing polyp multiplicity, NSAIDs have substantial adverse side-effect profiles (Trujillo et al., 1994) that may be overcome by using two or more drugs from different classes at lower doses. This strategy of combinational chemoprevention in Apc^{Min}-induced intestinal neoplasia is illustrated by Torrance and colleagues (Torrance et al., 2000). They used inhibitors of the epidermal growth factor receptor kinase in combination with the NSAID sulindac. Their results showed complete eradication of intestinal polyp formation in nearly 47% of $Apc^{Min/+}$ mice (Torrance et al., 2000).

Another study showed a similar eradication of intestinal polyp formation when $Apc^{Min/+}$ mice were treated with piroxicam and difluoromethylornithine, an ornithine decarboxylase inhibitor (Jacoby et al., 2000a). Reduction in polyp numbers in $Apc^{Min/+}$ mice was also shown with administration of uroguanylin (a local regulator of intestinal secretion), which activates the cGMP signaling pathway in vitro (Shailubhai et al., 2000). Studies have shown that administration of 5-fluorouracil (5-FU) reduces polyp number in $Apc^{Min/+}$ mice, although polyps returned after cessation of treatment (Tucker et al., 2002). However, an absence of folic acid in the diet not only lowered polyp number in 5-FU-treated mice but also inhibited polyp recovery (Tucker et al., 2002). Thus, there may be several mechanisms by which different compounds effectively inhibit polyp formation. Mutant *Apc* mice provide important and useful models for testing the safety and assessing the efficacy of chemotherapeutic agents as well as for investigating the molecular pathways to cancer.

ETHICAL ISSUES OF CANCER PREVENTION

The ability to genotype individuals and determine whether they carry genes that will make them susceptible to cancer is the first step in the prevention of cancer. This knowledge can be used potentially to tailor specific regimens to prevent and/or delay the onset of cancer. Ethical issues arise not with genotyping individuals per se but with where and how that information is used. Would employers use such knowledge to determine whom to hire, fire, promote, etc.? Would health care companies avoid insuring cancer-prone individuals? Who would bear the cost of testing and would every individual have equal access to such testing? Most importantly, would parents raise children differently if one were cancer prone and one were not? These questions are just a sample of the issues facing society now and in the future, and they are not easy to resolve. It is our hope that education will encourage an understanding of the benefits of cancer-prevention strategies to enhance quality of life without bringing about discrimination in economic spheres.

CONCLUSIONS

The usefulness of gene discovery is to uncover multiple avenues to detect, treat and reduce the occurrence of cancer. The results of research studies will successfully identify new modifier loci affecting cancer initiation, growth, and progression in mammals. More importantly, we will better understand the role of modifier genes in contributing to human cancer and treatment outcomes. New strategies involving gene and/or protein expression profile testing can be specifically designed to assess an individual's probability of developing cancer. The ultimate goal of preventing cancer may be realized with a combination of early intervention, dietary regimens, and chemopreventive agents made possible by identification of individuals at risk and physiological understanding of the genotypes of more and less susceptible individuals.

REFERENCES

Bailey, D. W. (1981). Recombinant inbred strains and bilineal strains. In *The Mouse in Biomedical Research*, H. L. Foster, J. D. Small, and J. G. Fox (eds.). New York: Academic Press.

Baker, S. M., Harris, A. C., Tsao J. L., Flath, T. J., Bronner, C. E., Gordon, M., Shibata, D., and Liskay, R. M. (1998). Enhanced intestinal adenomatous polyp formation in Pms2 − /−; Min mice. *Cancer Res 58*, 1087–1089.

Balmain, A. (2002). Cancer as a complex genetic trait: Tumor susceptibility in humans and mouse models. *Cell 108*, 145–152.

Balmain, A., and Nagase, H. (1998). Cancer resistance genes in mice: Models for the study of tumour modifiers. *Trends Genet 14*, 139–144.

Barnes, C. J., and Lee, M. (1998). Chemoprevention of spontaneous intestinal adenomas in the adenomatous polyposis coli Min mouse model with aspirin. *Gastroenterology 114*, 873–877.

Beazer-Barclay, Y., Levy, D. B., Moser, A. R., Dove, W. F., Hamilton, S. R., Vogelstein, B., and Kinzler, K. W. (1996). Sulindac suppresses tumorigenesis in the Min mouse. *Carcinogenesis 17*, 1757–1760.

Bedell, M. A., Jenkins, N. A., and Copeland, N. G. (1997a). Mouse models of human disease. Part I: Techniques and resources for genetic analysis in mice. *Genes Dev 11*, 1–10.

Bedell, M. A., Largaespada, D. A., Jenkins, N. A., and Copeland, N. G. (1997b). Mouse models of human disease. Part II: Recent progress and future directions. *Genes Dev 11*, 11–43.

Belknap, J. K., Hitzemann, R., Crabbe, J. C., Phillips, T. J., Buck, K. J., and Williams, R. W. (2001). QTL analysis and genomewide mutagenesis in mice: Complementary genetic approaches to the dissection of complex traits. *Behav Genet 31*, 5–15.

Beroud, C., and Soussi, T. (1996). APC gene: Database of germline and somatic mutations in human tumors and cell lines. *Nucleic Acids Res 24*, 121–124.

Blake, J. A., Richardson, J. E., Bult, C. J., Kadin, J. A., and Eppig, J. T. (2002). The Mouse Genome Database (MGD): The model organism database for the laboratory mouse. *Nucleic Acids Res 30*, 113–115.

Boolbol, S. K., Dannenberg, A. J., Chadburn, A., Martucci, C., Guo, X. J., Ramonetti, J. T., Abreu-Goris, M., Newmark, H. L., Lipkin, M. L., DeCosse, J. J., and Bertagnolli, M. M. (1996). Cyclooxygenase-2 overexpression and tumor formation are blocked by sulindac in a murine model of familial adenomatous polyposis. *Cancer Res 56*, 2556–2560.

Brookes, A. J. (1999). The essence of SNPs. *Gene 234*, 177–186.

Bruce, W. R., Wolever, T. M., and Giacca, A. (2000). Mechanisms linking diet and colorectal cancer: The possible role of insulin resistance. *Nutr Cancer 37*, 19–26.

Buchberg, A. M., and Siracusa, L. D. (1995). The Genetics of Cancer Susceptibility: Secretory Phospholipase A2 and Intestinal Neoplasia. In *General Motors Cancer Research Foundation, Accomplishments in Cancer Research 1995*, J. G. Fortner and J. E. Rhoads (eds.). Philadelphia: J.B. Lippincott Company, pp. 159–168.

Chiu, C. H., McEntee, M. F., and Whelan, J. (1997). Sulindac causes rapid regression of pre-existing tumors in Min/+ mice independent of prostaglandin biosynthesis. *Cancer Res 57*, 4267–4273.

Chiu, C. H., McEntee, M. F., and Whelan, J. (2000). Discordant effect of aspirin and indomethacin on intestinal tumor burden in Apc(Min/+) mice. *Prostaglandins Leukot Essent Fatty Acids 62*, 269–275.

Chulada, P. C., Thompson, M. B., Mahler, J. F., Doyle, C. M., Gaul, B. W., Lee, C., Tiano, H. F., Morham, S. G., Smithies, O., and Langenbach, R. (2000). Genetic disruption of Ptgs-1, as well as Ptgs-2, reduces intestinal tumorigenesis in Min mice. *Cancer Res 60*, 4705–4708.

Churchill, M., Chadburn, A., Bilinski, R. T., and Bertagnolli, M. M. (2000). Inhibition of intestinal tumors by curcumin is associated with changes in the intestinal immune cell profile. *J Surg Res 89*, 169–175.

Clarke, A. R., Cummings, M. C., and Harrison, D. J. (1995). Interaction between murine germline mutations in p53 and APC predisposes to pancreatic neoplasia but not to increased intestinal malignancy. *Oncogene 11*, 1913–1920.

Cormier, R. T., Hong, K. H., Halberg, R. B., Hawkins, T. L., Richardson, P., Mulherkar, R., Dove, W. F., and Lander, E. S. (1997). Secretory phospholipase Pla2g2a confers resistance to intestinal tumorigenesis. *Nat Genet 17*, 88–91.

Cormier, R. T., and Dove, W. F. (2000). Dnmt1N/+ reduces the net growth rate and multiplicity of intestinal adenomas in C57BL/6-multiple intestinal neoplasia (Min)/+ mice independently of p53 but demonstrates strong synergy with the modifier of Min 1(AKR) resistance allele. *Cancer Res 60*, 3965–3970.

Cormier, R. T., Bilger, A., Lillich, A. J., Halberg, R. B., Hong, K. H., Gould, K. A., Borenstein, N., Lander, E. S., and Dove, W. F. (2000). The Mom1AKR intestinal tumor resistance region consists of Pla2g2a and a locus distal to D4Mit64. *Oncogene 19*, 3182–3192.

Crabtree, M. D., Tomlinson, I. P., Hodgson, S. V., Neale, K., Phillips, R. K., and Houlston, R. S. (2002). Explaining variation in familial adenomatous polyposis: Relationship between genotype and phenotype and evidence for modifier genes. *Gut 51*, 420–423.

Darvasi, A. (1998). Experimental strategies for the genetic dissection of complex traits in animal models. *Nat Genet 18*, 19–24.

Demant, P., and Hart, A. A. (1986). Recombinant congenic strains—a new tool for analyzing genetic traits determined by more than one gene. *Immunogenetics 24*, 416–422.

Dietrich, W. F., Lander, E. S., Smith, J. S., Moser, A. R., Gould, K. A., Luongo, C., Borenstein, N., and Dove, W. (1993). Genetic identification of Mom-1, a major modifier locus affecting Min-induced intestinal neoplasia in the mouse. *Cell 75*, 631–639.

Dietrich, W. F., Copeland, N. G., Gilbert, D. J., Miller, J. C., Jenkins, N. A., and Lander, E. S. (1995). Mapping the mouse genome: Current status and future prospects. *Proc Natl Acad Sci USA 92*, 10849–10853.

Dobbie, Z., Heinimann, K., Bishop, D. T., Muller, H., and Scott, R. J. (1997). Identification of a modifier gene locus on chromosome 1p35–36 in familial adenomatous polyposis. *Hum Genet 99*, 653–657.

Dudley, M. E., Sundberg, J. P., and Roopenian, D. C. (1996). Frequency and histological appearance of adenomas in multiple intestinal neoplasia mice are unaffected by severe combined immunodeficiency (scid) mutation. *Int J Cancer 65*, 249–253.

Dunlop, M. G. (1997). Colorectal cancer. *Br Med J 314*, 1882–1885.

Eads, C. A., Nickel, A. E., and Laird, P. W. (2002). Complete genetic suppression of polyp formation and reduction of CpG-island hypermethylation in Apc(Min/+) Dnmt1-hypomorphic mice. *Cancer Res 62*, 1296–1299.

Edelmann, W., Yang, K., Kuraguchi, M., Heyer, J., Lia, M., Kneitz, B., Fan, K., Brown, A. M., Lipkin, M., and Kucherlapati, R. (1999). Tumorigenesis in Mlh1 and Mlh1/Apc1638N mutant mice. *Cancer Res 59*, 1301–1307.

Fazeli, A., Steen, R. G., Dickinson, S. L., Bautista, D., Dietrich, W. F., Bronson, R. T., Bresalier, R. S., Lander, E. S., Costa, J., and Weinberg, R. A. (1997). Effects of p53 mutations on apoptosis in mouse intestinal and human colonic adenomas. *Proc Natl Acad Sci USA 94*, 10199–10204.

Fearnhead, N. S., Britton, M. P., and Bodmer, W. F. (2001). The ABC of APC. *Hum Mol Genet 10*, 721–733.

Fearon, E. R., Cho, K. R., Nigro, J. M., Kern, S. E., Simons, J. W., Ruppert, J. M., Hamilton, S. R., Preisinger, A. C., Thomas, G., Kinzler, K. W., and Vogelstein, B. (1990). Identification of a chromosome 18q gene that is altered in colorectal cancers. *Science 247*, 49–56.

Ferguson, L. R., Chavan, R. R., and Harris, P. J. (2001). Changing concepts of dietary fiber: Implications for carcinogenesis. *Nutr Cancer 39*, 155–169.

Ficari, F., Cama, A., Valanzano, R., Curia, M. C., Palmirotta, R., Aceto, G., Esposito, D. L., Crognale, S., Lombardi, A., Messerini, L., Mariani-Costantini, R., Tonelli, F., and Battista, P. (2000). APC gene mutations and colorectal adenomatosis in familial adenomatous polyposis. *Br J Cancer 82*, 348–353.

Fishel, R. (1998). Mismatch repair, molecular switches, and signal transduction. *Genes Dev 12*, 2096–2101.

Fishel, R. (1999). Signaling mismatch repair in cancer. *Nat Med 5*, 1239–1241.

Fodde, R., and Khan, P. M. (1995). Genotype-phenotype correlations at the adenomatous polyposis coli (APC) gene. *Crit Rev Oncogenet 6*, 291–303.

Fodde, R., Edelmann, W., Yang, K., van Leeuwen, C., Carlson, C., Renault, B., Breukel, C., Alt, E., Lipkin, M., Khan, P. M., and Kucherlapati, R. (1994). A targeted chain-termination mutation in the mouse Apc gene results in multiple intestinal tumors. *Proc Natl Acad Sci USA 91*, 8969–8973.

Fodde, R., and Smits, R. (2001). Disease model: Familial adenomatous polyposis. *Trends Mol Med 7*, 369–373.

Fodde, R., Kuipers, J., Rosenberg, C., Smits, R., Kielman, M., Gaspar, C., van Es, J. H., Breukel, C., Wiegant, J., Giles, R. H., and Clevers, H. (2001a). Mutations in the APC tumour suppressor gene cause chromosomal instability. *Nat Cell Biol 3*, 433–438.

Fodde, R., Smits, R., and Clevers, H. (2001b). APC, signal transduction and genetic instability in colorectal cancer. *Nat Rev Cancer 1*, 55–67.

Frankel, W. N. (1995). Taking stock of complex trait genetics in mice. *Trends Genet 11*, 471–477.

Gardner, E. J., and Richards, E. C. (1953). Multiple cutaneous and sub-cutaneous lesions occurring simultaneously with hereditary polyposis and osteomatosis. *Am J Hum Genet 5*, 139–147.

Giardiello, F. M., Krush, A. J., Petersen, G. M., Booker, S. V., Kerr, M., Tong, L. L., and Hamilton, S. R. (1994). Phenotypic variability of familial adenomatous polyposis in 11 unrelated families with identical APC gene mutation. *Gastroenterology 106*, 1542–1547.

Glazier, A. M., Nadeau, J. H., and Aitman, T. J. (2002). Finding genes that underlie complex traits. *Science 298*, 2345–2349.

Glinghammar, B., and Rafter, J. (1999). Carcinogenesis in the colon: Interaction between luminal factors and genetic factors. *Eur J Cancer Prev 8*, suppl 1, S87–94.

Gould, K. A., and Dove, W. F. (1998). Analysis of the Mom1 modifier of intestinal neoplasia in mice. *Exp Lung Res 24*, 437–453.

Gould, K. A., Dietrich, W. F., Borenstein, N., Lander, E. S., and Dove, W. F. (1996a). Mom1 is a semi-dominant modifier of intestinal adenoma size and multiplicity in Min/+ mice. *Genetics 144*, 1769–1776.

Gould, K. A., Luongo, C., Moser, A. R., McNeley, M. K., Borenstein, N., Shedlovsky, A., Dove, W. F., Hong, K., Dietrich, W. F., and Lander, E. S. (1996b). Genetic evaluation of candidate genes for the Mom1 modifier of intestinal neoplasia in mice. *Genetics 144*, 1777–1785.

Goss, K. H., Risinger, M. A., Kordich, J. J., Sanz, M. M., Straughen, J. E., Slovek, L. E., Capibianco, A. J., German, J., Boivin, G. P., and Groden, J. (2002). Enhanced tumor formation in mice heterozygotes for *Blm* mutation. *Science 297*, 2051–2053.

Greenlee, R. T., Murray, T., Bolden, S., and Wingo, P. A. (2000). Cancer statistics, 2000. *CA Cancer J Clin 50*, 7–33.

Griffioen, G., Bus, P. J., Vasen, H. F., Verspaget, H. W., and Lamers, C. B. (1998). Extracolonic manifestations of familial adenomatous polyposis: Desmoid tumours, and upper gastrointestinal adenomas and carcinomas. *Scand J Gastroenterol*, suppl 225, 85–91.

Groden, J., Thliveris, A., Samowitz, W., Carlson, M., Gelbert, L., Albertsen, H., Joslyn, G., Stevens, J., Spirio, L., Robertson, M., Sargeant, L., Krapcho, K., Wolff, E., Burt, R., Hughes, J. P., Warrington, J., McPherson, J., Wasmuth, J., Le Paslier, D., Abderrahion, H., Cohen, D., Leppert, M., and White, R. (1991). Identification and characterization of the familial adenomatous polyposis coli gene. *Cell 66*, 589–600.

Halberg, R. B., Katzung, D. S., Hoff, P. D., Moser, A. R., Cole, C. E., Lubet, R. A., Donehower, L. A., Jacoby, R. F., and Dove, W. F. (2000). Tumorigenesis in the multiple intestinal neoplasia mouse: redundancy of negative regulators and specificity of modifiers. *Proc Natl Acad Sci USA 97*, 3461–3466.

Haluska, F. G., Thiele, C., Goldstein, A., Tsao, H., Benoit, E. P., and Housman, D. (1997). Lack of phospholipase A2 mutations in neuroblastoma, melanoma and colon cancer cell lines. *Int J Cancer 72*, 337–339.

Hamilton, S. R., Liu, B., Parsons, R. E., Papadopoulos, N., Jen, J., Powell, S. M., Krush, A. J., Berk, T., Cohen, Z., Tetu, B., Burger, P. C., Wood, P. A., Tagi, F., Booker, S. V., Petersen, G. M., Offerhaus, G. J. A., Tersmette, A. C., Giardiello, F. M., Vogelstein, B., and Kinzler, K. W. (1995). The molecular basis of Turcot's syndrome. *N Engl J Med 332*, 839–847.

Hansen-Petrik, M. B., McEntee, M. F., Jull, B., Shi, H., Zemel, M. B., and Whelan, J. (2002). Prostaglandin E(2) protects intestinal tumors from nonsteroidal antiinflammatory drug-induced regression in Apc(Min/+) mice. *Cancer Res 62*, 403–408.

Hart, M. J., de los Santos, R., Albert, I. N., Rubinfeld, B., and Polakis, P. (1998). Downregulation of beta-catenin by human Axin and its association with the APC tumor suppressor, beta-catenin and GSK3 beta. *Curr Biol 8*, 573–581.

Hassan, A. B., and Howell, J. A. (2000). Insulin-like growth factor II supply modifies growth of intestinal adenoma in Apc(Min/+) mice. *Cancer Res 60*, 1070–1076.

Hioki, K., Shivapurkar, N., Oshima, H., Alabaster, O., Oshima, M., and Taketo, M. M. (1997). Suppression of intestinal polyp development by low-fat and high-fiber diet in Apc(delta716) knockout mice. *Carcinogenesis 18*, 1863–1865.

Hong, K. H., Bonventre, J. C., O'Leary, E., Bonventre, J. V., and Lander, E. S. (2001). Deletion of cytosolic phospholipase A(2) suppresses Apc(Min)-induced tumorigenesis. *Proc Natl Acad Sci USA 98*, 3935–3939.

Houlston, R., Crabtree, M., Phillips, R., and Tomlinson, I. (2001). Explaining differences in the severity of familial adenomatous polyposis and the search for modifier genes. *Gut 48*, 1–5.

Howe, J. R., Ringold, J. C., Summers, R. W., Mitros, F. A., Nishimura, D. Y., and Stone, E. M. (1998). A gene for familial juvenile polyposis maps to chromosome 18q21.1. *Am J Hum Genet 62*, 1129–1136.

Huerta, S., Irwin, R. W., Heber, D., Go, V. L., Koeffler, H. P., Uskokovic, M. R., and Harris, D. M. (2002). 1alpha,25-(OH)(2)-D(3) and its synthetic analogue decrease tumor load in the Apc(min) mouse. *Cancer Res 62*, 741–746.

Ilyas, M., Straub, J., Tomlinson, I. P., and Bodmer, W. F. (1999). Genetic pathways in colorectal and other cancers. *Eur J Cancer 35*, 1986–2002.

Jacoby, R. F., Marshall, D. J., Newton, M. A., Novakovic, K., Tutsch, K., Cole, C. E., Lubet, R. A., Kelloff, G. J., Verma, A., Moser, A. R., and Dove, W. F. (1996). Chemoprevention of spontaneous intestinal adenomas in the Apc Min mouse model by the nonsteroidal anti-inflammatory drug piroxicam. *Cancer Res 56*, 710–714.

Jacoby, R. F., Cole, C. E., Tutsch, K., Newton, M. A., Kelloff, G., Hawk, E. T., and Lubet, R. A. (2000a). Chemopreventive efficacy of combined piroxicam and difluoromethylornithine treatment of Apc mutant Min mouse adenomas, and selective toxicity against Apc mutant embryos. *Cancer Res 60*, 1864–1870.

Jacoby, R. F., Seibert, K., Cole, C. E., Kelloff, G., and Lubet, R. A. (2000b). The cyclooxygenase-2 inhibitor celecoxib is a potent preventive and therapeutic agent in the min mouse model of adenomatous polyposis. *Cancer Res 60*, 5040–5044.

Johnson, G. C., and Todd, J. A. (2000). Strategies in complex disease mapping. *Curr Opin Genet Dev 10*, 330–334.

Johnson, I. T. (2002). Anticarcinogenic effects of diet-related apoptosis in the colorectal mucosa. *Food Chem Toxicol 40*, 1171–1178.

Joslyn, G., Carlson, M., Thliveris, A., Albertsen, H., Gelbert, L., Samowitz, W., Groden, J., Stevens, J., Spirio, L., Robertson, M., et al. (1991). Identification of deletion mutations and three new genes at the familial polyposis locus. *Cell 66*, 601–613.

Justice, M. J. (2000). Mutagenesis of the mouse germline. In *Mouse Genetics and Transgenics: A Practical Approach*, I. J. Jackson, and C. M. Abbott (eds.). New York: Oxford University Press.

Justice, M. J., Noveroske, J. K., Weber, J. S., Zheng, B., and Bradley, A. (1999). Mouse ENU mutagenesis. *Hum Mol Genet 8*, 1955–1963.

Kakuni, M., Morimura, K., Wanibuchi, H., Ogawa, M., Min, W., Hayashi, S., and Fukushima, S. (2002). Food restriction inhibits the growth of intestinal polyps in multiple intestinal neoplasia mouse. *Jpn J Cancer Res 93*, 236–241.

Kaplan, K. B., Burds, A. A., Swedlow, J. R., Bekir, S. S., Sorger, P. K., and Nathke, I. S. (2001). A role for the adenomatous polyposis coli protein in chromosome segregation. *Nat Cell Biol 3*, 429–432.

Kawasaki, Y., Senda, T., Ishidate, T., Koyama, R., Morishita, T., Iwayama, Y., Higuchi, O., and Akiyama, T. (2000). Asef, a link between the tumor suppressor APC and G-protein signaling. *Science 289*, 1194–1197.

Kennedy, A. R., Beazer-Barclay, Y., Kinzler, K. W., and Newberne, P. M. (1996). Suppression of carcinogenesis in the intestines of min mice by the soybean-derived Bowman-Birk inhibitor. *Cancer Res 56*, 679–682.

Kennedy, B. P., Payette, P., Mudgett, J., Vadas, P., Pruzanski, W., Kwan, M., Tang, C., Rancourt, D. E., and Cromlish, W. A. (1995). A natural disruption of the secretory group II phospholipase A2 gene in inbred mouse strains. *J Biol Chem 270*, 22378–22385.

Kinzler, K. W., Nilbert, M. C., Su, L. K., Vogelstein, B., Bryan, T. M., Levy, D. B., Smith, K. J., Preisinger, A. C., Hedge, P., McKechnie, D., Finniear, R., Markham, A., Groffen, J., Boguski, M. S., Altschul, S. F., Horii, A., Ando, H., Miyoshi, Y., Miki, Y., Nishisho, I., and Nakamura, Y. (1991a). Identification of FAP locus genes from chromosome 5q21. *Science 253*, 661–665.

Kinzler, K. W., Nilbert, M. C., Vogelstein, B., Bryan, T. M., Levy, D. B., Smith, K. J., Preisinger, A. C., Hamilton, S. R., Hedge, P., Markham, A., Carlson, M., Joslyn, G., Groden, J., White, R., Miki, Y., Miyoshi, Y., Nishisho, I., and Nakamura, Y. (1991b). Identification of a gene located at chromosome 5q21 that is mutated in colorectal cancers. *Science 251*, 1366–1370.

Kitamura, T., Kawamori, T., Uchiya, N., Itoh, M., Noda, T., Matsuura, M., Sugimura, T., and Wakabayashi, K. (2002). Inhibitory effects of mofezolac, a cyclooxygenase-1 selective inhibitor, on intestinal carcinogenesis. *Carcinogenesis 23*, 1463–1466.

Klausner, R. D. (1999). Studying cancer in the mouse. *Oncogene 18*, 5249–5252.

Korstanje, R., and Paigen, B. (2002). From QTL to gene: The harvest begins. *Nat Genet 31*, 235–236.

Koh, T. J., Bulitta, C. J., Fleming, J. V., Dockray, G. J., Varro, A., and Wang, T. C. (2000). Gastrin is a target of the beta-catenin/TCF-4 growth-signaling pathway in a model of intestinal polyposis. *J Clin Invest 106*, 533–539.

Koyama, M., Ito, M., Nagai, H., Emi, M., and Moriyama, Y. (1999). Inactivation of both alleles of the DPC4/SMAD4 gene in advanced colorectal cancers: Identification of seven novel somatic mutations in tumors from Japanese patients. *Mutat Res 406*, 71–77.

Kuraguchi, M., Yang, K., Wong, E., Avdievich, E., Fan, K., Kolodner, R. D., Lipkin, M., Brown, A. M., Kucherlapati, R., and Edelmann, W. (2001). The distinct spectra of tumor-associated Apc mutations in mismatch repair-deficient Apc 1638N mice define the roles of MSH3 and MSH6 in DNA repair and intestinal tumorigenesis. *Cancer Res 61*, 7934–7942.

Laird, P. W., Jackson-Grusby, L., Fazeli, A., Dickinson, S. L., Jung, W. E., Li, E., Weinberg, R. A., and Jaenisch, R. (1995). Suppression of intestinal neoplasia by DNA hypomethylation. *Cell 81*, 197–205.

Lal, G., and Gallinger, S. (2000). Familial adenomatous polyposis. *Semin Surg Oncol 18*, 314–323.

Lal, G., Ash, C., Hay, K., Redston, M., Kwong, E., Hancock, B., Mak, T., Kargman, S., Evans, J. F., and Gallinger, S. (2001). Suppression of intestinal polyps in Msh2-deficient and non-Msh2-deficient multiple intestinal neoplasia mice by a specific cyclooxygenase-2 inhibitor and by a dual cyclooxygenase-1/2 inhibitor. *Cancer Res 61*, 6131–6136.

Lamprecht, S. A., and Lipkin, M. (2001). Cellular mechanisms of calcium and vitamin D in the inhibition of colorectal carcinogenesis. *Ann NY Acad Sci 952*, 73–87.

Leister, I., Weith, A., Bruderlein, S., Cziepluch, C., Kangwanpong, D., Schlag, P., and Schwab, M. (1990). Human colorectal cancer: High frequency of deletions at chromosome 1p35. *Cancer Res 50*, 7232–7235.

Leppert, M., Dobbs, M., Scambler, P., O'Connell, P., Nakamura, Y., Stauffer, D., Woodward, S., Burt, R., Hughes, J., Gardner, E., Lathrop, M., Wasmuth, J., Lalouel, J.-M., and White, R. (1987). The gene for familial polyposis coli maps to the long arm of chromosome 5. *Science 238*, 1411–1413.

Leppert, M., Burt, R., Hughes, J. P., Samowitz, W., Nakamura, Y., Woodward, S., Gardner, E., Lalouel, J. M., and White, R. (1990). Genetic analysis of an inherited predisposition to colon cancer in a family with a variable number of adenomatous polyps. *N Engl J Med 322*, 904–908.

Levy, D. B., Smith, K. J., Beazer-Barclay, Y., Hamilton, S. R., Vogelstein, B., and Kinzler, K. W. (1994). Inactivation of both APC alleles in human and mouse tumors. *Cancer Res 54*, 5953–5958.

Lipkin, M. (1997). New rodent models for studies of chemopreventive agents. *J Cell Biochem*, suppl *29*, 144–147.

Luo, G., Santoro, I. M., McDaniel, L. D., Nishijima, I., Mills, M., Youssoufian, H., Vogel, H., Schultz, R. A., and Bradley, A. (2000). Cancer predisposition caused by elevated mitotic recombination in Bloom mice. *Nat Genet 26*, 424–429.

Luongo, C., Moser, A. R., Gledhill, S., and Dove, W. F. (1994). Loss of Apc+ in intestinal adenomas from Min mice. *Cancer Res 54*, 5947–5952.

Lynch, H. T., and Lynch, J. (2000). Lynch syndrome: Genetics, natural history, genetic counseling, and prevention. *J Clin Oncol 18*, 19S–31S.

MacPhee, M., Chepenik, K. P., Liddell, R. A., Nelson, K. K., Siracusa, L. D., and Buchberg, A. M. (1995). The secretory phospholipase A2 gene is a candidate for the Mom1 locus, a major modifier of ApcMin-induced intestinal neoplasia. *Cell 81*, 957–966.

Mahmoud, N. N., Boolbol, S. K., Dannenberg, A. J., Mestre, J. R., Bilinski, R. T., Martucci, C., Newmark, H. L., Chadburn, A., and Bertagnolli, M. M. (1998a). The sulfide metabolite of sulindac prevents tumors and restores enterocyte apoptosis in a murine model of familial adenomatous polyposis. *Carcinogenesis 19*, 87–91.

Mahmoud, N. N., Dannenberg, A. J., Mestre, J., Bilinski, R. T., Churchill, M. R., Martucci, C., Newmark, H., and Bertagnolli, M. M. (1998b). Aspirin prevents tumors in a murine model of familial adenomatous polyposis. *Surgery 124*, 225–231.

Mahmoud, N. N., Carothers, A. M., Grunberger, D., Bilinski, R. T., Churchill, M. R., Martucci, C., Newmark, H. L., and Bertagnolli, M. M. (2000). Plant phenolics decrease intestinal tumors in an animal model of familial adenomatous polyposis. *Carcinogenesis 21*, 921–927.

Markowitz, S., Wang, J., Myeroff, L., Parsons, R., Sun, L., Lutterbaugh, J., Fan, R. S., Zborowska, E., Kinzler, K. W., Vogelstein, B., Brattain, M., and Willson, J. K. V. (1995). Inactivation of the type II TGF-beta receptor in colon cancer cells with microsatellite instability. *Science 268*, 1336–1338.

Martin-Denavit, T., Duthel, S., Giraud, S., Olschwang, S., Saurin, J. C., and Plauchu, H. (2001). Phenotype variability of two FAP families with an identical APC germline mutation at codon 1465: A potential modifier effect? *Clin Genet 60*, 125–131.

Matsumine, A., Ogai, A., Senda, T., Okumura, N., Satoh, K., Baeg, G. H., Kawahara, T., Koba-yashi, S., Okada, M., Toyoshima, K., and Akiyama, T. (1996). Binding of APC to the human homolog of the Drosophila discs large tumor suppressor protein. *Science 272*, 1020–1023.

McPeek, M. S. (2000). From mouse to human: Fine mapping of quantitative trait loci in a model organism. *Proc Natl Acad Sci USA 97*, 12389–12390.

Midgley, C. A., White, S., Howitt, R., Save, V., Dunlop, M. G., Hall, P. A., Lane, D. P., Wyl-lie, A. H., and Bubb, V. J. (1997). APC expression in normal human tissues. *J Pathol 181*, 426–433.

Millar, C. B., Guy, J., Sansom, O. J., Selfridge, J., MacDougall, E., Hendrich, B., Keightley, P. D., Bishop, S. M., Clarke, A. R., and Bird, A. (2002). Enhanced CpG mutability and tumorigenesis in MBD4-deficient mice. *Science 297*, 403–405.

Miyaki, M., Konishi, M., Kikuchi-Yanoshita, R., Enomoto, M., Igari, T., Tanaka, K., Muraoka, M., Takahashi, H., Amada, Y., and Fukayama, M. (1994). Characteristics of somatic mutation of the adenomatous polyposis coli gene in colorectal tumors. *Cancer Res 54*, 3011–3020.

Miyaki, M., Iijima, T., Kimura, J., Yasuno, M., Mori, T., Hayashi, Y., Koike, M., Shitara, N., Iwama, T., and Kuroki, T. (1999a). Frequent mutation of beta-catenin and APC genes in pri-mary colorectal tumors from patients with hereditary nonpolyposis colorectal cancer. *Cancer Res 59*, 4506–4509.

Miyaki, M., Iijima, T., Konishi, M., Sakai, K., Ishii, A., Yasuno, M., Hishima, T., Koike, M., Shitara, N., Iwama, T., Utsunomiya, J., Kuroki, T., and Mori, T. (1999b). Higher frequency of Smad4 gene mutation in human colorectal cancer with distant metastasis. *Oncogene 18*, 3098–3103.

Miyoshi, Y., Ando, H., Nagase, H., Nishisho, I., Horii, A., Miki, Y., Mori, T., Utsunomiya, J., Baba, S., Petersen, G., Hamilton, S. R., Kinzler, K. W., Vogelstein, B., and Nakamura, Y. (1992a). Germ-line mutations of the APC gene in 53 familial adenomatous polyposis patients. *Proc Natl Acad Sci USA 89*, 4452–4456.

Miyoshi, Y., Nagase, H., Ando, H., Horii, A., Ichii, S., Nakatsuru, S., Aoki, T., Miki, Y., Mori, T., and Nakamura, Y. (1992b). Somatic mutations of the APC gene in colorectal tumors: Mutation cluster region in the APC gene. *Hum Mol Genet 1*, 229–233.

Moore, K. J., and Nagle, D. L. (2000). Complex trait analysis in the mouse: The strengths, the limitations and the promise yet to come. *Annu Rev Genet 34*, 653–686.

Moser, A. R., Pitot, H. C., and Dove, W. F. (1990). A dominant mutation that predisposes to multiple intestinal neoplasia in the mouse. *Science 247*, 322–324.

Moser, A. R., Dove, W. F., Roth, K. A., and Gordon, J. I. (1992). The Min (multiple intestinal neoplasia) mutation: Its effect on gut epithelial cell differentiation and interaction with a modifier system. *J Cell Biol 116*, 1517–1526.

Moser, A. R., Mattes, E. M., Dove, W. F., Lindstrom, M. J., Haag, J. D., and Gould, M. N. (1993). ApcMin, a mutation in the murine Apc gene, predisposes to mammary carcinomas and focal alveolar hyperplasias. *Proc Natl Acad Sci USA 90*, 8977–8981.

Moser, A. R., Luongo, C., Gould, K. A., McNeley, M. K., Shoemaker, A. R., and Dove, W. F. (1995). ApcMin: A mouse model for intestinal and mammary tumorigenesis. *Eur J Cancer 31 A*, 1061–1064.

Moser, A. R., Hegge, L. F., and Cardiff, R. D. (2001). Genetic background affects susceptibility to mammary hyperplasias and carcinomas in Apc(min)/+ mice. *Cancer Res 61*, 3480–3485.

Mott, R., Talbot, C. J., Turri, M. G., Collins, A. C., and Flint, J. (2000). From the cover: A method for fine mapping quantitative trait loci in outbred animal stocks. *Proc Natl Acad Sci USA 97*, 12649–12654.

Mutanen, M., Pajari, A. M., and Oikarinen, S. I. (2000). Beef induces and rye bran prevents the formation of intestinal polyps in Apc(Min) mice: Relation to beta-catenin and PKC isozymes. *Carcinogenesis 21*, 1167–1173.

Nadeau, J. H., Singer, J. B., Matin, A., and Lander, E. S. (2000). Analysing complex genetic traits with chromosome substitution strains. *Nat Genet 24*, 221–225.

Nagase, H., and Nakamura, Y. (1993). Mutations of the APC (adenomatous polyposis coli) gene. *Hum Mutat 2*, 425–434.

Nakatsugi, S., Fukutake, M., Takahashi, M., Fukuda, K., Isoi, T., Taniguchi, Y., Sugimura, T., and Wakabayashi, K. (1997). Suppression of intestinal polyp development by nimesulide, a selective cyclooxygenase-2 inhibitor, in Min mice. *Jpn J Cancer Res 88*, 1117–1120.

Nathke, I. S., Adams, C. L., Polakis, P., Sellin, J. H., and Nelson, W. J. (1996). The adenomatous polyposis coli tumor suppressor protein localizes to plasma membrane sites involved in active cell migration. *J Cell Biol 134*, 165–179.

Neufeld, K. L., and White, R. L. (1997). Nuclear and cytoplasmic localizations of the adenomatous polyposis coli protein. *Proc Natl Acad Sci USA 94*, 3034–3039.

Newmark, H. L., Yang, K., Lipkin, M., Kopelovich, L., Liu, Y., Fan, K., and Shinozaki, H. (2001). A Western-style diet induces benign and malignant neoplasms in the colon of normal C57Bl/6 mice. *Carcinogenesis 22*, 1871–1875.

Nishisho, I., Nakamura, Y., Miyoshi, Y., Miki, Y., Ando, H., Horii, A., Koyama, K., Utsunomiya, J., Baba, S., and Hedge, P. (1991). Mutations of chromosome 5q21 genes in FAP and colorectal cancer patients. *Science 253*, 665–669.

Nugent, K. P., Phillips, R. K., Hodgson, S. V., Cottrell, S., Smith-Ravin, J., Pack, K., and Bodmer, W. F. (1994). Phenotypic expression in familial adenomatous polyposis: Partial prediction by mutation analysis. *Gut 35*, 1622–1623.

Oshima, M., Murai, N., Kargman, S., Arguello, M., Luk, P., Kwong, E., Taketo, M. M., and Evans, J. F. (2001). Chemoprevention of intestinal polyposis in the Apcdelta716 mouse by rofecoxib, a specific cyclooxygenase-2 inhibitor. *Cancer Res 61*, 1733–1740.

Oshima, M., Oshima, H., Kitagawa, K., Kobayashi, M., Itakura, C., and Taketo, M. (1995). Loss of Apc heterozygosity and abnormal tissue building in nascent intestinal polyps in mice carrying a truncated Apc gene. *Proc Natl Acad Sci USA 92*, 4482–4486.

Oshima, M., Oshima, H., Tsutsumi, M., Nishimura, S., Sugimura, T., Nagao, M., and Taketo, M. M. (1996). Effects of 2-amino-1-methyl-6-phenylimidazo[4,5-b]pyridine on intestinal polyp development in Apc delta 716 knockout mice. *Mol Carcinog 15*, 11–17.

Oshima, H., Oshima, M., Kobayashi, M., Tsutsumi, M., and Taketo, M. M. (1997). Morphological and molecular processes of polyp formation in Apc(delta716) knockout mice. *Cancer Res 57*, 1644–1649.

Ouyang, H., Shiwaku, H. O., Hagiwara, H., Miura, K., Abe, T., Kato, Y., Ohtani, H., Shiiba, K., Souza, R. F., Meltzer, S. J., and Horii, A. (1997). The insulin-like growth factor II receptor gene is mutated in genetically unstable cancers of the endometrium, stomach, and colorectum. *Cancer Res 57*, 1851–1854.

Paul, P., Letteboer, T., Gelbert, L., Groden, J., White, R., and Coppes, M. J. (1993). Identical APC exon 15 mutations result in a variable phenotype in familial adenomatous polyposis. *Hum Mol Genet 2*, 925–931.

Paulsen, J. E. (2000). Modulation by dietary factors in murine FAP models. *Toxicol Lett 112–113*, 403–409.

Paulsen, J. E., and Alexander, J. (2001). Growth stimulation of intestinal tumours in Apc(Min/+) mice by dietary L-methionine supplementation. *Anticancer Res 21*, 3281–3284.

Paulsen, J. E., Elvsaas, I. K., Steffensen, I. L., and Alexander, J. (1997). A fish oil derived concentrate enriched in eicosapentaenoic and docosahexaenoic acid as ethyl ester suppresses the formation and growth of intestinal polyps in the Min mouse. *Carcinogenesis 18*, 1905–1910.

Peifer, M., and Polakis, P. (2000). Wnt signaling in oncogenesis and embryogenesis—a look outside the nucleus. *Science 287*, 1606–1609.

Perkins, S., Verschoyle, R. D., Hill, K., Parveen, I., Threadgill, M. D., Sharma, R. A., Williams, M. L., Steward, W. P., and Gescher, A. J. (2002). Chemopreventive efficacy and pharmacokinetics of curcumin in the min/+ mouse, a model of familial adenomatous polyposis. *Cancer Epidemiol Biomarkers Prev 11*, 535–540.

Petrik, M. B., McEntee, M. F., Johnson, B. T., Obukowicz, M. G., and Whelan, J. (2000). Highly unsaturated (n-3) fatty acids, but not alpha-linolenic, conjugated linoleic or gamma-linolenic acids, reduce tumorigenesis in Apc(Min/+) mice. *J Nutr 130*, 2434–2443.

Pierre, F., Perrin, P., Champ, M., Bornet, F., Meflah, K., and Menanteau, J. (1997). Short-chain fructo-oligosaccharides reduce the occurrence of colon tumors and develop gut-associated lymphoid tissue in Min mice. *Cancer Res 57*, 225–228.

Polakis, P. (1997). The adenomatous polyposis coli (APC) tumor suppressor. *Biochim Biophys Acta 1332*, F127–147.

Polakis, P. (1999). The oncogenic activation of beta-catenin. *Curr Opin Genet Dev 9*, 15–21.

Polakis, P., Hart, M., and Rubinfeld, B. (1999). Defects in the regulation of beta-catenin in colorectal cancer. *Adv Exp Med Biol 470*, 23–32.

Potter, J. D. (1995). Risk factors for colon neoplasia—epidemiology and biology. *Eur J Cancer 31 A*, 1033–1038.

Powell, S. M., Zilz, N., Beazer-Barclay, Y., Bryan, T. M., Hamilton, S. R., Thibodeau, S. N., Vogelstein, B., and Kinzler, K. W. (1992). APC mutations occur early during colorectal tumorigenesis. *Nature 359*, 235–237.

Praml, C., Savelyeva, L., Le Paslier, D., Siracusa, L. D., Buchberg, A. M., Schwab, M., and Amler, L. C. (1995). Human homologue of a candidate for the Mom1 locus, the secretory type II phospholipase A2 (PLA2S-II), maps to 1p35–36.1/D1S199. *Cancer Res 55*, 5504–5506.

Quesada, C. F., Kimata, H., Mori, M., Nishimura, M., Tsuneyoshi, T., and Baba, S. (1998). Piroxicam and acarbose as chemopreventive agents for spontaneous intestinal adenomas in APC gene 1309 knockout mice. *Jpn J Cancer Res 89*, 392–396.

Radice, G. L. (2000). Chromosome 18. *Chromosome Committee Reports*, Mouse Genome Database (MGD), Mouse Genome Informatics, The Jackson Laboratory, Bar Harbor, Maine.

Rampino, N., Yamamoto, H., Ionov, Y., Li, Y., Sawai, H., Reed, J. C., and Perucho, M. (1997). Somatic frameshift mutations in the BAX gene in colon cancers of the microsatellite mutator phenotype. *Science 275*, 967–969.

Rao, C. V., Cooma, I., Rodriguez, J. G., Simi, B., El-Bayoumy, K., and Reddy, B. S. (2000). Chemoprevention of familial adenomatous polyposis development in the APC(min) mouse model by 1,4-phenylene bis(methylene)selenocyanate. *Carcinogenesis 21*, 617–621.

Reitmair, A. H., Cai, J. C., Bjerknes, M., Redston, M., Cheng, H., Pind, M. T., Hay, K., Mitri, A., Bapat, B. V., Mak, T. W., and Gallinger, S. (1996). MSH2 deficiency contributes to accelerated APC-mediated intestinal tumorigenesis. *Cancer Res 56*, 2922–2926.

Reuter, B. K., Zhang, X. J., and Miller, M. J. (2002). Therapeutic utility of aspirin in the ApcMin/+ murine model of colon carcinogenesis. *BMC Cancer 2*, 19.

Riboli, E., and Norat, T. (2001). Cancer prevention and diet: Opportunities in Europe. *Public Health Nutr 4*, 475–484.

Riggins, G. J., Markowitz, S., Wilson, J. K., Vogelstein, B., and Kinzler, K. W. (1995). Absence of secretory phospholipase A2 gene alterations in human colorectal cancer. *Cancer Res 55*, 5184–5186.

Rikke, B. A., and Johnson, T. E. (1998). Towards the cloning of genes underlying murine QTLs. *Mamm Genome 9*, 963–968.

Ritland, S. R., and Gendler, S. J. (1999). Chemoprevention of intestinal adenomas in the ApcMin mouse by piroxicam: Kinetics, strain effects and resistance to chemosuppression. *Carcinogenesis 20*, 51–58.

Ritland, S. R., Leighton, J. A., Hirsch, R. E., Morrow, J. D., Weaver, A. L., and Gendler, S. J. (1999). Evaluation of 5-aminosalicylic acid (5-ASA) for cancer chemoprevention: Lack of efficacy against nascent adenomatous polyps in the Apc(Min) mouse. *Clin Cancer Res 5*, 855–863.

Roberts, R. B., Min, L., Washington, M. K., Olsen, S. J., Settle, S. H., Coffey, R. J., and Threadgill, D. W. (2002). Importance of epidermal growth factor receptor signaling in establishment of adenomas and maintenance of carcinomas during intestinal tumorigenesis. *Proc Natl Acad Sci USA 99*, 1521–1526.

Rustgi, A. K. (1994). Hereditary gastrointestinal polyposis and nonpolyposis syndromes [see comments]. *N Engl J Med 331*, 1694–1702.

Ryan, B. M., and Weir, D. G. (2001). Relevance of folate metabolism in the pathogenesis of colorectal cancer. *J Lab Clin Med 138*, 164–176.

Sanabria, J. R., Croxford, R., Berk, T. C., Cohen, Z., Bapat, B. V., and Gallinger, S. (1996). Familial segregation in the occurrence and severity of periampullary neoplasms in familial adenomatous polyposis. *Am J Surg 171*, 136–140.

Sansom, O. J., Stark, L. A., Dunlop, M. G., and Clarke, A. R. (2001). Suppression of intestinal and mammary neoplasia by lifetime administration of aspirin in Apc(Min/+) and Apc(Min/+), Msh2(−/−) mice. *Cancer Res 61*, 7060–7064.

Sasai, H., Masaki, M., and Wakitani, K. (2000). Suppression of polypogenesis in a new mouse strain with a truncated Apc(Delta474) by a novel COX-2 inhibitor, JTE-522. *Carcinogenesis 21*, 953–958.

Schimenti, J., and Bucan, M. (1998). Functional genomics in the mouse: Phenotype-based mutagenesis screens. *Genome Res 8*, 698–710.

Schmelz, E. M., Roberts, P. C., Kustin, E. M., Lemonnier, L. A., Sullards, M. C., Dillehay, D. L., and Merrill, A. H., Jr. (2001). Modulation of intracellular beta-catenin localization and intestinal tumorigenesis in vivo and in vitro by sphingolipids. *Cancer Res 61*, 6723–6729.

Schneider, Y., Duranton, B., Gosse, F., Schleiffer, R., Seiler, N., and Raul, F. (2001). Resveratrol inhibits intestinal tumorigenesis and modulates host-defense-related gene expression in an animal model of human familial adenomatous polyposis. *Nutr Cancer 39*, 102–107.

Schwartz, S., Jr., Yamamoto, H., Navarro, M., Maestro, M., Reventos, J., and Perucho, M. (1999). Frameshift mutations at mononucleotide repeats in caspase-5 and other target genes in endometrial and gastrointestinal cancer of the microsatellite mutator phenotype. *Cancer Res 59*, 2995–3002.

Seeling, J. M., Miller, J. R., Gil, R., Moon, R. T., White, R., and Virshup, D. M. (1999). Regulation of beta-catenin signaling by the B56 subunit of protein phosphatase 2A. *Science 283*, 2089–2091.

Shailubhai, K., Yu, H. H., Karunanandaa, K., Wang, J. Y., Eber, S. L., Wang, Y., Joo, N. S., Kim, H. D., Miedema, B. W., Abbas, S. Z., Boddupalli, S. S., Currie, M. G., and Forte, L. R. (2000). Uroguanylin treatment suppresses polyp formation in the Apc(Min/+) mouse and induces apoptosis in human colon adenocarcinoma cells via cyclic GMP. *Cancer Res 60*, 5151–5157.

Shibata, H., Toyama, K., Shioya, H., Ito, M., Hirota, M., Hasegawa, S., Matsumoto, H., Takano, H., Akiyama, T., Toyoshima, K., Kanamaru, R., Kanegae, Y., Saito, I., Nakamura, Y., Shiba, K., and Noda, T. (1997). Rapid colorectal adenoma formation initiated by conditional targeting of the Apc gene. *Science 278*, 120–123.

Shoemaker, A. R., Haigis, K. M., Baker, S. M., Dudley, S., Liskay, R. M., and Dove, W. F. (2000). Mlh1 deficiency enhances several phenotypes of Apc(Min)/+ mice. *Oncogene 19*, 2774–2779.

Sibani, S., Melnyk, S., Pogribny, I. P., Wang, W., Hiou-Tim, F., Deng, L., Trasler, J., James, S. J., and Rozen, R. (2002). Studies of methionine cycle intermediates (SAM, SAH), DNA methylation and the impact of folate deficiency on tumor numbers in Min mice. *Carcinogenesis 23*, 61–65.

Silver, L. M. (1995). *Mouse Genetics, Concepts and Applications*. New York: Oxford University Press.

Silverman, K. A., Koratkar, R., Siracusa, L. D., and Buchberg, A. M. (2002). Identification of the modifier of Min 2 (Mom2) locus, a new mutation that influences Apc-induced intestinal neoplasia. *Genome Res 12*, 88–97.

Slattery, M. L. (2000). Diet, lifestyle, and colon cancer. *Semin Gastrointest Dis 11*, 142–146.

Smith, K. J., Johnson, K. A., Bryan, T. M., Hill, D. E., Markowitz, S., Willson, J. K., Paraskeva, C., Petersen, G. M., Hamilton, S. R., Vogelstein, B., and Kinzler, K. W. (1993). The APC gene product in normal and tumor cells. *Proc Natl Acad Sci USA 90*, 2846–2850.

Smits, R., Kielman, M. F., Breukel, C., Zurcher, C., Neufeld, K., Jagmohan-Changur, S., Hofland, N., van Dijk, J., White, R., Edelmann, W., Kucherlapati, R., Khan, P. M., and Fodde, R. (1999). Apc1638T: a mouse model delineating critical domains of the adenomatous polyposis coli protein involved in tumorigenesis and development. *Genes Dev 13*, 1309–1321.

Smits, R., Ruiz, P., Diaz-Cano, S., Luz, A., Jagmohan-Changur, S., Breukel, C., Birchmeier, C., Birchmeier, W., and Fodde, R. (2000a). E-cadherin and adenomatous polyposis coli mutations are synergistic in intestinal tumor initiation in mice. *Gastroenterology 119*, 1045–1053.

Smits, R., Hofland, N., Edelmann, W., Geugien, M., Jagmohan-Changur, S., Albuquerque, C., Breukel, C., Kucherlapati, R., Kielman, M. F., and Fodde, R. (2000b). Somatic Apc mutations are selected upon their capacity to inactivate the beta-catenin downregulating activity. *Genes Chromosomes Cancer 29*, 229–239.

Smits, R., van der Houven van Oordt, W., Luz, A., Zurcher, C., Jagmohan-Changur, S., Breukel, C., Khan, P. M., and Fodde, R. (1998). Apc1638N: A mouse model for familial adenomatous polyposis–associated desmoid tumors and cutaneous cysts. *Gastroenterology 114*, 275–283.

Song, J., Medline, A., Mason, J. B., Gallinger, S., and Kim, Y. I. (2000). Effects of dietary folate on intestinal tumorigenesis in the Apc^{Min} mouse. *Cancer Res 60*, 5434–5440.

Sorensen, I. K., Kristiansen, E., Mortensen, A., Nicolaisen, G. M., Wijnands, J. A., van Kranen, H. J., and van Kreijl, C. F. (1998). The effect of soy isoflavones on the development of intestinal neoplasia in ApcMin mouse. *Cancer Lett 130*, 217–225.

Sparks, A. B., Morin, P. J., Vogelstein, B., and Kinzler, K. W. (1998). Mutational analysis of the APC/beta-catenin/Tcf pathway in colorectal cancer. *Cancer Res 58*, 1130–1134.

Spirio, L., Otterud, B., Stauffer, D., Lynch, H., Lynch, P., Watson, P., Lanspa, S., Smyrk, T., Cavalieri, J., Howard, L., Burt, R., White, R., and Leppert, M. (1992). Linkage of a variant or attenuated form of adenomatous polyposis coli to the adenomatous polyposis coli (APC) locus. *Am J Hum Genet 51*, 92–100.

Spirio, L., Olschwang, S., Groden, J., Robertson, M., Samowitz, W., Joslyn, G., Gelbert, L., Thliveris, A., Carlson, M., Otterud, B., Lynch, H., Watson, P., Lynch, P., Laurent-Puig, P., Burt, R., Hughes, J. P., Thomas, G., Leppert, M., and White, R. (1993). Alleles of the APC gene: An attenuated form of familial polyposis. *Cell 75*, 951–957.

Strachan, T., and Read, A. P. (1996). *Human Molecular Genetics*. New York: Bios Scientific Publishers and Wiley-Liss Publication.

Su, L. K., Kinzler, K. W., Vogelstein, B., Preisinger, A. C., Moser, A. R., Luongo, C., Gould, K. A., and Dove, W. F. (1992). Multiple intestinal neoplasia caused by a mutation in the murine homolog of the APC gene [published erratum appears in *Science* 1992 May 22;256(5060):1114]. *Science 256*, 668–670.

Su, L. K., Vogelstein, B., and Kinzler, K. W. (1993). Association of the APC tumor suppressor protein with catenins. *Science 262*, 1734–1737.

Su, L. K., Burrell, M., Hill, D. E., Gyuris, J., Brent, R., Wiltshire, R., Trent, J., Vogelstein, B., and Kinzler, K. W. (1995). APC binds to the novel protein EB1. *Cancer Res 55*, 2972–2977.

Takagi, Y., Kohmura, H., Futamura, M., Kida, H., Tanemura, H., Shimokawa, K., and Saji, S. (1996). Somatic alterations of the DPC4 gene in human colorectal cancers in vivo. *Gastroenterology 111*, 1369–1372.

Tarafa, G., Villanueva, A., Farre, L., Rodriguez, J., Musulen, E., Reyes, G., Seminago, R., Olmedo, E., Paules, A. B., Peinado, M. A., Bachs, O., and Capella, G. (2000). DCC and SMAD4 alterations in human colorectal and pancreatic tumor dissemination. *Oncogene 19*, 546–555.

Takaku, K., Oshima, M., Miyoshi, H., Matsui, M., Seldin, M. F., and Taketo, M. M. (1998). Intestinal tumorigenesis in compound mutant mice of both Dpc4 (Smad4) and Apc genes. *Cell 92*, 645–656.

Taylor, B. A. (2000). Mapping phenotypic trait loci. In *Mouse Genetics and Transgenics: A Practical Approach*, I. J. Jackson and C. M. Abbott (eds.). New York: Oxford University Press, pp. 87–120.

Thiagalingam, S., Lengauer, C., Leach, F. S., Schutte, M., Hahn, S. A., Overhauser, J., Willson, J. K., Markowitz, S., Hamilton, S. R., Kern, S. E., Kinzler, K. W., and Vogelstein, B. (1996). Evaluation of candidate tumour suppressor genes on chromosome 18 in colorectal cancers. *Nat Genet 13*, 343–346.

Tomlinson, I. P., Beck, N. E., Neale, K., and Bodmer, W. F. (1996a). Variants at the secretory phospholipase A2 (PLA2G2A) locus: Analysis of associations with familial adenomatous polyposis and sporadic colorectal tumours. *Ann Hum Genet 60*, 369–376.

Tomlinson, I. P., Neale, K., Talbot, I. C., Spigelman, A. D., Williams, C. B., Phillips, R. K., and Bodmer, W. F. (1996b). A modifying locus for familial adenomatous polyposis may be present on chromosome 1p35-p36. *J Med Genet 33*, 268–273.

Torrance, C. J., Jackson, P. E., Montgomery, E., Kinzler, K. W., Vogelstein, B., Wissner, A., Nunes, M., Frost, P., and Discafani, C. M. (2000). Combinatorial chemoprevention of intestinal neoplasia. *Nat Med 6*, 1024–1028.

Trujillo, M. A., Garewal, H. S., and Sampliner, R. E. (1994). Nonsteroidal antiinflammatory agents in chemoprevention of colorectal cancer. At what cost? *Dig Dis Sci 39*, 2260–2266.

Tucker, J. M., Davis, C., Kitchens, M. E., Bunni, M. A., Priest, D. G., Spencer, H. T., and Berger, F. G. (2002). Response to 5-fluorouracil chemotherapy is modified by dietary folic acid deficiency in Apc(Min/+) mice. *Cancer Lett 187*, 153–162.

Ushida, Y., Sekine, K., Kuhara, T., Takasuka, N., Iigo, M., and Tsuda, H. (1998). Inhibitory effects of bovine lactoferrin on intestinal polyposis in the Apc(Min) mouse. *Cancer Lett 134*, 141–145.

van Es, J. H., Giles, R. H., and Clevers, H. C. (2001). The many faces of the tumor suppressor gene APC. *Exp Cell Res 264*, 126–134.

van Kranen, H. J., van Iersel, P. W., Rijnkels, J. M., Beems, D. B., Alink, G. M., and van Kreijl, C. F. (1998). Effects of dietary fat and a vegetable-fruit mixture on the development of intestinal neoplasia in the ApcMin mouse. *Carcinogenesis 19*, 1597–1601.

Wakeland, E., Morel, L., Achey, K., Yui, M., and Longmate, J. (1997). Speed congenics: A classic technique in the fast lane (relatively speaking). *Immunol Today 18*, 472–477.

Wasan, H. S., Novelli, M., Bee, J., and Bodmer, W. F. (1997). Dietary fat influences on polyp phenotype in multiple intestinal neoplasia mice. *Proc Natl Acad Sci USA 94*, 3308–3313.

Watson, M. A., Zehnbauer, B., Kodner, I., and Milbrandt, J. (1995). Genetic diagnosis of familial adenomatous polyposis. *Laboratory Medicine Newsletter 3*, 10.

Wechter, W. J., Kantoci, D., Murray, E. D., Jr., Quiggle, D. D., Leipold, D. D., Gibson, K. M., and McCracken, J. D. (1997). R-flurbiprofen chemoprevention and treatment of intestinal adenomas in the APC(Min)/+ mouse model: Implications for prophylaxis and treatment of colon cancer. *Cancer Res 57*, 4316–4324.

Wechter, W. J., Murray, E. D., Jr., Kantoci, D., Quiggle, D. D., Leipold, D. D., Gibson, K. M., and McCracken, J. D. (2000). Treatment and survival study in the C57BL/6J-APC(Min)/+(Min) mouse with R-flurbiprofen. *Life Sci 66*, 745–753.

Weyant, M. J., Carothers, A. M., Dannenberg, A. J., and Bertagnolli, M. M. (2001). (+)-Catechin inhibits intestinal tumor formation and suppresses focal adhesion kinase activation in the min/+ mouse. *Cancer Res 61*, 118–125.

Wilson, C. L., Heppner, K. J., Labosky, P. A., Hogan, B. L., and Matrisian, L. M. (1997). Intestinal tumorigenesis is suppressed in mice lacking the metalloproteinase matrilysin. *Proc Natl Acad Sci USA 94*, 1402–1407.

Xu, X., Brodie, S. G., Yang, X., Im, Y. H., Parks, W. T., Chen, L., Zhou, Y. X., Weinstein, M., Kim, S. J., and Deng, C. X. (2000). Haploid loss of the tumor suppressor Smad4/Dpc4 initiates gastric polyposis and cancer in mice. *Oncogene 19*, 1868–1874.

Yamamoto, H., Sawai, H., and Perucho, M. (1997). Frameshift somatic mutations in gastrointestinal cancer of the microsatellite mutator phenotype. *Cancer Res 57*, 4420–4426.

Yamamoto, H., Sawai, H., Weber, T. K., Rodriguez-Bigas, M. A., and Perucho, M. (1998). Somatic frameshift mutations in DNA mismatch repair and proapoptosis genes in hereditary nonpolyposis colorectal cancer. *Cancer Res 58*, 997–1003.

Yang, W. C., Mathew, J., Velcich, A., Edelmann, W., Kucherlapati, R., Lipkin, M., Yang, K., and Augenlicht, L. H. (2001). Targeted inactivation of the p21(WAF1/cip1) gene enhances Apc-initiated tumor formation and the tumor-promoting activity of a Western-style high-risk diet by altering cell maturation in the intestinal mucosal. *Cancer Res 61*, 565–569.

Yu, C. F., Whiteley, L., Carryl, O., and Basson, M. D. (2001). Differential dietary effects on colonic and small bowel neoplasia in C57BL/6J Apc Min/+ mice. *Dig Dis Sci 46*, 1367–1380.

Zeng, L., Fagotto, F., Zhang, T., Hsu, W., Vasicek, T. J., Perry, W. L., III, Lee, J. J., Tilghman, S. M., Gumbiner, B. M., and Costantini, F. (1997). The mouse Fused locus encodes Axin, an inhibitor of the Wnt signaling pathway that regulates embryonic axis formation. *Cell 90*, 181–192.

Zwick, M. E., Cutler, D. J., and Chakravarti, A. (2000). Patterns of genetic variation in Mendelian and complex traits. *Annu Rev Genomics Hum Genet 1*, 387–407.

Section IV

MOLECULARLY TARGETED DRUGS

13

PROTEIN KINASES AS TARGETS IN CANCER THERAPY: VALIDATED AND EMERGING APPROACHES

Paul Nghiem, Yong-son Kim, and Stuart L. Schreiber

INTRODUCTION

Protein kinase signaling is abnormal in a large proportion of human cancers. We discuss progress in targeting kinases that serve in each of four distinct functional classes relevant to cancer: (1) promitotic kinases (c-abl, c-kit, cyclin-dependent kinases, and epidermal growth factor receptor kinases including Her2/neu/ErbB2); (2) proangiogenic kinases (vascular endothelial growth factor and platelet-derived growth factor receptor kinases). The third and fourth classes involve emerging concepts relating to kinases involved in sensing cellular stresses: (3) DNA replication checkpoint kinases (ATR and Chk-1) that normally prevent entry into mitosis if replication is inhibited by DNA damage or insufficient nucleotides and (4) kinases involved in nutrient sensing and regulating metabolic pathways (FRAP/mTOR and Her2). In each of these four cases, the underlying biological pathways are outlined schematically, the unique features of targeting kinases in these pathways are highlighted, and the status of development of inhibitors is described.

Oncogenomics: Molecular Approaches to Cancer, Edited by Charles Brenner and David Duggan
ISBN 0-471-22592-4 © 2004 John Wiley & Sons, Inc.

The discovery of hundreds of protein kinases since the 1980s gave rise to a bewildering proposal that 1001 kinases may exist to carry out diverse functions within our cells and tissues (reviewed in Blume-Jensen and Hunter, 2001). The fact that each of these enzymes uses adenosine triphosphate (ATP) as a substrate to phosphorylate protein targets suggests that specificity of kinase inhibitors would be a major challenge. Indeed, for many years, kinase-selective small-molecule inhibitors did not exist and the pharmacologic manipulation of kinases appeared to be an unlikely approach to successful therapy for cancer. After all, if a cell required hundreds of protein kinases for normal function, a nonselective inhibitor would be expected to have diverse unintended toxicities.

For these reasons, the approval of Gleevec (STI571/imatinib), a small-molecule inhibitor of the BCR-ABL tyrosine kinase, served as a very welcome proof of principle for this class of therapeutics. Gleevec demonstrated impressive efficacy in controlling chronic myelogenous leukemia as well as surprisingly low toxicity from a small molecule that inhibits several kinases other than the intended target, BCR-ABL. This agent, together with the approval of Herceptin (trastuzumab), an antibody that targets the Her2 tyrosine kinase, has generated an explosion of interest in kinases as therapeutic targets. These developments coincide with a greatly expanded understanding of how kinases normally function and are abnormally regulated in cancer cells. Indeed, according to the Pharmaceutical Research and Manufacturers Association, approximately 400 cancer-targeted drugs were under development or investigation in 2002, many of which target kinases (Box 13-1).

We review the biological rationale and development of four major protein kinase classes. (1) promitotic kinases (growth factor tyrosine kinases and cyclin-dependent kinases); (2) proangiogenic kinases, which are required for the increased vascular supply that tumors need to grow beyond about 2 mm; (3) DNA replication checkpoint kinases, which appear to be more important for cancer cells than normal cells; and (4) kinases involved in nutrient sensing and metabolic regulation. Throughout the chapter we have highlighted particular small molecules or agents in development because of the interesting pathways they target or their more advanced status in clinical

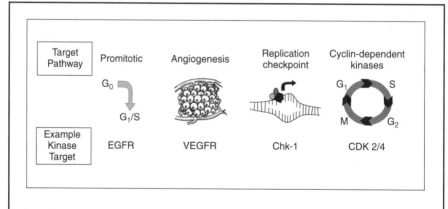

Box 13-1. Four major biological processes that are promising targets of small molecule inhibition in cancer therapy.

trials. This chapter is not, however, intended to be an exhaustive review of the many kinase inhibitors in development.

PROMITOTIC KINASES

The Epidermal Growth Factor Receptor Family

The epidermal growth factor receptors (EGFRs) are a family of signaling kinases implicated in a large fraction of carcinomas (cancers of the epithelial tissues such as breast, colon, stomach, and prostate). The EGF receptor family is composed of 4 transmembrane receptor subunits and at least 11 ligands that bind and activate them in various combinations, depending on the tissue. These receptors are membrane tyrosine kinases that bind to another family member upon ligand binding. They include the EGF receptor (ErbB1), Her2/neu (ErbB2), ErbB3, and ErbB4. Of these, ErbB2 is of special interest because it is overexpressed in many human cancers, and this overexpression is correlated with resistance to chemotherapy and poor prognosis (Harari and Yarden, 2000). Upon activation by a ligand, EGFR family members form dimers that lead to autophosphorylation of their cytoplasmic kinase domains. This in turn activates an array of downstream signaling pathways affecting cell survival and division. The exact nature of the activated downstream signaling pathways is determined by several factors including the expression pattern of receptors on the cell, the number of receptors expressed, and the amount and type of ligand that stimulates the cell.

Two-thirds of solid cancers are derived from epithelia, and EGF receptor signaling alterations are heavily implicated in a large fraction of these. Multiple mechanisms allow aberrant EGFR/ErbB signaling: Receptor mutations that constitutively activate the function of the receptor occur in glioma, non-small-cell lung cancer, prostate, ovary, breast, and stomach carcinomas; overexpression of normal ligands can induce activation of normal EGFR—for example TGF-alpha is overproduced by many tumor types and activates EGFR signaling in an autocrine loop; overexpression of wild-type EGFR family members occurs as a result of increased transcription or gene amplification and is associated with invasiveness, frequency of relapse, and prognosis in a variety of carcinomas (reviewed in Harari and Yarden, 2000).

The first agent to be approved that targets this pathway is an antibody directed against Her2 called Herceptin (trastuzumab; see Table 13-1). This antibody is approved for use in a subset of breast cancers that demonstrate ErbB2 overexpression (roughly 25–30% of breast cancers; Slamon et al., 2001). The clinical efficacy of this antibody is significant: It roughly doubles the response rate of Taxol (paclitaxel) in breast cancer as first-line therapy (from 15% for Taxol to 38% with Taxol and Herceptin).

When Herceptin was added to chemotherapy in metastatic Her2-overexpressing breast cancer, overall survival improved to 25.1 months versus 20.3 months, and time to disease progression improved (7.4 vs. 4.6 months; $p < 0.001$) relative to chemotherapy alone (Slamon et al., 2001). The major side effect from this therapy was heart disease. Specifically, Herceptin was associated with decreased left ventricular function, especially in patients who also received cardiotoxic anthracycline chemotherapy simultaneously.

In patients who received Herceptin and anthracyclines, 27% developed significant heart defects. This is a much higher number than among those receiving Taxol and Herceptin, of which 13% developed heart disease. Only 1% of Taxol-treated patients experienced this major side effect (Slamon et al., 2001). There is strong evidence that

TABLE 13-1. Summary of Kinase Inhibitors[a]

Name	Alternate Name	Target	Type of Inhibition	Class	Biological Mechanism
Herceptin	Trastuzumab	HER2/Neu/ErbB2	Antibody	Promitotic	Blocks signaling in HER2 overexpressing carcinomas
2 C-4		ErbB$_2$	Antibody	Promitotic	Blocks ErbB2 signaling
Cetuximab	IMC-C225	ErbB$_1$/EGFR/HER$_1$	Antibody	Promitotic	Binds/inhibits transmembrane receptor
Iressa	ZD 1839	EGFR	Small molecule	Angiogenic	Blocks EGFR tyrosine kinases
Gleevec	STI 571 or imatinib mesylate	bcr-abl Tyrosine kinase	Small molecule	Promitotic	Inhibits BCR-ABL, c-kit, PDGFR
Flavopiridol		Cyclin D$_1$/CDK$_{4/6}$	Small molecule	Promitotic	Blocks multiple cyclin-dependent kinases
SU 5416		KDR/VEGF-R$_2$/Flk-1	Small molecule	Angiogenic	Blocks the VEGF receptor—most important in tumor vessels
SU 6668		VEGF/PDGF/FGF receptor + c-kit	Small molecule	Angiogenic	Blocks kinase activity of VEGFR and PDGFR
Bevacizumab		pan-VEGF	Antibody-fusion protein	Angiogenic	Binds and disables VEGF
Rapamycin ester	CCI-779	FRAP/mTOR/RAFT1	Small molecule	Nutrient sensing and angiogenic	Counteracts loss of PTEN
UCN-01		Chk-1 and protein kinase C	Small molecule	Replication checkpoint	Inhibits Chk-1

[a]Presented in order discussed in chapter.

this cardiotoxicity is related to the actual mechanism of Her2-signaling inhibition by Herceptin: Transgenic animals in which Her2 was selectively deleted from the heart developed marked cardiac abnormalities (Crone et al., 2002). These mice developed thinning of the ventricular wall and decreased contractility, suggesting that ongoing Her2 expression and function is required for cardiac function.

A further point of interest about Herceptin is that it has shown marked antiangiogenic effects in a mouse model of human breast cancer, possibly by downregulating the vascular endothelial growth factor (VEGF) as well as other proangiogenic factors (Izumi et al., 2002). In summary, Herceptin, the first approved agent to target a receptor tyrosine kinase in cancer, does show significant efficacy over standard chemotherapy but also has a surprising mechanism-based cardiotoxicity as well as an additional unexpected therapeutic mechanism (angiogenesis inhibition).

A new antibody-based inhibitor of Her2 activity, called 2C4, works by a distinct mechanism to target the recruitment of Her2 into EGFR-ligand complexes. Unlike Herceptin, 2C4 blocks signaling mediated by Her2 by interfering with dimerization of Her2 to other members of the EGF receptor family (Her2 cannot dimerize with itself or bind to a ligand directly, so it must interact with another member of this family). Importantly, when Her2 does form an active dimer with ErbB1, ErbB3, or ErbB4, it signals very potently to activate the cell and is less sensitive to downregulation than when the dimer does not contain Her2. These effects are believed to underlie the potent oncogenic activity of Her2 (Harari and Yarden, 2000). A major advantage of the mechanism of 2C4 is that it allows a broader range of efficacy among carcinomas including those of the breast and prostate that do not overexpress Her2 (Agus et al., 2002). Cetuximab (IMC-C225) is an antibody that binds ErbB1 and has also shown preliminary promise in a variety of epithelial cancers.

Several small-molecule inhibitors of the entire EGFR family are in development as cancer therapies. Iressa (ZD1839) is currently the most advanced of these drugs. Iressa works as a competitive inhibitor of ATP binding by EGFR tyrosine kinases and has shown antitumor activity in multiple tumor types in humans in a phase I trial (Herbst et al., 2002b). Toxicities in this trial were minimal and mostly involved diarrhea and an acne-like rash. Interestingly, Iressa also has antiangiogenic properties that may support its efficacy in cancer therapy via inhibition of EGFR function in vascular proliferation (Hirata et al., 2002).

BCR-ABL and Gleevec

Chronic myelogenous leukemia is rare among malignancies in that it is highly dependent on a single genetic mutation: a translocation between chromosomes 9 and 22, often resulting in a distinct cytogenetic phenotype known as the Philadelphia chromosome. It is present in over 95% of patients with chronic myelogenous leukemia (CML) and leads to production of the BCR-ABL oncogene. BCR-ABL is a tyrosine kinase with aberrant regulation of the kinase domain derived from the normal cellular version of the Abl tyrosine kinase. Expression of BCR-ABL can induce a CML-like disease in mouse models, an observation that contributed to great interest in developing inhibitors of its kinase activity.

Gleevec (imatinib, STI571) was approved by the FDA in 2001 after demonstration of marked efficacy in early and late stages of CML (Druker et al., 2001a, 2001b). Of 54 patients with CML who had been unresponsive to interferon-alpha treatment, 53 experienced a complete hematologic response with Gleevec treatment (Druker et al., 2001b). The success of this small-molecule inhibitor has provided great encouragement to the idea that selective kinase inhibitors can be effective therapy for cancer.

In the case of Gleevec, a lack of specificity (it also inhibits the c-kit and PDGF receptor tyrosine kinases) in fact has led to its utility in two other rare malignancies. Gastrointestinal stromal tumors (GISTs) and chronic myeloproliferative diseases have also been effectively treated with Gleevec. GI stromal tumors depend on overexpression of c-kit activity and are highly refractory to conventional therapies (Demetri et al., 2002). In a trial of 147 patients with advanced GIST, over half had a sustained objective response in the form of stable or diminished disease (there were, however, no complete responses; Demetri et al., 2002). For a subset of patients with myeloproliferative diseases associated with a constitutively active platelet-derived growth factor receptor beta (PDGFB), Gleevec has proved effective in controlling their disease in four of four cases (Apperley et al., 2002). Strikingly, the side-effect profile of Gleevec is quite mild, including skin rashes and edema that rarely require discontinuation of the drug.

The major limitation of Gleevec appears to be the onset of resistance. In the case of CML, this appears to be mostly related to the emergence of mutations in the BCR-ABL kinase itself, rather than in the acquisition of efflux pumps for the drug in cancer cells (Shah et al., 2002). The mechanism of Gleevec's inhibition of BCR-ABL has been studied at the structural level. Like most kinase inhibitors, Gleevec binds the kinase in the ATP-binding pocket/catalytic domain. Most kinases are very similar in structure when they are in their active conformation, as they all must bind ATP and act as a phosphotransferase when in this active shape. In contrast, there are many mechanisms by which their activity is switched to an "off" position in which they do not bind ATP and substrate (Shah et al., 2002). The significance of this concept is that small molecules that bind to the kinase catalytic domain when it is in the active state are likely to have minimal specificity for a particular kinase. In contrast, there are more opportunities for specificity when small molecules bind to the inactive state of a kinase.

Indeed, in the case of Gleevec, elegant structural studies have demonstrated that this drug binds to the catalytic domain only in the inactive state, stabilizes this state, and thus prevents kinase function (Schindler et al., 2000). Thirty-two patients whose disease relapsed after an initial response to Gleevec were studied for mutations in the coding sequence of BCR-ABL. The 15 mutations were grouped into two classes: (1) those that alter the amino acids that directly interact with Gleevec, presumably interfering with binding to the drug; and (2) those that alter the kinase so that it cannot adopt its inactive (Gleevec-binding) state, hence locking it in an active state and causing Gleevec-resistant, constitutive activity of BCR-ABL (Shah et al., 2002). These detailed structural/molecular/clinical studies being performed on Gleevec are aiding in the development of second-generation drugs. Such modified Gleevec-like drugs will hopefully have less propensity for resistance, or could be used in a cocktail (much as HIV drugs are now administered) to minimize emergence of resistance.

Cyclin-Dependent Kinase Inhibitors

Because all dividing cells depend on the function of cyclin-dependent kinases to progress through the cell cycle, inhibition of this class of kinases would certainly be effective in controlling cancer if toxicity were acceptable. Flavopiridol is the only agent of this class that is currently in clinical trials for cancer (Zhai et al., 2002). Initially known as an inhibitor of protein kinase A and EGF receptor tyrosine kinase, flavopiridol emerged from the anticancer drug screening program at the National Cancer Institute as a potent inhibitor of cell proliferation. Although it is a nonspecific inhibitor of multiple cyclin-dependent kinases (CDK2, CDK4, CDK6; see Fig. 13-1), it has shown activity against gastric and renal cancers in early clinical trials (Zhai et al., 2002). Future agents in this class will no doubt demonstrate some level of specificity for individual cyclin-dependent protein kinases, which will likely improve the therapeutic index.

Why Does Inhibiting Oncoprotein Signaling Often Kill Cancer Cells? The Addiction Model

On initial consideration, pharmacologic inhibition of a signaling pathway that promotes cell division might be expected to temporarily slow the progression of cancer and have few other effects. In the terminology used for antibiotics, such drugs are cytostatic rather than cytocidal. A major reason for excitement about inhibitors of oncoproteins is the surprising observation that temporarily blocking the signaling activity of these molecules can lead to death and/or loss of the malignant phenotype, rather than merely a temporary mitotic arrest. This has been observed in a variety of pathways required for cancer cell proliferation and likened to the cancer cell becoming "addicted" to the activity of the pathway (Weinstein, 2002).

Many of these observations have been made in mouse models of cancer involving hyperactivity of promitotic oncoproteins such as Myc and Ras. These studies made use of genetic switches to specifically turn on and off the expression of an oncogene temporarily (akin to having a totally specific small molecule targeting only one oncoprotein). In diverse examples, temporarily switching off the activity of the target caused the tumor to undergo extensive apoptosis, as though the cancerous "house of cards" collapsed when one key support was temporarily removed. In the case of Ras (Chin et al., 1999), the temporary loss of Ras expression caused regression of tumor vasculature and cancer cell death. In the case of osteosarcomas (bone tumors) induced by ongoing Myc overexpression, the temporary discontinuation of Myc expression in these tumors led to longstanding differentiation into mature bone tissue (Jain et al., 2002).

Using an elegant chemical genetic approach, Fan and co-workers transformed fibroblasts with a modified version of v-erbB. They used an engineered version of the v-erbB kinase that is constitutively active but also mutated so that it can be specifically inhibited by an ATP-competitive inhibitor that has no effect on other kinases. Addition of the inhibitor to cells that express this v-erbB kinase caused the cells to arrest. As expected, withdrawal of the inhibitor allowed v-erbB kinase activity to become constitutive again. However, unexpectedly the cells failed to reenter the cell cycle after temporary inhibition of this pathway (Fan et al., 2002), again suggesting that a temporary disruption of promitotic signaling can have a long-lasting effect on the malignant phenotype.

In addition to these studies of the "addiction" paradigm in mouse and in vitro models, there is now excellent evidence that human cancers behave similarly in many cases. Gleevec serves as an important example, with tumors such as chronic myelogenous leukemia addicted to BCR-ABL signaling (Druker et al., 2001b) and gastrointestinal

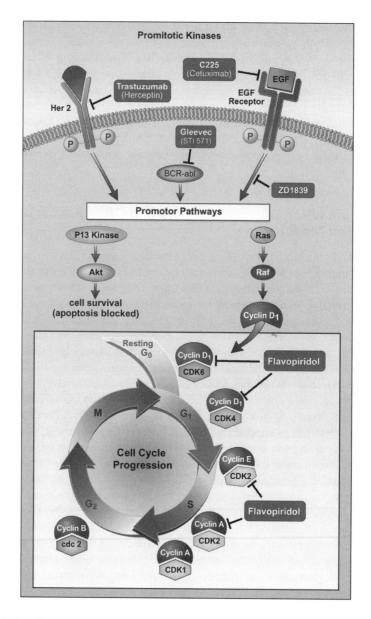

Figure 13-1. Promitotic kinases. Complex signaling networks link growth factors to survival and cellular proliferation. Tyrosine kinases are heavily represented in these pathways and their function is directly or indirectly upregulated in many cancers. These tyrosine kinases are activated when they bind ligand, dimerize, and phosphorylate each other to form an actively signaling complex. Several tyrosine kinases have been selected as targets for cancer therapy. As shown, the two recently approved protein kinase inhibitors, Herceptin and Gleevec, both target proteins in these pathways that promote cell survival and mitosis. In addition, a nonselective first-generation cyclin-dependent kinase inhibitor, flavopiridol, targets the kinases required for progression of the cell cycle. EGF = epidermal growth factor; CDK = cyclin-dependent kinase; Her2 = ErbB2 = Neu = a member of the epidermal growth factor family that is often misregulated or upregulated in cancer. See insert for color representation of this figure.

stromal tumors addicted to c-kit signaling (Demetri et al., 2002). In each of these cases, the majority of the malignant cells are not merely arrested in mitotic activity but also depleted in their numbers by many orders of magnitude when deprived of the oncogenic kinase activity to which they have become addicted.

PROANGIOGENIC KINASES

The concept that tumors depend on angiogenesis (recruitment of blood vessels) for their growth has received extensive attention in the past few years in the scientific and lay press. This basic concept has been championed for three decades by Folkman and his colleagues, and has gained general acceptance. There is, however, much controversy over how effective this approach will ultimately be and when it may show efficacy. Phase I human trials using the initially described peptides (endostatin and angiostatin; Herbst et al., 2002a) are not meeting the high expectations created by the prior mouse studies (O'Reilly et al., 1997) and extensive media coverage. The field is now maturing beyond initial excitement and beyond these inhibitory peptides. The most active and promising areas of antiangiogenesis research are now based on antibodies and small molecules targeted against kinases.

A key concept underlying the approach of targeting cancer by depriving its blood supply is that the blood vessels that feed malignant tumors are unstable and highly immature relative to those of normal tissues. Tumor-associated vessels appear to depend on ongoing growth factor stimulation from the tumor in a manner that is different from blood vessels elsewhere in normal mature tissues. In particular, tumor vessels express high levels of vascular endothelial growth factor (VEGF) receptors. Such high-level expression of VEGF receptors is not characteristic of mature vessels (Brown et al., 1993). In support of the functional significance of this expression, inhibition of VEGF signaling causes rapid apoptosis of tumor-associated endothelial cells but not normal endothelial cells (Laird et al., 2002). These concepts have added enthusiasm to the possibility of transiently inhibiting VEGF signaling and inducing selective toxicity to tumor tissue while sparing normal tissue.

The VEGF family of transmembrane tyrosine kinase receptors is composed of three subtypes of receptors bound in different combinations by seven ligands. VEGF-receptor function is highly similar in nature to that of other tyrosine kinase growth factor receptors in signaling and activation. As shown in Figure 13-2, VEGF/ligand binding to the receptor causes dimerization of two receptor subunits and autotransphosphorylation of defined tyrosine residues on the intracellular portion of the receptor, leading to activation of signal transduction pathways including src and ras-MAP kinases (Arbiser et al., 1997; Kroll and Waltenberger, 1997).

One VEGF receptor of particular interest is KDR (VEGF-R-2/FLK1), which is important in endothelial cell proliferation and angiogenesis, facilitating tumor progression. A small molecule called SU-5416 specifically inhibits this target (Fong et al., 1999). Relative to other VEGF-receptor subtypes, inhibition of the KDR receptor (via genetic approaches) in particular shuts down tumor growth and causes regression in animal models (Brekken et al., 2000; Yoshiji et al., 1999). These observations argue that the VEGF-R-2/KDR receptor is of particular importance as a cancer therapeutic. In addition, an anti-KDR/flk receptor antibody is being developed (Zhu et al., 1999).

Several approaches are being developed to more broadly inhibit the signaling from all VEGF receptors. SU6668 is a small molecule that targets the catalytic activity of a

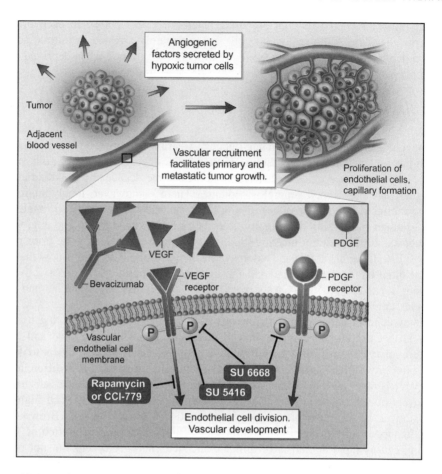

Figure 13-2. Angiogenesis-related kinases. Unlike the normal blood vessels that supply mature tissues in our bodies, the blood vessels that supply malignant tumors require ongoing growth factor stimulation to avoid apoptosis as well as to expand. For these reasons, inhibiting proangiogenic kinase pathways has shown great promise in preclinical and early clinical trials. Small molecules and antibodies that disrupt key steps in these pathways are described in the text. See insert for color representation of this figure.

wide variety of tyrosine kinases including all three VEGF receptors: PDGF receptor, FGF receptor, and c-kit (see Fig. 13-2). Bevacizumab is a monoclonal antibody that binds the VEGF ligand, hence acting like a sponge to bind up VEGF and prevent it from interacting with VEGF receptor present on vascular endothelial cells. An initial trial of this antibody in metastatic renal cell carcinoma showed a decrease in average time to cancer progression among 37 patients treated with Bevacizumab (5 months to progression) compared with 38 patients who received placebo (<2 months to progression; Yang et al., 2002).

Rapamycin is a small molecule that is currently approved for prevention of rejection of transplanted kidneys via its inhibitory effects on the activation of lymphocytes. Recently, however, both rapamycin and the closely related rapamycin ester, CCI-779, have been shown to inhibit the intracellular signaling pathway leading from the VEGF receptor to proliferation in endothelial cells (Guba et al., 2002). There are also other mechanisms by which rapamycin appears to act against cancer, as described next in the section on kinases involved in metabolism and nutrient sensing.

As with many other approaches to cancer therapy, the combination of antiangiogenic treatments with other established therapies appears promising (Klement et al., 2000) and will be extensively investigated once these agents become readily available.

KINASES INVOLVED IN NUTRIENT SENSING AND METABOLIC PATHWAYS

Since the early 1990s, great progress has been made in understanding the mechanism of action of the immune suppressant and anticancer agent called rapamycin. The relevant cellular target for rapamycin is a large protein kinase known as FRAP (mTOR/RAFT1; Brown et al., 1994; Sabatini et al., 1994). FRAP/mTOR is not directly bound by rapamycin but instead is complexed when rapamycin binds a small cellular protein called FKBP12; this FKBP12-rapamycin complex inhibits FRAP/mTOR function. The rapamycin ester CCI-779 (cell cycle inhibitor-779) has an altered stability and solubility profile but functions in the exact same manner within cells. CCI-779 is on the fast track for clinical development in renal cell carcinoma through the National Cancer Institute.

Through studies in yeast (where the FRAP/mTOR ortholog is known as the target of rapamycin or TOR) and in mammalian cells, it now appears that the normal cellular role of FRAP/mTOR is to serve as a nutrient sensor, regulating transcription and translation in order to optimally respond to the abundance or paucity of nutrients such as amino acids and glucose (Hardwick et al., 1999; Peng et al., 2002; see Fig. 13-3). To a first approximation, rapamycin's ability to inhibit lymphocyte activation is due to the signal it seems to send cells: "Nutrient supply is inadequate—do not proliferate or grow."

Given this background, it came as something of a surprise to find that rapamycin has anticancer effects as cancer cells have typically lost their sensitivity to most growth controls. Recent work has identified the molecular basis of why a major subset of cancers shows sensitivity to rapamycin. Using mouse and human cell approaches, several independent laboratories have concluded that the loss of a tumor suppressor called Pten (phosphatase and tensin homolog) is characteristic of cancer cells with rapamycin sensitivity (Mills et al., 2001; Neshat et al., 2001).

Figure 13-3 puts our knowledge of this pathway into a perspective that allows us to explain why rapamycin would have this "synthetic lethal" effect when combined with the loss of Pten function. As discussed in Chapter 10, yeast geneticists define synthetic lethality as a combination of individually nonessential mutations that lead to inviability. Similarly, a single chemical inhibitor that is tolerated by wild-type cells but not tolerated by mutants deficient in another protein target can reveal synthetic lethal relationships. Interestingly, as shown in Figure 13-3, a tumor suppressor lies on each arm of these two converging pathways. In the arm leading down from mitogens (e.g., insulin), Pten has now been established as an important tumor suppressor. People with a mutant copy of the *PTEN* tumor suppressor develop Cowden's disease, which is characterized by benign tumors called hamartomas, which often occur on the skin as hair follicle tumors called trichilemomas (Li et al., 1997). In contrast, tuberous sclerosis results when the *TSC* tumor suppressor is mutated (Cheadle et al., 2000).

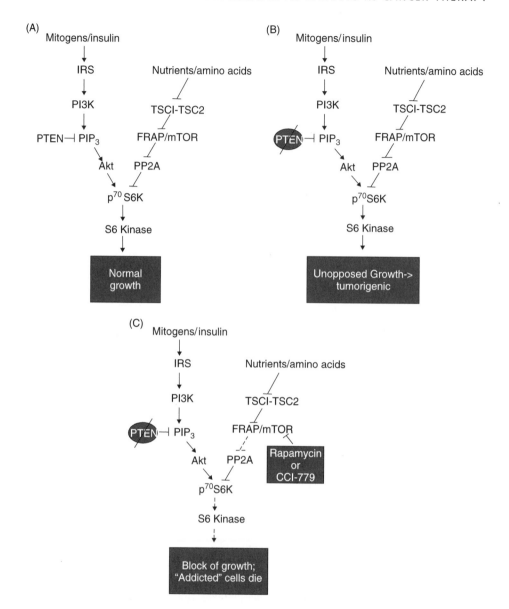

Figure 13-3. PTEN and FRAP/mTOR interactions in cancer. As shown in A (normal state), PTEN is a phosphatase that regulates the activation of the pivotal kinases, Akt and p70S6 kinase, by decreasing production of PIP₃. An opposing pathway integrates information about the nutrient status of the cell via the tuberous sclerosis tumor suppressors (TSC1 and TSC2), FRAP/mTOR, and PP2A, a phosphatase that is normally restrained by FRAP/mTOR (Peterson et al., 1999). As shown in B, a large subset of cancers have decreased PTEN activity, causing unopposed activation of Akt, p70S6 kinase, and cell growth. Panel C shows how the addition of rapamycin (or the closely related rapamycin ester, CCI-779) inhibits this pathway. Rapamycin leads to death of the cancer cells that have grown "addicted" to signaling via the PTEN pathway.

This tumor suppressor functions on the arm of the pathway that integrates information about nutrient status (Gao et al., 2002; Fig. 13-3). When this TSC tumor suppressor is lost, the net effect is again numerous benign hamartomas, which often manifest in skin as oil gland tumors called sebaceous adenomas. Cowden's disease and tuberous sclerosis are inherited in an autosomal-dominant pattern and behave as classic tumor suppressors according to the Knudson hypothesis: All somatic cells have lost one copy of the tumor suppressor and the loss of the other copy in a random manner leads to preneoplastic progression. For both *Pten* (Cowden's disease) and *TSC* (tuberous sclerosis), loss of the tumor suppressor leads to benign tumors and a predisposition for more serious malignancies of epithelia such as gastrointestinal and breast cancer.

It appears that a key readout of these two pathways relates to the signals for growth and cell survival that are mediated by the protein kinases Akt and p70S6 kinase. As shown in Figure 13-3, in the normal state the mitogen-activated pathway is held in check by Pten and by the inhibitory signals from the nutrient-sensing pathway involving Tsc. In cancers that have lost Pten function, there is unopposed activity of Akt and p70S6 kinase, leading to more rapid growth in cell size and protein translation (Vivanco and Sawyers, 2002). In a strong analogy to the addiction model presented in the promitotic kinase section, it appears that Pten-deficient cancer cells become highly dependent on this augmented level of Akt and p70S6 kinase activity. Indeed, when rapamycin is used to shut down the activity of p70S6 kinase (rapamycin inactivation is dominant over Akt hyperactivation for this pathway), these Pten-deficient tumor cells are far more sensitive than normal cells to this agent. We are still in the early days of investigating this type of cancer therapy, and it is likely that rapamycin (or other more promising "rapalogs" under development) will be capable of synergy with other, established cancer treatments.

Of significance to a large population of organ transplant recipients, rapamycin has allowed a dissection of the process of immune suppression from tumor promotion—that is, most immune suppressants that have been used for preventing the rejection of transplanted organs (cyclosporine and azathioprine) have shown a marked increase in the incidence of malignancies in the rapidly growing segment of our population that requires immune suppression. This has led to a hypothesis that immune suppression *per se* may lead to increased cancer incidence. A strong indication that this is not the case came in 1999 when cyclosporine was shown to promote cancer growth directly, even in mice that had no immune system (Hojo et al., 1999). In contrast to cyclosporine, at doses that prevent organ rejection, rapamycin has been associated with a *suppression* of malignant progression (Guba et al., 2002; Luan et al., 2002). Because malignancies that develop during prolonged immune suppression are now a cause of major morbidity and mortality (affecting up to half of transplant recipients by 10 years after transplant), rapamycin may become the immune suppressant of choice in this population.

REVISITING THE WARBURG EFFECT WITH MODERN MOLECULAR BIOLOGY

In the mid-1950s, Warburg believed he had solved the problem of cancer by applying principles he had discovered relating to the metabolism of sugars (Warburg, 1956). Recall that ATP can be produced by anaerobic glycolysis or aerobic respiration. In an observation that has held up quite well over time, Warburg noted that cancer cells frequently displayed an unusual metabolic process known as aerobic glycolysis, or lactic acid production from glucose, despite the presence of oxygen. Normal cells, in contrast, use oxygen when it is present to metabolize pyruvate fully to carbon dioxide and water, leading to respiration-derived ATP production.

In a jump of logic that did not turn out to be accurate, Warburg promoted the idea that it was merely the process of aerobic glycolysis (primary ATP production by an anaerobic process even under aerobic conditions) that was solely responsible for malignancy. He then reasoned that inhibiting this glycolytic process would have selective toxicity to cancer cells. Many decades later, as shown in Figure 13-4, we finally have the beginnings of a molecular understanding of the factors that regulate cellular metabolism. These factors switch cells between anaerobic and aerobic ATP production.

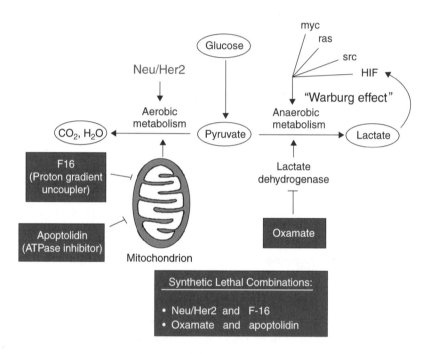

Figure 13-4. A modern model of the Warburg effect and cancer. In the presence of oxygen, most normal cells break down glucose to pyruvate, then proceed to the left side of this figure, using mitochondrial oxidative metabolism to produce carbon dioxide and water. In 1956, Otto Warburg noted that many cancer cells instead produced lactate from pyruvate and suggested this pathway could be inhibited, leading to cell death. Recent studies have revived this notion after the observation that the Warburg effect is promoted by certain oncogenes (myc, ras, src) as well as HIF (hypoxia inducible factor; Lu et al., 2002a). In contrast, overexpression of Her2 has been shown to promote aerobic metabolism as judged by increased transmembrane potential across the mitochondrion. Synthetic lethality has been observed with agents that inhibit one of these pathways in cells that have been made to be dependent on that pathway. For example, Her2 overexpression promotes aerobic metabolism and makes cells selectively sensitive to killing by F16, a small-molecule proton gradient uncoupler. By inhibiting lactate dehydrogenase (and hence forcing cells to use aerobic metabolism), oxamate sensitizes cells to apoptolidin and other ATPase inhibitors. See text for details.

Overactivity of the Her2 kinase promotes aerobic ATP production, whereas the myc oncoprotein and HIF (hypoxia inducible factor) promote anaerobic ATP production (Lu et al., 2002a).

Several recent publications suggest that it is now time to revisit the Warburg effect to explain the antitumor activity of several small molecules. Fantin and co-workers searched for small molecules that would selectively kill cells that overexpressed the Her2 kinase but would not damage an isogenic clone of cells that did not overexpress this protein kinase (Fantin et al., 2002). This unbiased approach yielded a small molecule called F16 that killed Her2-overexpressing cells, had little effect on normal cells, and appeared to act by uncoupling the proton gradient within the mitochondria necessary for aerobic ATP production (Fantin et al., 2002).

In an analogous study, Salomon and co-workers found that a class of small molecules that act as F_0F_1 ATPase inhibitors had a striking pattern of selectivity among the 60 cancer cell lines established by the National Cancer Institute (Salomon et al., 2000), discussed in Chapter 7. A subset of the cancer cell lines were highly sensitive to inhibition of ATPase function by each of the three ATPase inhibitors used: apoptolidin, oligomycin, and ossamycin. The simplest explanation for this observation is that these cell lines were highly dependent on aerobic production of ATP through mitochondrial function such that inhibiting the mitochondrial ATPase produced toxicity in these cells.

Salomon and co-workers then found that the cell lines that were resistant to the mitochondrial F_0F_1 ATPase inhibitors could be made sensitive by inhibiting anaerobic ATP production using a variety of small molecules. Taken together, the data from these two distinct studies suggest that cancer cells (1) often have abnormal regulation of glucose metabolism that makes them sensitive to certain metabolic inhibitors; and (2) can be shifted in their metabolism so that they are selectively sensitive to such inhibitors.

Metabolism in cancer is only recently reemerging into the limelight, and the possibilities for characterization of the oncogenes that regulate these energy utilization pathways and the small molecules that can disable them are truly exciting. We anticipate that studies of the interactions of metabolic and oncogenic signaling networks will be a fertile area for cancer biology in the future.

DNA REPLICATION CHECKPOINT KINASES: ATR AND CHK-1

Human cells encounter major challenges in maintaining genomic fidelity as they divide in the presence of environmental and endogenous DNA-damaging agents such as chemicals, oxygen radicals, and radiation. When DNA is damaged or DNA synthesis is otherwise delayed, a cell requires additional time to ensure complete DNA replication prior to cell division. The replication checkpoint is the mechanism by which a cell ensures that DNA replication is complete prior to initiating chromatin condensation, an initial stage of mitosis. Studies in yeast and more recently mammalian cells have elucidated many of the key players in the replication checkpoint pathway. In humans, the protein kinase ATR and its downstream target, Chk-1, are required for the replication checkpoint and for survival after DNA damage (see Fig. 13-5). A major reason for the interest in therapeutically targeting this pathway is that cancer cells appear to be especially sensitive to inhibition of this pathway.

Why would cancer cells need ATR or Chk-1 more than normal cells? Many cancer cells have defects in regulation of the G0/G1 transition—that is, they tend to progress

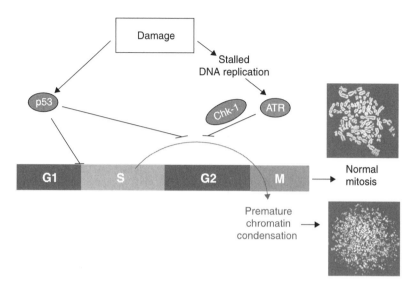

Figure 13-5. The replication checkpoint and p53 in the cell cycle. DNA damage activates p53 and causes DNA replication to stall, which in turn activates ATR. A major role for ATR is to activate Chk-1 and hence ensure that DNA replication (S phase) is complete before a cell enters mitosis (Nghiem et al., 2001). The curved arrow represents premature chromatin condensation (PCC), typically a lethal cellular event. PCC occurs when cells that have not completed DNA synthesis (S phase) undergo chromatin condensation. p53 is activated independently of ATR (Nghiem et al., 2002) and plays an important role in the replication checkpoint, synergizing with ATR and Chk-1 (Wang et al., 1996). (*Source:* Figure modified from Nghiem et al., 2002.).

into the cell division cycle more rapidly than normal cells, especially through its early phases. This is often caused by loss of the tumor suppressors retinoblastoma (Rb) or p53 or other components of these pathways. There are many mechanisms through which p53 function is inhibited in various cancers, including overexpression of the normal cellular protein MDM2 (which inhibits p53 function), direct genetic mutation of the p53 gene, or expression of the human papilloma virus protein E6, which degrades cellular p53 (Levine, 1997). Through loss of p53 or other tumor suppressors, the net effect is that many cancer cells are defective in early cell cycle checkpoints.

We have demonstrated in vitro that many of these cancer-associated mutations make cells more sensitive to death following the combination of low-dose DNA damage and ATR inhibition (Nghiem et al., 2001; see Fig. 13-6). Similar observations of increased killing of p53-negative cells have been made for Chk-1 inhibition by UCN-01 (a staurosporine analog; Wang et al., 1996) or for methylxanthines (caffeine and pentoxyfylline) at high concentrations (Fingert et al., 1986; Powell et al., 1995). It is now known that methylxanthines inactivate ATR as a key target in sensitization of p53-negative cells to DNA damage (Nghiem et al., 2001; Sarkaria et al., 1999). The simplest explanation is that in cells that have already lost cell cycle checkpoint function, further checkpoint inhibition is especially toxic or synthetically lethal when combined with the underlying functional defect.

How might replication checkpoint inhibition be used therapeutically? Caution will be required in approaching this problem as complete loss of function of the replication

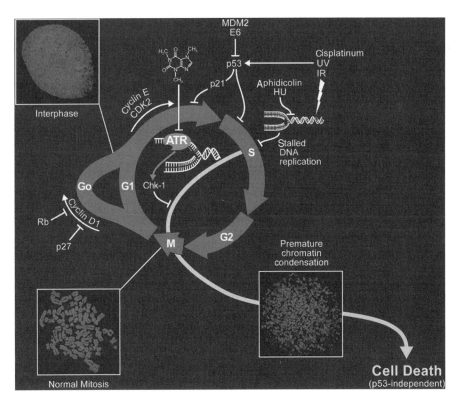

Figure 13-6. A model of ATR and Chk-1 function in the cell cycle of normal and cancer cells. DNA damage promotes cell cycle arrest via multiple mechanisms including activation of p53 and p21, but these checkpoints are defective in cancer cells (Levine, 1997). In addition, DNA-damaging agents (UV, ultraviolet; IR, ionizing radiation and cisplatinum, a DNA cross-linking agent) and DNA synthesis inhibitors (aphidicolin and hydroxyurea) increase the number of stalled replication forks (i.e., regions where DNA synthesis has halted abnormally). Naturally, such problems prolong the time required for DNA synthesis.

The signal that DNA replication is not complete is sent by ATR (bound to a stalled DNA replication fork). When ATR detects that replication is incomplete/stalled, it phosphorylates Chk-1, leading to the delay of mitosis while DNA remains incompletely replicated. The net effect is that the cell avoids a lethal error (represented by the white line that short-circuits the DNA synthesis [S]/G2 phases, leading directly to mitosis [M], premature chromatin condensation and death). Less severe defects can occur when premature chromatin condensation takes place at only a few sites in the genome, leading to gaps, breaks, and translocations that can be found in cancer cells at chromosomal fragile sites (Casper et al., 2002; Huebner and Croce, 2001). The chemical structure of a small-molecule inhibitor of ATR (caffeine) is depicted blocking ATR activity. For an interactive, animated version of this model, see www.schreiber.chem.harvard.edu/home/animation.html.

checkpoint by genetic deletion of either ATR or Chk-1 is rapidly lethal to a developing embryo or to dividing cells in culture. In contrast, partial inhibition of the replication checkpoint by small-molecule inhibitors or by expression of dominant negative ATR or Chk-1 is tolerated for many cell divisions in unstressed cells. In cells that have lost other G0-G1 checkpoint pathways that are typically lost in cancer, partial inhibition of ATR by genetic or chemical approaches has been shown selectively to induce premature chromatin condensation, leading to cell death (Nghiem et al., 2001, 2002). Several studies of Chk-1 demonstrated similar effects (Wang et al., 1996; Graves et al., 2000).

Subsequent studies have shown that one of ATR's key roles is to safeguard chromosomal stability at so-called fragile sites within the genome (Casper et al., 2002). This observation is of significant interest in cancer biology because of extensive evidence that cancer cells show frequent breaks and translocations at these same fragile sites as normal cells (Huebner and Croce, 2001). This suggests that cancer cells have previously experienced sublethal replication checkpoint insufficiency: "battle scars," as it were, of premature chromatin condensation. On the one hand, it suggests that cancer cells are already deficient in replication checkpoint function and hence would be very susceptible to inhibition of this checkpoint by small molecules. On the other hand, it is plausible that inhibiting this replication checkpoint may cause genomic instability at these sites, disrupt known tumor suppressors at these sites, and promote carcinogenesis. One likely mechanism for such an effect would be loss of the Fhit tumor suppressor that lies on chromosome 3 within the most common fragile site in the human genome (Huebner and Croce, 2001).

Several approaches will be required in order to address the feasibility of inhibiting the replication checkpoint as a therapy for cancer. First and foremost, there is a great need for selective small-molecule inhibitors of these kinases. The best-known inhibitor of ATR is caffeine (Nghiem et al., 2001; Sarkaria et al., 1999), which has been used extensively for in vitro studies of this checkpoint. Interestingly, topical application of caffeine to the skin has recently been used to markedly suppress the development of carcinomas in mouse skin that arise after ultraviolet radiation treatment (Lu et al., 2002b). Unfortunately, in order to inhibit ATR systemically, caffeine must be administered in doses that are too high to be tolerated in humans due to its unintended inhibition of phosphodiesterases and other targets, leading to seizures and cardiac arrythmias (Stewart et al., 1987). For Chk-1, the best-known inhibitor is a small molecule called UCN-01 that was initially identified due to its potent inhibition of protein kinase C. Indeed, UCN-01 is currently in clinical trials with some evidence of efficacy in phase I studies (Sausville et al., 2001).

The future of this approach of inhibiting the replication checkpoint depends on development of new small-molecule inhibitors and on studies that illuminate the effects of replication checkpoint inhibition on normal tissues. The characterization of the three-dimensional structure of the human Chk-1 kinase serves as a solid working point to determine and improve upon small-molecule inhibitors of this kinase (Chen et al., 2000). The crystal structure suggests that the amino-terminal kinase domain may be controlled by interaction with the carboxyl terminus of Chk-1, as deletion of the carboxyl terminus increases kinase activity (Chen et al., 2000). Efficacy of these agents will likely require combination with other DNA-damaging or replication inhibitors but may well provide a novel mode of selectively targeting cancer cells based on common defects in their cell cycle checkpoint regulation.

SUMMARY

The past decade has brought great excitement and promise to the concept of targeting protein kinases for the therapy of cancer. The four general classes of protein kinases were presented roughly in the order of their realization. Exemplified by Gleevec and Herceptin, inhibitors of promitotic kinases are already available in the clinic and more will soon be available. For the angiogenic kinases, rationally designed inhibitors are now in clinical trials. In addition, several kinase inhibitors that were approved based on other known mechanisms (rapamycin and Herceptin) have demonstrated significant antiangiogenic properties. FRAP/mTOR, a key kinase that regulates nutrient-sensing pathways, can be inhibited by rapamycin or the closely related CCI-779, which selectively kills cancer cells deficient in the Pten tumor suppressor. Regarding the ability to target cancer selectively via a newly acquired understanding of the Warburg effect relating to cancer cell metabolism, studies are still in the preclinical phase, but good small-molecule leads exist. The class of replication checkpoint kinases, the least advanced class presented here, has one agent, UCN-01, in clinical trials. Many questions remain to be answered, however, regarding the risk/benefit profile of inhibiting the ability of a cell to sense whether it has completed DNA replication.

A major challenge for the future remains the discovery of novel inhibitors that demonstrate specificity toward the desired kinases and acceptable side-effect profiles. It is now clear, however, that in many cases this will be both possible and therapeutically effective.

REFERENCES

Agus, D. B., Akita, R. W., Fox, W. D., Lewis, G. D., Higgins, B., Pisacane, P. I., Lofgren, J. A., Tindell, C., Evans, D. P., Maiese, K., et al. (2002). Targeting ligand-activated ErbB2 signaling inhibits breast and prostate tumor growth. *Cancer Cell 2*, 127.

Apperley, J. F., Gardembas, M., Melo, J. V., Russell-Jones, R., Bain, B. J., Baxter, E. J., Chase, A., Chessells, J. M., Colombat, M., Dearden, C. E., et al. (2002). Response to imatinib mesylate in patients with chronic myeloproliferative diseases with rearrangements of the platelet-derived growth factor receptor beta. *N Engl J Med 347*, 481–487.

Arbiser, J. L., Moses, M. A., Fernandez, C. A., Ghiso, N., Cao, Y., Klauber, N., Frank, D., Brownlee, M., Flynn, E., Parangi, S., et al. (1997). Oncogenic H-ras stimulates tumor angiogenesis by two distinct pathways. *Proc Natl Acad Sci USA 94*, 861–866.

Blume-Jensen, P., and Hunter, T. (2001). Oncogenic kinase signalling. *Nature 411*, 355–365.

Brekken, R. A., Overholser, J. P., Stastny, V. A., Waltenberger, J., Minna, J. D., and Thorpe, P. E. (2000). Selective inhibition of vascular endothelial growth factor (VEGF) receptor 2 (KDR/Flk-1) activity by a monoclonal anti-VEGF antibody blocks tumor growth in mice. *Cancer Res 60*, 5117–5124.

Brown, E. J., Albers, M. W., Shin, T. B., Ichikawa, K., Keith, C. T., Lane, W. S., and Schreiber, S. L. (1994). A mammalian protein targeted by G1-arresting rapamycin-receptor complex. *Nature 369*, 756–758.

Brown, L. F., Berse, B., Jackman, R. W., Tognazzi, K., Manseau, E. J., Senger, D. R., and Dvorak, H. F. (1993). Expression of vascular permeability factor (vascular endothelial growth factor) and its receptors in adenocarcinomas of the gastrointestinal tract. *Cancer Res 53*, 4727–4735.

Casper, A., Nghiem, P., Arlt, M., and Glover, T. (2002). ATR regulates fragile site stability. *Cell 111*, 779–789.

Cheadle, J. P., Reeve, M. P., Sampson, J. R., and Kwiatkowski, D. J. (2000). Molecular genetic advances in tuberous sclerosis. *Hum Genet 107*, 97–114.

Chen, P., Luo, C., Deng, Y., Ryan, K., Register, J., Margosiak, S., Tempczyk-Russell, A., Nguyen, B., Myers, P., Lundgren, K., et al. (2000). The 1.7 A crystal structure of human cell cycle checkpoint kinase Chk1: Implications for Chk1 regulation. *Cell 100*, 681–692.

Chin, L., Tam, A., Pomerantz, J., Wong, M., Holash, J., Bardeesy, N., Shen, Q., O'Hagan, R., Pantginis, J., Zhou, H., et al. (1999). Essential role for oncogenic Ras in tumour maintenance. *Nature 400*, 468–472.

Crone, S. A., Zhao, Y. Y., Fan, L., Gu, Y., Minamisawa, S., Liu, Y., Peterson, K. L., Chen, J., Kahn, R., Condorelli, G., et al. (2002). ErbB2 is essential in the prevention of dilated cardiomyopathy. *Nat Med 8*, 459–465.

Demetri, G. D., von Mehren, M., Blanke, C. D., Van den Abbeele, A. D., Eisenberg, B., Roberts, P. J., Heinrich, M. C., Tuveson, D. A., Singer, S., Janicek, M., et al. (2002). Efficacy and safety of imatinib mesylate in advanced gastrointestinal stromal tumors. *N Engl J Med 347*, 472–480.

Druker, B. J., Sawyers, C. L., Kantarjian, H., Resta, D. J., Reese, S. F., Ford, J. M., Capdeville, R., and Talpaz, M. (2001a). Activity of a specific inhibitor of the BCR-ABL tyrosine kinase in the blast crisis of chronic myeloid leukemia and acute lymphoblastic leukemia with the Philadelphia chromosome. *N Engl J Med 344*, 1038–1042.

Druker, B. J., Talpaz, M., Resta, D. J., Peng, B., Buchdunger, E., Ford, J. M., Lydon, N. B., Kantarjian, H., Capdeville, R., Ohno-Jones, S., and Sawyers, C. L. (2001b). Efficacy and safety of a specific inhibitor of the BCR-ABL tyrosine kinase in chronic myeloid leukemia. *N Engl J Med 344*, 1031–1037.

Fan, Q., Zhang, C., Shokat, K., and Weiss, W. (2002). Chemical genetic blockade of transformation reveals dependence on aberrant oncogenic signaling. *Curr Biol 12*, 1386.

Fantin, V. R., Berardi, M. J., Scorrano, L., Korsmeyer, S. J., and Leder, P. (2002). A novel mitochondriotoxic small molecule that selectively inhibits tumor cell growth. *Cancer Cell 2*, 29–42.

Fingert, H. J., Chang, J. D., and Pardee, A. B. (1986). Cytotoxic, cell cycle, and chromosomal effects of methylxanthines in human tumor cells treated with alkylating agents. *Cancer Res 46*, 2463–2467.

Fong, T. A., Shawver, L. K., Sun, L., Tang, C., App, H., Powell, T. J., Kim, Y. H., Schreck, R., Wang, X., Risau, W., et al. (1999). SU5416 is a potent and selective inhibitor of the vascular endothelial growth factor receptor (Flk-1/KDR) that inhibits tyrosine kinase catalysis, tumor vascularization, and growth of multiple tumor types. *Cancer Res 59*, 99–106.

Gao, X., Zhang, Y., Arrazola, P., Hino, O., Kobayashi, T., Yeung, R. S., Ru, B., and Pan, D. (2002). Tsc tumour suppressor proteins antagonize amino-acid#150;TOR signalling. *Nat Cell Biol 4*, 699–704.

Graves, P. R., Yu, L., Schwarz, J. K., Gales, J., Sausville, E. A., O'Connor, P. M., and Piwnica-Worms, H. (2000). The Chk1 protein kinase and the Cdc25C regulatory pathways are targets of the anticancer agent UCN-01. *J Biol Chem 275*, 5600–5605.

Guba, M., von Breitenbuch, P., Steinbauer, M., Koehl, G., Flegel, S., Hornung, M., Bruns, C. J., Zuelke, C., Farkas, S., Anthuber, M., et al. (2002). Rapamycin inhibits primary and metastatic tumor growth by antiangiogenesis: Involvement of vascular endothelial growth factor. *Nat Med 8*, 128–135.

Harari, D., and Yarden, Y. (2000). Molecular mechanisms underlying ErbB2/HER2 action in breast cancer. *Oncogene 19*, 6102–6114.

Hardwick, J. S., Kuruvilla, F. G., Tong, J. K., Shamji, A. F., and Schreiber, S. L. (1999). Rapamycin-modulated transcription defines the subset of nutrient-sensitive signaling pathways directly controlled by the Tor proteins. *Proc Natl Acad Sci USA 96*, 14866–14870.

Herbst, R. S., Hess, K. R., Tran, H. T., Tseng, J. E., Mullani, N. A., Charnsangavej, C., Madden, T., Davis, D. W., McConkey, D. J., O'Reilly, M. S., et al. (2002a). Phase I study of recombinant human endostatin in patients with advanced solid tumors. *J Clin Oncol 20*, 3792–3803.

Herbst, R. S., Maddox, A. M., Rothenberg, M. L., Small, E. J., Rubin, E. H., Baselga, J., Rojo, F., Hong, W. K., Swaisland, H., Averbuch, S. D., et al. (2002b). Selective oral epidermal growth factor receptor tyrosine kinase inhibitor ZD1839 is generally well-tolerated and has activity in non-small-cell lung cancer and other solid tumors: Results of a phase I trial. *J Clin Oncol 20*, 3815–3825.

Hirata, A., Ogawa, S., Kometani, T., Kuwano, T., Naito, S., Kuwano, M., and Ono, M. (2002). ZD1839 (Iressa) induces antiangiogenic effects through inhibition of epidermal growth factor receptor tyrosine kinase. *Cancer Res 62*, 2554–2560.

Hojo, M., Morimoto, T., Maluccio, M., Asano, T., Morimoto, K., Lagman, M., Shimbo, T., and Suthanthiran, M. (1999). Cyclosporine induces cancer progression by a cell-autonomous mechanism. *Nature 397*, 530–534.

Huebner, K., and Croce, C. M. (2001). FRA3B and other common fragile sites: The weakest links. *Nat Rev Cancer 1*, 214–221.

Izumi, Y., Xu, L., di Tomaso, E., Fukumura, D., and Jain, R. K. (2002). Tumour biology: Herceptin acts as an anti-angiogenic cocktail. *Nature 416*, 279–280.

Jain, M., Arvanitis, C., Chu, K., Dewey, W., Leonhardt, E., Trinh, M., Sundberg, C. D., Bishop, J. M., and Felsher, D. W. (2002). Sustained loss of a neoplastic phenotype by brief inactivation of MYC. *Science 297*, 102–104.

Klement, G., Baruchel, S., Rak, J., Man, S., Clark, K., Hicklin, D. J., Bohlen, P., and Kerbel, R. S. (2000). Continuous low-dose therapy with vinblastine and VEGF receptor-2 antibody induces sustained tumor regression without overt toxicity. *J Clin Invest 105*, R15–24.

Kroll, J., and Waltenberger, J. (1997). The vascular endothelial growth factor receptor KDR activates multiple signal transduction pathways in porcine aortic endothelial cells. *J Biol Chem 272*, 32521–32527.

Laird, A. D., Christensen, J. G., Li, G., Carver, J., Smith, K., Xin, X., Moss, K. G., Louie, S. G., Mendel, D. B., and Cherrington, J. M. (2002). SU6668 inhibits Flk-1/KDR and PDGFRbeta in vivo, resulting in rapid apoptosis of tumor vasculature and tumor regression in mice. *Faseb J 16*, 681–690.

Levine, A. J. (1997). p53, the cellular gatekeeper for growth and division. *Cell 88*, 323–331.

Li, J., Yen, C., Liaw, D., Podsypanina, K., Bose, S., Wang, S. I., Puc, J., Miliaresis, C., Rodgers, L., McCombie, R., et al. (1997). PTEN, a putative protein tyrosine phosphatase gene mutated in human brain, breast, and prostate cancer. *Science 275*, 1943–1947.

Lu, H., Forbes, R. A., and Verma, A. (2002a). Hypoxia-inducible factor 1 activation by aerobic glycolysis implicates the Warburg effect in carcinogenesis. *J Biol Chem 277*, 23111–23115.

Lu, Y. P., Lou, Y. R., Xie, J. G., Peng, Q. Y., Liao, J., Yang, C. S., Huang, M. T., and Conney, A. H. (2002b). Topical applications of caffeine or (−)-epigallocatechin gallate (EGCG) inhibit carcinogenesis and selectively increase apoptosis in UVB-induced skin tumors in mice. *Proc Natl Acad Sci USA 99*, 12455–12460.

Luan, F. L., Hojo, M., Maluccio, M., Yamaji, K., and Suthanthiran, M. (2002). Rapamycin blocks tumor progression: Unlinking immunosuppression from antitumor efficacy. *Transplantation 73*, 1565–1572.

Mills, G. B., Lu, Y., and Kohn, E. C. (2001). Linking molecular therapeutics to molecular diagnostics: Inhibition of the FRAP/RAFT/TOR component of the PI3K pathway preferentially blocks PTEN mutant cells in vitro and in vivo. *Proc Natl Acad Sci USA 98*, 10031–10033.

Neshat, M. S., Mellinghoff, I. K., Tran, C., Stiles, B., Thomas, G., Petersen, R., Frost, P., Gibbons, J. J., Wu, H., and Sawyers, C. L. (2001). Enhanced sensitivity of PTEN-deficient tumors to inhibition of FRAP/mTOR. *Proc Natl Acad Sci USA 98*, 10314–10319.

Nghiem, P., Park, P. K., Kim, Y., Vaziri, C., and Schreiber, S. L. (2001). ATR inhibition selectively sensitizes G1 checkpoint-deficient cells to lethal premature chromatin condensation. *Proc Natl Acad Sci USA 98*, 9092–9097.

Nghiem, P., Park, P. K., Kim, Y., Desai, B. N., and Schreiber, S. L. (2002). ATR is not required for p53 activation but synergizes with p53 in the replication checkpoint. *J Biol Chem 277*, 4428–4434.

O'Reilly, M. S., Boehm, T., Shing, Y., Fukai, N., Vasios, G., Lane, W. S., Flynn, E., Birkhead, J. R., Olsen, B. R., and Folkman, J. (1997). Endostatin: An endogenous inhibitor of angiogenesis and tumor growth. *Cell 88*, 277–285.

Peng, T., Golub, T. R., and Sabatini, D. M. (2002). The immunosuppressant rapamycin mimics a starvation-like signal distinct from amino acid and glucose deprivation. *Mol Cell Biol 22*, 5575–5584.

Peterson, R. T., Desai, B. N., Hardwick, J. S., and Schreiber, S. L. (1999). Protein phosphatase 2A interacts with the 70-kDa S6 kinase and is activated by inhibition of FKBP12-rapamycin-associated protein. *Proc Natl Acad Sci USA 96*, 4438–4442.

Powell, S. N., DeFrank, J. S., Connell, P., Eogan, M., Preffer, F., Dombkowski, D., Tang, W., and Friend, S. (1995). Differential sensitivity of p53(−) and p53(+) cells to caffeine-induced radiosensitization and override of G2 delay. *Cancer Res 55*, 1643–1648.

Sabatini, D. M., Erdjument-Bromage, H., Lui, M., Tempst, P., and Snyder, S. H. (1994). RAFT1: A mammalian protein that binds to FKBP12 in a rapamycin-dependent fashion and is homologous to yeast TORs. *Cell 78*, 35–43.

Salomon, A. R., Voehringer, D. W., Herzenberg, L. A., and Khosla, C. (2000). Understanding and exploiting the mechanistic basis for selectivity of polyketide inhibitors of F(0)F(1)-ATPase. *Proc Natl Acad Sci USA 97*, 14766–14771.

Sarkaria, J. N., Busby, E. C., Tibbetts, R. S., Roos, P., Taya, Y., Karnitz, L. M., and Abraham, R. T. (1999). Inhibition of ATM and ATR kinase activities by the radiosensitizing agent, caffeine. *Cancer Res 59*, 4375–4382.

Sausville, E. A., Arbuck, S. G., Messmann, R., Headlee, D., Bauer, K. S., Lush, R. M., Murgo, A., Figg, W. D., Lahusen, T., Jaken, S., et al. (2001). Phase I trial of 72-hour continuous infusion UCN-01 in patients with refractory neoplasms. *J Clin Oncol 19*, 2319–2333.

Schindler, T., Bornmann, W., Pellicena, P., Miller, W. T., Clarkson, B., and Kuriyan, J. (2000). Structural mechanism for STI-571 inhibition of abelson tyrosine kinase. *Science 289*, 1938–1942.

Shah, N., Nicoll, J., Nagar, B., Gorre, M., Paquette, R., Kuriyan, J., and Sawyers, C. (2002). Multiple BCR-ABL kinase domain mutations confer polyclonal resistance to the tyrosine kinase inhibitor imatinib (STI571) in chronic phase and blast crisis chronic myeloid leukemia. *Cancer Cell 2*, 117.

Slamon, D. J., Leyland-Jones, B., Shak, S., Fuchs, H., Paton, V., Bajamonde, A., Fleming, T., Eiermann, W., Wolter, J., Pegram, M., et al. (2001). Use of chemotherapy plus a monoclonal antibody against HER2 for metastatic breast cancer that overexpresses HER2. *N Engl J Med 344*, 783–792.

Stewart, D. J., Hugenholtz, H., DaSilva, V., Benoit, B., Richard, M., Russell, N., Maroun, J., and Verma, S. (1987). Cytosine arabinoside plus cisplatin and other drugs as chemotherapy for gliomas. *Semin Oncol 14*, 110–115.

Vivanco, I., and Sawyers, C. L. (2002). The phosphatidylinositol 3-kinase AKT pathway in human cancer. *Nat Rev Cancer 2*, 489–501.

Wang, Q., Fan, S., Eastman, A., Worland, P. J., Sausville, E. A., and O'Connor, P. M. (1996). UCN-01: A potent abrogator of G2 checkpoint function in cancer cells with disrupted p53. *J Natl Cancer Inst 88*, 956–965.

Warburg, O. (1956). On the origin of cancer cells. *Science 123*, 309–314.

Weinstein, I. B. (2002). Cancer. Addiction to oncogenes—the Achilles heal of cancer. *Science 297*, 63–64.

Yang, J., Haworth, L., and Steinberg, S. (2002). A randomized double-blind placebo-controlled trial of bevacizumab (anti-VEGF antibody) demonstrating a prolongation in time to progression in patients with metastatic renal cancer. Proceedings from the 38th Annual Meeting of the American Society of Clinical Oncology 21: Abstract 15.

Yoshiji, H., Kuriyama, S., Hicklin, D. J., Huber, J., Yoshii, J., Miyamoto, Y., Kawata, M., Ikenaka, Y., Nakatani, T., Tsujinoue, H., and Fukui, H. (1999). KDR/Flk-1 is a major regulator of vascular endothelial growth factor–induced tumor development and angiogenesis in murine hepatocellular carcinoma cells. *Hepatology 30*, 1179–1186.

Zhai, S., Senderowicz, A. M., Sausville, E. A., and Figg, W. D. (2002). Flavopiridol, a novel cyclin-dependent kinase inhibitor, in clinical development. *Ann Pharmacother 36*, 905–911.

Zhu, Z., Lu, D., Kotanides, H., Santiago, A., Jimenez, X., Simcox, T., Hicklin, D. J., Bohlen, P., and Witte, L. (1999). Inhibition of vascular endothelial growth factor induced mitogenesis of human endothelial cells by a chimeric anti-kinase insert domain-containing receptor antibody. *Cancer Lett 136*, 203–213.

14

RAS SUPERFAMILY-DIRECTED COMPOUNDS

George C. Prendergast

INTRODUCTION

Activated *Ras* genes are among the most frequent genetic changes in solid tumors. Ras superfamily proteins are small GTPases that regulate many cellular processes including division, adhesion, survival, motility, and secretion. We consider some of the tactics that have been explored to block Ras function as a strategy to treat cancer, focusing in part on the significant effort that has been put into developing farnesyltransferase inhibitors (FTIs) for this purpose. FTIs were designed to block the critical posttranslational modification that Ras proteins require to drive neoplasia. These drugs are among the leading wave of rationally targeted anticancer agents to enter the clinic. Extensive preclinical studies have demonstrated that FTIs can target the proliferation and survival of cancer cells with limited toxicities to normal cells. Interestingly, proteins other than Ras have been implicated in the antineoplastic activity of FTIs, including most notably RhoB, a member of the Rho subgroup of the Ras superfamily that regulates cytoskeletal actin organization. In clinical trials, FTIs have been largely well tolerated, but their efficacy has been limited. How best to refine the selectivity of these compounds and to apply them based on our evolving understanding of their mechanisms of action remain

Oncogenomics: Molecular Approaches to Cancer, Edited by Charles Brenner and David Duggan
ISBN 0-471-22592-4 © 2004 John Wiley & Sons, Inc.

important questions. Other strategies to inhibit Ras that have been explored are blocking its insertion into membranes or its interaction with key effector molecules, while other approaches target downstream effector molecules themselves. The frequency of alterations in the *Ras* pathway and the fact that some such alterations are sufficient to maintain the malignant phenotype suggest that drugs targeted to this pathway will be critically important to the new cancer pharmacopeia.

Despite the investment of major intellectual and financial resources in cancer research, malignancies remain the second leading cause of death in the developed world. While improved surgical and radiotherapy techniques permit the cure of most patients who present with localized tumors, only approximately 10% of patients with disseminated cancer are cured by existing treatments (DeVita et al., 1997). Clearly, more effective treatments are needed. The past decade witnessed a significant change in drug discovery approaches, changing the focus from biology-based systems to molecule-based systems. This shift has been driven by advances in identifying the fundamental molecular mechanisms responsible for malignant cell transformation. The new approaches aim at exploiting the explosion in understanding of the biochemical, cell biological, and genetic bases of cancer. Will the new strategies be fruitful in clinical treatment of the disease? While this question has yet to be answered, it is clear that these strategies provide new directions and hopes to address cancer.

We now know that cancer is driven by both genetic and epigenetic changes. Mutations in at least three classes of genes underlie cancer pathogenesis, including oncogenes, tumor suppressor genes, and genes that govern the faithful replication of DNA (e.g., DNA repair enzymes and cellular checkpoint genes). These genes are central players in cancer initiation and development. More recently, it has become evident that changes in the expression pattern of certain genes (epigenetic changes) contribute significantly to cancer progression. There is emerging evidence that epigenetic events may limit or modify the clinical consequences of mutational events. Epigenetic events include contributions from tumor stromal cells as well as tumor cells themselves. Realms where epigenetic influences predominate include immunity and the "3 A's of cancer": apoptosis, angiogenesis, and adhesion. These realms figure centrally into whether and how early neoplastic lesions progress to clinically significant cancers. However, given questions of redundancy and necessity for various target genes in these processes, genes that are genetically altered in cancer may be more appealing for therapeutic exploitation.

Cancer-causing mutations that abolish the activity of tumor suppressor gene products and DNA repair enzymes typically cause loss-of-function changes. As discussed in Chapter 10, proteins harboring such changes offer poor targets for traditional drug therapy, because small molecules are rarely capable of restoring biological activity to mutated proteins. In contrast, mutations in pro-oncogenic proteins that cause gain-of-function changes can offer useful targets for small-molecule therapeutics. Similarly, certain proteins that are overexpressed in cancer are tractable to pharmaceutical intervention because one can readily screen for small molecules that block the enhanced activities of enzymes or receptor ligands (Gibbs and Oliff, 1994). As an example of a mutated protein in cancer, which is sufficient to initiate and maintain a malignant phenotype, Ras has gained significant attention as a focus for drug development activity.

Ras GENETICS AND CANCER BIOLOGY

Among cancer genes, the *Ras* oncogenes have attracted as much attention as any target for the creation of cancer therapeutics. Mutated *Ras* genes exist in 20–30% of all human cancers but are most commonly found in cancers of the pancreas, colon, and lung (Bollag and McCormick, 1991; Bos, 1990; Clarke and Der, 1995; Lowy and Willumsen, 1993). While three *Ras* genes are transcribed in human cells (*H-Ras, K-Ras,* and *N-Ras*), the *K-Ras* gene is by far the most commonly mutated *Ras* gene in human cancers. This fact is of special relevance to the development of farnesyltransferase inhibitors (FTIs) as anticancer drugs (Box 14-1; see below). Nevertheless, all mutated *Ras* genes can transform mammalian cells in culture and can drive the formation of spontaneous cancer in transgenic animals (Mangues et al., 1990; Sinn et al., 1987). Moreover, mutated *Ras* was among the first oncogenes to be shown by genetic proofs to be required to maintain the malignant status of tumor cells (Chin et al., 1999; Shirasawa et al., 1993). Taken together, the evidence strongly supports the notion that drugs directed against *Ras* or *Ras*-induced cell physiology would comprise an effective attack on some human cancers. A more skeptical view suggests that such compounds might not be desirable, because Ras functions are also required for many aspects of normal cell physiology. However, a determination of the breadth of any therapeutic window always depends on animal and clinical testing.

Ras BIOCHEMISTRY

Ras proteins are small GTP-binding proteins that participate in the regulation of many cellular functions including cell growth, differentiation, and intracellular signal transduction. Ras proteins cycle between GTP and GDP bound states. The GDP bound state is converted to a GTP bound state through interaction with guanine nucleotide exchange factors (Bollag and McCormick, 1991; Chardin et al., 1993; Shih et al., 1980). In the GTP bound state, Ras is activated and sends signals that stimulate key downstream effector molecules including Raf kinase, phosphotidylinositol 3'kinase (PI3K), and others. These signals are attenuated by interaction with GTPase-activating proteins that stimulate GTP hydrolysis and return Ras to its GDP bound form. Cancer cell mutations destroy the intrinsic GTPase activity of Ras proteins. Mutant proteins cannot hydrolyze GTP, so they remain trapped in the GTP bound state. Therefore, they continuously send signals for cell division.

In principle, two approaches can be considered to fight tumors that arise from activated *Ras* genes. Conceptually, the simplest therapeutic strategy to target Ras would be to restore GTPase activity of mutated proteins to normal. However, although *Ras* mutations induce a gain of biological activity (i.e., stimulation of cell division), at the biochemical level, their primary defect is loss of GTPase activity. Because loss-of-function alterations are largely intractable to pharmacological invention, this feature of Ras biochemistry frustrated efforts to develop anti-Ras drugs in the 1980s.

Advances regarding posttranslational modifications of Ras proteins stimulated new approaches to block Ras function in the 1990s (Gibbs et al., 1994). Because Ras proteins undergo multiple posttranslational modifications needed to localize to the

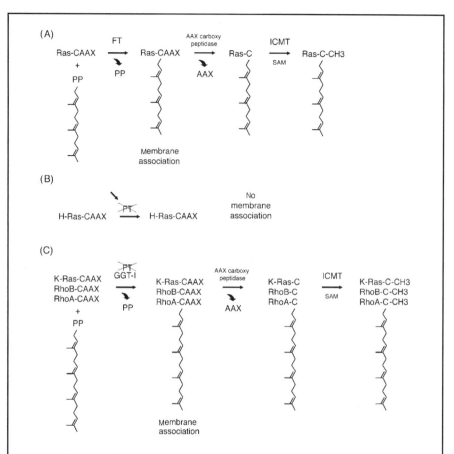

Box 14-1. Ras modification and the effects of farnesyltransferase inhibition. (A) Ras proteins are posttranslationally modified in three steps. The first step is catalyzed by farnesyltransferase (FT), which transfers the C15 isoprenyl moiety of farnesyl pyrophosphate to the cysteine residue in the CAAX-box amino acid sequence motif at the C-terminus of all Ras proteins. The required farnesylation is sufficient for membrane association, oncogenic activity, and subsequent modifications of Ras proteins, which include proteolysis of the three C-terminal amino acids and carboxymethylation of the free C-terminus. (B) Suppression of the activity of FT by small-molecule inhibitors of FT (FTI) leads to a loss of posttranslation modification of H-Ras, which relies on FT for posttranslational modification. (C) In the absence of FT activity, farnesylated K-Ras and RhoB proteins are isoprenylated by geranylgeranyl transferase type I (GGT-I). Geranylgeranylated proteins such as RhoA are unaffected by FT inhibition. For K-Ras, this event constitutes a "shunt pathway" that allows the protein to associate with membranes in FTI-treated cells. For RhoB, this event promotes a gain-of-function that is important for certain FTI responses (see text).

plasma membrane, mediate intracellular signal transduction, and stimulate cell division, these same modifications could be targeted as new strategies to attack Ras function (Gibbs and Oliff, 1997). Three successive enzymatic modifications occur at the C-terminal tetrapeptide, or CaaX box (where C = cysteine, a = any aliphatic residue, and X = the terminal residue). The γ-sulfur atom of the cysteine residue is first prenylated (modified by addition of a 15- or 20-carbon acyl chain). The three carboxy-terminal aaX residues are then proteolyzed and the carboxyl group of the newly isoprenylated and C-terminal cysteine residue is methylated. Prenylation is essential for the other reactions and crucial for Ras biological activity (Kato et al., 1992).

Thus, interference with Ras prenylation offered a new strategy to interfere with Ras-driven malignancy. In 1990, the enzyme that catalyzes Ras prenylation, farnesyl-transferase (FT), was identified; its cloning provided a source of recombinant enzyme for drug-screening assays (Gibbs et al., 1993; Omer et al., 1993; Reiss et al., 1990). The discovery and characterization of FT opened up the area of protein prenylation, which has grown to encompass a large field beyond its roots in Ras signaling and cancer biology.

PRENYLTRANSFERASES

In addition to FT, Ras studies revealed a second prenyltransferase called geranyl-geranyltransferase type I (GGT-I). These heterodimeric enzymes are composed of a common alpha subunit plus a unique but related beta subunit (Chen et al., 1991; Omer et al., 1993). FT catalyzes the transfer of the 15-carbon isoprenyl group on farnesyl diphosphate (FPP) to specific protein substrates via formation of a covalent thioether bond. GGT-I similarly transfers a 20-carbon isoprenyl group to its target proteins. The sequence of the CaaX box on the target protein generally dictates prenyltransferase specificity, with FT preferring CaaX sequences that terminate in serine, methionine, or glutamine, and GGT preferring CaaX sequences that end in leucine (Moores et al., 1991). However, these preferences are not absolute and there is no definitive rule to predict the CaaX specificity for prenyltransferases.

All Ras proteins are preferentially farnesylated by FT, but if FT activity is inhibited, K-Ras and N-Ras can be geranylgeranylated by GGT-I (Lerner et al., 1997; Whyte et al., 1997). The reason the latter Ras proteins are preferentially farnesylated has been explained by the fact that the k_{cat}/K_m values for in vitro prenylation by recombinant FT exceed the corresponding values for prenylation by recombinant GGT-I. However, when FT activity is depressed, K-Ras and N-Ras are modified by GGT-I (Zhang et al., 1997). A third prenyltransferase also exists, geranylgeranyl transferase type II (GGT-II), but this enzyme is structurally and mechanistically distinct from the others, and it only prenylates Rab proteins, not Ras or Rho proteins, or other members of the Ras superfamily.

The biochemical data suggested that a combination of FT and GGT-I inhibitors would be needed to inhibit prenylation of K-Ras or N-Ras proteins. However, FT inhibitors are sufficient to achieve growth suppression in cancer cells and coapplication of GGT-I inhibitors does not increase this effect (Sun et al., 1998). Mutated Ras proteins remain active when geranylgeranylated but normal H-Ras protein exerts growth-suppressive effects when geranylgeranylated (Cox et al., 1992). Therefore, the type of *Ras* gene driving cancer cell proliferation may be a factor in the degree of tumor growth suppression that can be achieved by FT inhibitors. Indeed, exactly how FT inhibitors block cancer cell growth remains a question of unresolved debate in the field.

FARNESYLTRANSFERASE INHIBITORS

The requirement of Ras proteins for modification by FT led many groups to seek small molecules that inhibited this enzyme. The goal of this project, which grew immensely in the 1990s, was to create potent and selective compounds that reversibly inhibit human FT, penetrate mammalian cells, and display appropriate properties of absorption, tissue distribution, metabolism, and elimination in animals. A number of structurally diverse molecules have been isolated that meet many of these criteria (reviewed in Gibbs and Oliff, 1997; Leonard, 1997). The reader interested in more than a general overview is directed to one of the many comprehensive reviews of FTIs in the recent literature that synthesize the wide diversity of viewpoints on these drugs (e.g., End, 1999; Sebti and Hamilton, 2000; Rowinsky, 2000; Adjei, 2001).

In general, FTIs have been derived from either random screening of natural products or rational design and modification of lead structures, using quantitative structure-activity relationships to guide incremental improvement of active compounds. The former strategy yielded such agents as manumycin or chaetomellic acids (Hara et al., 1993; Lingham et al., 1993) that are structurally related to FPP. The latter strategy generated molecules that were CaaX-peptidomimetic in character—that is, they competed with FT protein substrates for binding to the enzyme (Augeri et al., 1998; Bishop et al., 1995; deSolms et al., 1998; Graham et al., 1994; Williams et al., 1996). Some work was aided by NMR spectroscopy to define the structure of inhibitors bound to FT (Koblan et al., 1995). Other work was assisted by X-ray crystallographic analysis of FT complexed with its FPP substrate (Dunten et al., 1998; Park et al., 1997). A notable feature of these studies was the definition of the hydrophobic cleft in FT that serves as the catalytic site for isoprenyl group transfer (Long et al., 1998).

Preclinical Evaluation

Initial cell culture studies established the ability of FTIs to prevent the farnesylation of Ras (James et al., 1993; Kohl et al., 1993). Strikingly, these biochemical events were associated in *Ras*-transformed cells with a loss of anchorage-independent growth capacity and with a rapid morphological reversion to a nontransformed phenotype (Prendergast et al., 1994). FTIs displayed selectivity in their inhibition of anchorage-independent cell growth: rodent cells transformed by oncoproteins that did not act via Ras and that did not undergo prenylation, such as v-*raf*, were not affected by FTI at concentrations that blocked growth of H-*Ras*-transformed cells (Kohl et al., 1993; Prendergast et al., 1994). Phenotypic reversion associated with FTI treatment was characterized by gross changes in morphology—i.e., cell enlargement and flattening—and by a robust induction of actin stress fibers, which replaced the actin membrane ruffles that predominate in transformed cells. Interestingly, normal cells treated with FTIs also display these effects but more subtly (Prendergast et al., 1994). The mechanism underlying actin reorganization was traced to alterations in the prenylation status of the Rho family small GTPase RhoB (Lebowitz et al., 1995; Liu et al., 2000).

The growth-inhibitory effects of FTIs were not limited to rodent cells. Initial work by Sepp-Lorenzino and Rosen and their colleagues showed that over 70% of a panel of 42 human tumor cell lines lost the ability to grow in an anchorage-independent fashion when treated with FTI at low micromolar concentrations sufficient to block Ras processing and transformation in rodent cells (Sepp-Lorenzino et al., 1995). Interestingly, the *Ras* gene mutational status in these cell lines did not correlate with response to treatment: cell lines with either wild-type or mutated *Ras* genes were equally susceptible to growth inhibition.

Other clues suggested a complex mechanism of action of FTI in cells. For example, in H-Ras-transformed rodent cells, the kinetics of phenotypic reversion outpaced the kinetics of depletion of processed H-Ras in cells (Prendergast et al., 1994). Also, ectopic expression of myristylated RhoB could block reversion and growth inhibition by FTIs in H-Ras-transformed cells (Lebowitz et al., 1995). Lastly, as mentioned, FTI treatment could suppress transformation by K-Ras, even though it could not block prenylation of K-Ras (due to its geranylgeranylation by GGT-I in FTI-treated cells; Lerner et al., 1997; Whyte et al., 1997). These observations provoked questions about the cell physiological mechanism underlying FTI effects: Was Ras a necessary target of FTI action, or were effects on other prenylated proteins important (Prendergast and Du, 1999)?

The mechanistic basis for the antiproliferative and apoptotic effects of FTIs on transformed cells has been widely investigated and debated. In most cases, both Ras-transformed rodent fibroblasts and human tumor cell lines undergo cell cycle arrest upon exposure to FTIs (Miquel et al., 1997; Sepp-Lorenzino and Rosen, 1998). Depending on the cell lines examined and the compound tested, either a G1 or a G2/M blockade is observed. FTIs have also been shown to induce apoptosis in transformed cell lines. Working in H-Ras-transformed rodent fibroblasts, Lebowitz and Prendergast discovered that FTIs—generally nontoxic in tissue culture settings—would trigger apoptosis if cells were denied substratum attachment (Lebowitz et al., 1997b). This finding revealed an interesting role for cell adhesion signals in modifying the FTI response. One implication of this work was that differences in the cell adhesion requirements of normal and transformed cells could distinguish the effects of FTIs on normal and transformed cells, possibly explaining tumor responses as well, as discussed elsewhere (Prendergast, 2000).

Other studies by Suzuki and Tamanoi demonstrated that cytokine depletion was similarly sufficient to shift the FTI response in K-Ras-transformed cells from growth inhibition to apoptosis (Suzuki et al., 1998). A common thread to these studies was provided by the finding that the status of the PI3K pathway determined whether Ras-transformed cells responded to FTI by growth inhibition or apoptosis (Du et al., 1999c). As both integrins and IGF1 activate PI3K, this observation explained how adhesion or the IGF1 component of serum could negate FTI-induced apoptosis, converting it to growth inhibition by activating PI3K. Evidence for Akt as the relevant target in this pathway was also provided in the same study (Du et al., 1999c).

However, subsequent studies have shown that the relationship between the FTI response and Akt depends on tissue context: in fibroblast models, Akt activation prevents FTI-induced cell death, but in certain epithelial cancer cells and endothelial cells, FTIs can directly inhibit Akt (Prendergast, 2001a). This issue is addressed further below. Apoptotic effects are desired in an anticancer drug, but while such effects are seen in transformed rodent cells, they are relatively rarer in frank tumor cell lines, with some exceptions (Jiang et al., 2000; Kainuma et al., 1996; Sepp-Lorenzino and Rosen, 1998; Ura et al., 1998). Given the impact of cell adhesion signals on the FTI response, it is tempting to speculate that the relative resistance of most human tumor lines to most of the FTIs that have been tested is related to the development of anoikis resistance in virtually all bona fide tumors.

In animal studies, as alluded to previously, FTIs have been found to block the growth of *Ras*-transformed rodent fibroblasts and human tumor cell lines when grown as tumor xenografts in nude mice (Kohl et al., 1994; Liu et al., 1998; Nagasu et al., 1995; Sun et al., 1995). Growth of rodent fibroblasts transformed by mutated H-, K- or N-*Ras* genes is inhibited by FTI treatment, in the absence of overt systemic toxicities, more robustly than doxorubicin applied at the maximum tolerated dose, where toxic side effects are pronounced (Kohl et al., 1994). Similar observations have been made using human tumor cell lines that represent a wide variety of tumor types (e.g., Liu et al., 1998), confirming the ability of FTIs to block tumor growth.

While classical tumor xenograft models are simple and inexpensive, drug studies in such models can be predictors of anticancer activity in people. In pursuit of improved cancer models, several groups have used transgenic mice to evaluate FTI responses in vivo. The first such model to be tested was an H-*Ras* "oncomouse" (Sinn et al., 1987) that employed a viral H-*Ras* gene under the control of the MMTV promoter, as described in Chapter 11. Although H-*Ras* is not frequently mutated in human breast carcinomas, these mice spontaneously develop mammary gland carcinomas that recapitulate the pathological and histological features of human cancers. Upon treatment of tumor-bearing mice with FTIs, not only was tumor growth suppressed but complete regressions of existing tumors were observed with response rates as high as 100% (Kohl et al., 1995). These very high response rates were obtained at drug doses that failed to elicit any laboratory or histological evidence of toxicity to normal tissues.

Doxorubicin, used in this model as a positive control at its maximally tolerated dose, yielded complete regressions in only 18% of mice. These findings were confirmed in transgenic mice harboring the H-*Ras* gene driven by the breast-specific *Wap* promoter (Liu et al., 1998) and the N-*Ras* gene driven by the MMTV promoter (Mangues et al., 1998). In each case, tumors were allowed to develop spontaneously and were then treated with an FTI. More recently, tumors in mice driven by an MMTV-K-*Ras* gene were shown to be growth inhibited by FTI treatment (Omer et al., 2000). Treatment also suppressed the development of new tumors during the study. Notably, histological examination of normal tissues at the conclusion of these studies was generally unremarkable, except for minimal evidence of bone marrow depression and intestinal crypt cell hypoplasia.

As discussed in Chapter 11, one deficiency in these transgenic models was their reliance on a single oncogene for the induction of cancer. Human tumors, by contrast, virtually always harbor multiple genetic changes. In an effort to further simulate the molecular pathology of human cancers in murine oncomouse models, animals bearing a mutated H-*Ras* gene were crossed with animals possessing either a mutated MMTV-c-*myc* gene or a deleted p53 gene. These animals again developed spontaneous breast or salivary gland tumors that grew more aggressively than the tumors found in animals possessing a single oncogenic mutation. However, these tumors responded to treatment with FTIs as well or better than the mice bearing mutated H-*Ras*-driven tumors (Barrington et al., 1998). Tumor growth was suppressed and existing tumors regressed on therapy. Interestingly, the mechanism of tumor regression involved apoptosis in both of the bitransgenic mouse strains tested. Cell cycle changes were also noted that were consistent with the findings of cell culture experiments (i.e., enhanced G1 arrest and reductions of cells in S-phase). These studies illustrate the ability of FTIs to attack Ras-dependent cancers that are formed in different genetic backgrounds by more than one mechanism.

Effects on Cellular Prenylation Patterns

The striking biological effects of FTIs in preclinical cancer trials suggested that the drugs probed some unique aspect of neoplastic pathophysiology, strongly promoting interest in their precise effects on cells. One interesting aspect of FTI treatment that has become apparent is that the drugs promote protein geranylgeranylation in cells. This counterintuitive effect is mediated by GGT-I, which can modify certain FT substrates when FT activity is blocked by drug treatment. The three different effects of FTIs on protein prenylation is illustrated in Box 14-1, using as examples H-Ras, K-Ras, and RhoB, three drug target proteins that have received the most attention in mechanistic analyses. FTIs cause loss of function of H-Ras by preventing its farnesylation. Unfarnesylated H-Ras is unstable and accumulates in cells at much lower steady-state levels than processed Ras (Prendergast et al., 1994). While unfarnesylated Ras proteins might act in a dominant inhibitory fashion, their low level of accumulation argues that such effects would be marginal at best.

In contrast to H-Ras, K-Ras is normally farnesylated but becomes geranylgeranylated in cells treated with FTIs (Lerner et al., 1997; Rowell et al., 1997; Whyte et al., 1997). This GGT-I "shunt pathway" allows K-Ras to remain prenylated and membrane bound. This alteration in prenylation status does not affect the oncogenic properties of mutated K-Ras (A. Cox, personal communication). The operation of this shunt pathway may help maintain the function of farnesylated proteins that would otherwise be inactivated by FTI treatment, possibly explaining why FTIs are relatively benign to normal cells.

Similar to the effects on K-Ras, but with a potentially different consequence on function, FTIs also alter the prenylation status of RhoB. This small GTPase is a short-lived member of the Rho family that is localized on endosomes, where it functions in receptor trafficking (Gampel et al., 1999). A unique feature of RhoB is that it is normally present in either farnesylated or geranylgeranylated populations in cells (Adamson et al., 1992). FTIs abolish the farnesylation but not the geranylgeranylation of newly synthesized RhoB (Lebowitz et al., 1997a). Thus, the GGT-I shunt pathway ensures that all the RhoB in cells treated with FTIs is geranylgeranylated. In contrast to K-Ras, this shift in prenylation status is correlated with a profound alteration in cellular localization and an increase in steady-state protein expression (Lebowitz et al., 1995, 1997a; H. Mellor, personal communication). Thus, in the case of RhoB, the operation of the GGT-I shunt pathway leads to a change- or gain-of-function effect. In summary, FTIs can elicit loss of function (H-Ras), altered prenylation but not loss of function (K-Ras), or change or gain of function (RhoB), depending on the target protein.

Cellular Mechanism of Action

As discussed, inhibition of Ras farnesylation correlates with inhibition of cell proliferation and antitumor activity. However, it has become clear that the correlation between the effects of FTI on Ras and FTI biology is not watertight. Indeed, an unanticipated turn in FTI research has emerged from evidence that the antineoplastic effects of these agents can be separated from their effects on Ras—that is, to inhibit tumor cell growth an inhibition of Ras farnesylation may be sufficient in principle but is unnecessary in practice. As mentioned, the clues that this was the case came from the earliest days of research into the cell biological mechanism of FTase inhibitor action. Using one of the first bioactive FTIs to be generated in the Merck group, I noticed that the kinetics of the phenotypic reversion induced by drug treatment was too rapid to be accounted for simply by depletion of processed H-Ras (Prendergast et al., 1994).

Fully modified H-Ras is long-lived, with a half-life of 24 hours (Shih et al., 1982). FTIs block modification of newly synthesized Ras but not its steady-state level or activity once Ras proteins have been prenylated. Therefore, 2 to 3 days of drug treatment are required to significantly deplete processed Ras from cells. In contrast, phenotypic reversion of H-Ras-transformed cells by FTIs was achieved within 18 to 24 hours of treatment. Steady-state Ras levels persisted at 50% of their pretreatment values in fully reverted cells. Moreover, once initiated by a single drug dose, the reverted phenotype persisted for several days after FTI activity had been restored and prenylated Ras had returned to normal levels (Prendergast et al., 1994). This long-lived phenotype was traced subsequently to upregulation of collagen Iα2 (Du et al., 1999b), a long-lived isoform of collagen that is growth inhibitory and that Ras must suppress to transform cells (Andreu et al., 1998; Travers et al., 1996). The kinetics of this genetic response suggested a Ras-independent effect.

Subsequent studies corroborated evidence that argued against a link between inhibition of Ras prenylation and anticancer activity. First, rodent fibroblasts transformed with N-myristoylated Ras remain susceptible to FTase inhibitors, despite the fact that N-myristoylated Ras does not require farnesylation to be biologically active (Lebowitz et al., 1995). Second, as already mentioned, $\sim$70% of human tumor cell lines are susceptible to growth inhibition by FTase inhibitors, although there was no correlation between susceptibility and Ras status (Nagasu et al., 1995; Sepp-Lorenzino et al., 1995). Lastly, FTase inhibitors could block the malignant growth induced by activated K-Ras or N-Ras, even though FTase inhibitors do not block prenylation of these proteins. While there is some difference in the susceptibility of fibroblasts transformed by K-Ras versus H-Ras, this is not the case in rat intestinal epithelial cells (Zeng et al., 2003). The "resistance" of K-Ras-transformed cells to FTI-induced growth inhibition is a tissue-specific phenomenon; this is contrasted with FTI-induced apoptosis, to which Tamanoi's group has shown K-Ras-transformed cells to be fully susceptible. The ability of FTIs to block K-Ras transformation (and the growth of >90% of human tumor cell lines) has suggested to many investigators that FTIs act, at least in part, via a Ras-independent mechanism.

Role of RhoB in the FTI Response

My laboratory has developed a significant body of evidence supporting a causal role for RhoB in the antineoplastic response to FTI treatment (Lebowitz and Prendergast, 1998; Prendergast, 2000). This link was first suggested by the ability of FTIs to drive stress fiber formation, even in normal cells, because Rho GTPases are responsible for actin cytoskeletal regulation. Most Rho proteins are geranylgeranylated, but RhoB is farnesylated, short-lived, and linked to cell growth regulation (Adamson et al., 1992;

Jahner and Hunter, 1991). Yet a further twist in the drug mechanism came with the finding that elevation of the geranylgeranylated RhoB isoform by itself is both necessary and sufficient to mediate antineoplastic responses to FTIs in transformed rodent cells (Du et al., 1999a; Liu et al., 2000). These effects are not confined to rodent models but are also seen in human tumor cells, where there is a good correlation between susceptibility to growth inhibition by FTI and by engineered elevation of geranylgeranylated RhoB (Du and Prendergast, 1999). More recent studies confirm that ectopic RhoB can phenocopy FTI suppression of K-Ras-transformed rat intestinal epithelial cells, RhoC-transformed human mammary epithelial cells, and even Rac1-transformed cells (van Golen et al., 2002; Zeng et al., 2003). Taken together, the results suggest that RhoB has an antioncogenic role in cells that may oppose the prooncogenic roles of other important Rho proteins, such as RhoA, RhoC, or Rac1 (Prendergast, 2001a).

Although still a question of some dispute in the field (Sebti and Hamilton, 2000), handled in detail elsewhere (Prendergast, 2001a), the strongest evidence of the role of RhoB in the FTI response comes from recent studies in a RhoB knockout mouse, where geranylgeranylated RhoB cannot be generated by drug treatment due to deletion of the *rhoB* gene. Notably, primary mouse fibroblasts transformed by E1A + Ras but lacking *rhoB* exhibit defects in the response to drug treatment, especially in the actin and apoptotic responses (Liu et al., 2000), establishing that elevation of geranylgeranylated RhoB has a necessary role in the drug mechanism. This study also showed that growth inhibition can occur by a RhoB-independent mechanism. Thus, while geranylgeranylated RhoB is sufficient to suppress growth and to phenocopy the FTI response, other targets may also be sufficient. However, the actin/apoptotic defects are crucial, as the antitumor efficacy of FTI is significantly compromised in −/− cells where geranylgeranylated RhoB cannot be elicited in response to drug treatment (Liu et al., 2000).

Recently, our laboratory has expanded the key role of RhoB in anticancer responses by showing that it is critical for apoptosis in transformed cells exposed to DNA-damaging agents or paclitaxel, two major arsenals of the clinical oncologist (Liu et al., 2001a). Notably, the latest work on the knockout mouse implicates RhoB as a negative modifier gene in cancer: −/− mice do not exhibit an elevated susceptibility to cancer but these mice are more prone to tumor formation if exposed to an oncogenic stimulus (Liu et al., 2001b). Taken together, drug and knockout mouse studies present a self-consistent picture of RhoB as a dominant susceptibility-reducing modifier as defined in Chapter 12 that suppresses tumor formation (Prendergast, 2001a).

Perhaps the most interesting implication of this work is that FTIs act in part by recruiting a tumor suppressor rather than blocking an oncoprotein. In summary, the RhoB gain-of-function elicited by FTI treatment has a major role in apoptotic and antineoplastic properties of these drugs. The best test of the utility of this mechanism will be illustrated by examining new clinical applications of FTIs that might not have been guessed at by simply following Ras connections, namely Rho-driven inflammatory breast cancer and age-associated blindness (Prendergast and Rane, 2001).

Additional FTI Target Proteins

The best-studied FTI targets so far are certainly the Ras and RhoB proteins. RhoB is the only FTI target that has been assessed critically for its involvement in the FTI response using a mouse knockout system. Some investigators have proposed that a loss of H-Ras function in tumor cells driven by K-Ras or N-Ras (which are not blocked directly by FTI treatment) might underlie the antiproliferative response to FTI (Feldkamp et al., 2001). H-Ras knockout mice, which are viable (Ise et al., 2000), offer an excellent model to assess this hypothesis.

Many other farnesylated proteins have been proposed as FTI targets, but whether inhibiting the farnesylation of these proteins is causally connected to the FTI response is generally not well established. A partial list of these candidate targets includes the lamin A and B proteins; the protein phosphatases PTP1 and PTP2; the peroxisomal protein PxF; the molecular chaperone HDJ-2; inositol trisphosphate 5'phosphatase; the small GTPases RhoD, RhoE/Rnd, and Rheb; the skeletal muscle α- and ß-phosphorylase kinases; and the centromere-binding proteins CENP-E and CENP-F. Unlike RhoB, which is dispensable for normal development and adult physiology (Liu et al., 2001b), many of these alternate FTI targets would seem to be important to normal cell physiology, making it more difficult to invoke their alteration as a way to explain the cancer-selective effects of FTIs.

CENP dysfunction may relate to G2/M-phase phenomena that have been described recently: FTIs may trigger apoptosis in susceptible cells via a terminal arrest in M-phase (Liu et al., 2001a), whereas in nonsusceptible cells M-phase arrest may be associated with chromosome nondisjunction and/or other abnormalities (Ashar et al., 2000; Crespo et al., 2001). If the target is hypothesized to be pro-oncogenic, then mechanistic criteria to validate a causal role in the drug response should minimally include demonstrations that the FTI response can be (1) blocked by maintaining target function (e.g., by engineering a farnesyl-independent function), and (2) phenocopied by genetic ablation (e.g., by RNAi, etc.).

Clinical Evaluation

Although our understanding of the cell biology and biochemistry of FTIs is increasing rapidly, questions remain concerning how best to use these agents in the clinic. As will be examined for other cancer drugs in Chapter 15, clinical researchers must ask, which patient populations and tumor types are most appropriate candidates for treatment? Should *Ras* gene mutational status guide choice of treatment? As noted, *Ras* status does not correlate with the response to FTIs in human tumor cell lines, yet transgenic models driven by *Ras* respond relatively well to FTIs. Given evidence of the role for Rho alteration in the drug response, tumors driven by Rho, such as inflammatory breast cancer, might respond well to FTI inhibitors. Indeed, recent work supports this notion (van Golen et al., 2002). Should FTIs be administered chronically or acutely? Xenograft studies argue that FTIs act primarily as cytostatic drugs, while transgenic mouse studies suggest apoptotic prowess. Cell biological experiments argue that cell adhesion environment and the status of the cell survival pathway regulated by PTEN-AKT may predict apoptotic susceptibility (Du et al., 1999c). Should FTIs be applied alone or in combinations with existing anticancer modalities? As with many other anticancer agents, preclinical studies of FTIs clearly demonstrate additive or even synergistic antitumor activities in cell culture and animal experiments with standard chemotherapeutics (Liu et al., 1998; Moasser et al., 1998; Sun et al., 1999) or irradiation (Bernhard et al., 1996, 1998).

Results from initial phase I and phase II clinical testing of several different FTIs are summarized here but have been considered in depth elsewhere (Adjei, 2001; Cox, 2001;

Karp et al., 2001; Prendergast and Rane, 2001; Purcell and Donehower, 2002). To date, several FTIs have been evaluated in such trials as single agents or as components of combinatorial regimens with approved cancer treatments. Reports indicate that two of the better-studied compounds, SCH-66336 and R115777, are generally well tolerated. Dose-limiting toxicities for R115777 were QTc prolongation, neutropenia, fatigue, and myelosuppression. A combination trial with radiotherapy of a total of 21 patients resulted in 2 complete and 4 partial responses. A general grade III diarrhea and grade IV hematological toxicity was seen.

In a study of relapsed and refractory acute leukemias, 21-day cycles repeated up to 4 times yielded stable disease in 4/20 patients. In another study, R115777 administration produced partial remission in 1 patient with dose-limiting toxicities at 400 mg, which included neutropenia, thrombocytopenia, and fever. In a phase II trial for breast cancer, 3/26 patients showed partial response, while 9 other patients showed stable disease at 3 months evaluation. This drug has entered into phase III trials for a wide variety of solid tumors; a combination regimen with either gemcitabine or capecitabine will be explored based on preliminary findings of efficacy and reduced toxicity.

Recently, a phase II study of SCH66336 was completed at doses up to 400 mg bid. Dose-limiting toxicity at 400 mg consisted of gastrointestinal toxicities, neutropenia, and thrombocytopenia. However, at 200 mg, SCH66336 was safely administered on long-term protocol without myelosuppression toxicity (Adjei et al., 2000). A combinatorial therapy with paclitaxel and gemcitabine was also evaluated as a phase I trial for solid tumors. Of 18 evaluable patients, 6 showed partial responses with minor toxicities for paclitaxel, whereas 2 partial and 2 minor responses were achieved with gemcitabine treatment. In addition, 11/25 patients showed stability of disease for greater than 6 months.

Other compounds are at earlier stages of development. BMS-214662 is an unusually proapoptotic compound (Rose et al., 2001). In phase I trials, BMS-214662 was given as a 1 hr infusion for 1 to 30 weeks of treatment. Toxicities were grade 3 neutropenia, vomiting, and hypotension. This compound has entered in phase II trials for pancreatic, head and neck, lung, and colorectal cancers. Two other compounds, CP-609754 and AZD-3409, have also entered into clinical trials, but no data are yet available. In general, researchers might judge the results of phase II trials of FTIs to be somewhat disappointing, based on the promising and in some cases dramatic preclinical results. However, combinatorial applications with other cancer chemotherapeutics are somewhat encouraging and the most susceptible tumors may have yet to be identified. Clearly, all of the technologies described in Section II of this book including genotyping, and expression-profiling at the RNA, protein, cell and tissue-levels will be essential to define the most susceptible neoplastic diseases for these drugs.

INHIBITORS OF Ras MEMBRANE INSERTION

As mentioned, Ras proteins undergo three steps of posttranslational modification: farnesylation, C-terminal proteolysis (to remove the aaX residues from the farnesylated CaaX terminus), and methylation of the farnesyl-cysteine C-terminus. H-Ras and N-Ras proteins also become palmitoylated immediately upstream of the farnesyl-cysteine residue, further increasing hydrophobicity of the C-terminus. Proteolysis and methylation steps are catalyzed; it is not yet clear whether palmitoylation is catalyzed. Initial studies highlighted the critical nature of farnesylation for Ras transformation activity (Kato et al., 1992), focusing therapeutic efforts on inhibition of FT.

Recently, other possible strategies to block Ras function have been prompted by studies of Ras aaX proteolysis, carboxymethylation, and membrane insertion. Interestingly, Young and colleagues have reported that a conditional deletion of the mouse gene for Rce1, which mediates Ras proteolysis and is necessary for Ras membrane localization (Kim et al., 1999), not only significantly reduces Ras transformation but also heightens the response of *Ras*-transformed cells to FTI treatment (Bergo et al., 2002). Efforts to identify specific peptidyl and nonpeptidyl inhibitors of Rce1 have been initiated (Dolence et al., 2000; Schlitzer et al., 2001). A deletion has also been made in the mouse gene for isoprenylcysteine carboxyl methyltransferase (ICMT), the enzyme responsible for C-terminal methylation of Ras and other Ras superfamily proteins (Bergo et al., 2001). The knockout displays an embryonic lethal phenotype, suggesting an important role in cell proliferation and survival. While little is known about the precise role of C-terminal methylation in Ras function, this processing step has been reported to be critical for K-Ras to achieve a specific association with microtubules (Chen et al., 2000). However, the lethal phenotype displayed in knockout mice suggests that ICMT might be problematic as a cancer therapeutic target because normal as well as malignant cells may depend on its activity.

Kloog and colleagues have developed this area from a different direction, starting with the notion that the membrane insertion of Ras is critical for its activity (Kloog and Cox, 2000; Kloog et al., 1999). This group has developed an interesting set of studies on S-trans, trans-farnesylthiosalicylic acid (FTS), a competitive inhibitor of a cellular prenylated protein methyltransferase that suppresses Ras transformation (Marom et al., 1995). FTS may act by dislodging Ras proteins from membranes, including K-Ras (Elad et al., 1999), leading to their degradation and loss of transforming activity. FTS has low micromolar activity in vitro but is sufficiently bioactive to be used in mouse studies, where significant antitumor activity has been demonstrated (Egozi et al., 1999; Jansen et al., 1999; Weisz et al., 1999).

Interestingly, FTS also has efficacy in mouse models for autoimmune diseases, such as lupus (Katzav et al., 2001), suggesting that membrane disruption of Ras superfamily proteins may have therapeutic utility beyond malignant settings. Whether some of the effects of FTS are mediated nonselectively via the immune system is prompted by the recent report that FTS can disrupt interactions of Ras with galectin-1 (Paz et al., 2001), a member of a class of glycoproteins that have diverse immunostimulatory effects (Rabinovich et al., 2002). Nevertheless, this line of work is intriguing and illustrates the possible strategy of targeting Ras membrane localization or prenylated protein methyltransferases such as ICMT for cancer therapy.

INHIBITORS OF Ras-EFFECTOR INTERACTIONS AND OTHER ANTI-Ras APPROACHES

An obvious strategy to block the function of Ras is to block its interaction with key downstream effectors. Indeed, the original efforts in this direction focused on the first Ras-binding protein to be discovered: the GTPase-activating protein GAP. However, this project faces an intrinsic challenge. Entropy is a major thermodynamic driver of protein-protein interactions, because of the energy released by disordering surface water molecules. From first principles, one would imagine it might be difficult to develop a small-molecule inhibitor of protein-protein interactions, because such an inhibitor could not disorder sufficient water to compete effectively with another protein interface. This problem might be attacked by screening for loss of *functional* interactions, rather than simply a general loss of interaction. A well-designed screen might make it possible to identify molecules that disrupt an interaction-dependent activation event. Few such screens have been reported to date.

One screen for Ras-Raf inhibitors identified 7 amino acid peptides with IC50s in the micromolar range (Barnard et al., 1998), but the findings of this study were not expanded. Despite the attention of many industrial groups, there have been few reliable reports of inhibitors of protein-protein interactions, including Ras-effector interactions. Nevertheless, there remains significant interest given the validation of key Ras effector pathways involving Raf kinase, PI3K-Akt, and Ral GDS. Guanine nucleotide exchange factors (GEFs) such as Ral GDS or Sos might be tractable to inhibitor development, based on evidence that the fungal inhibitor brefeldin A acts by inhibiting guanine nucleotide exchange on the Ras superfamily protein Arf1 (Donaldson et al., 1992; Helms and Rothman, 1992). Undoubtedly, Ras interactions will continue to get the attention of therapeutic development groups.

Efforts to target Ras-effector pathways instead of Ras itself may ultimately prove more successful. As discussed in Chapter 13, kinases are attractive oncology targets and thus, projects to target Raf, MEK, and MAPK have led to the identification of moderately selective kinase inhibitors that may have cancer potential. These projects generally have been burdened with issues of specificity and nonselective toxicity, however. Interest in the PI3K-Akt pathway, a major oncogenic pathway in cancer cells, has stimulated significant efforts in the pharmaceutical industry to define inhibitors of Akt kinase. Anecdotal reports suggest that inhibitors of Akt are relatively difficult to identify by high-throughput screening, relative to other kinases, although this may prove to be good news with regard to selectivity issues. Another kinase that has gotten some attention from the Ras field is the Rho-effector kinase ROCK, which like Rho (Qiu et al., 1995) is required for Ras transformation and invasive growth (Itoh et al., 1999). The compound Y-27632, which inhibits ROCK activity, effectively suppresses Rho-dependent Ras transformation (Sahai et al., 1999).

Other strategies to target Ras-signaling pathways by genetic routes continue to be explored. One advantage to such strategies is their ability in principle to distinguish mutant and wild-type proteins or functions. Evolving antisense technologies continue to be investigated. For example, hammerhead ribozymes have been developed that can target mutant K-Ras RNAs (e.g., Tsuchida et al., 1998). While published reports represent only proof-of-concept experiments, efforts to optimize the pharmacokinetic properties of ribozymes for in vivo application have been undertaken in the biotechnology industry, and, in fact, phase I and II clinical trials with such ribozymes are being conducted currently by Ribozyme Pharmaceuticals Inc., which holds rights to this technology.

With the recent explosion of interest in RNA interference and the coming exploration of its in vivo applications, Ras and its effector molecules will again become a focus of attention in the field. Other genetic technologies that have yet to be fully exploited for drug screening are knockout and gene chip technologies. A novel utility for knockout technology was recently illustrated by a screen for compounds that selectively interfere with K-Ras-driven human cancers (Torrance et al., 2001). This approach compared the cytotoxic response of DLD-1 colon cancer cells that were targeted for K-ras deletion with parental DLD-1 cells, in the same tissue culture well, by using green fluorescence protein technology to distinguish the two populations. Similarly, gene-chip fingerprinting approaches have been used to identify chemotherapeutic compounds that are more active against cells that harbor mutant K-Ras (Koo et al., 2000).

Such top-down approaches for drug screening, which rely on more traditional cell-based screens instead of molecule-based screens to identify compounds (Prendergast, 2001b), may turn up novel targets and directions. Indeed, given the somewhat disappointing results of the molecular biology revolution for the discovery of effective new clinical agents (Rees, 2002)—a situation reflected in the relatively poor pipelines of many pharmaceutical companies—specialized niches for new discovery based on biological *systems* rather than *molecules* should be welcomed. Few areas have been founded and developed as fully as Ras signaling in cancer. Thus, no matter what the approach, the foundation provided by this area to assess novel technologies for drug development will likely remain attractive in the long run.

REFERENCES

Adamson, P., Marshall, C. J., Hall, A., and Tilbrook, P. A. (1992). Post-translational modification of p21rho proteins. *J Biol Chem 267*, 20033–20038.

Adjei, A. A. (2001). Blocking oncogenic Ras signaling for cancer therapy, *J Natl Cancer Inst 93*, 1062–1074.

Adjei, A. A., Erlichman, C., Davis, J. N., Cutler, D. L., Sloan, J. A., Marks, R. S., Hanson, L. J., Svingen, P. A., Atherton, P., Bishop, W. R., et al. (2000). A phase I trial of the farnesyl transferase inhibitor SCH66336: Evidence for biological and clinical activity. *Cancer Res 60*, 1871–1877.

Andreu, T., Beckers, T., Thoenes, E., Hilgard, P., and von Melchner, H. (1998). Gene trapping identifies inhibitors of oncogenic transformation: The tissue inhibitor of metalloproteinases-3 (TIMP3) and collagen type I–alpha-2 (COL1A2) are epidermal growth factor–regulated growth repressors. *J Biol Chem 273*, 13848–13854.

Ashar, H. R., James, L., Gray, K., Carr, D., Black, S., Armstrong, L., Bishop, W. R., and Kirschmeier, P. (2000). Farnesyl transferase inhibitors block the farnesylation of CENP-E and CENP-F and alter the association of CENP-E with the microtubules. *J Biol Chem 275*, 30451–30457.

Augeri, D. J., O'Connor, S. J., Janowick, D., Szczepankiewicz, B., Sullivan, G., Larsen, J., Kalvin, D., Cohen, J., Devine, B., Zhang, H., et al. (1998). Potent and selective non-cysteine-containing inhibitors of protein farnesyltransferase. *J Med Chem 41*, 4288–4300.

Barnard, D., Sun, H., Baker, L., and Marshall, M. S. (1998). In vitro inhibition of Ras-Raf association by short peptides. *Biochem Biophys Res Commun 247*, 176–180.

Barrington, R. E., Subler, M. A., Rands, E., Omer, C. A., Miller, P. J., Hundley, J. E., Koester, S. K., Troyer, D. A., Bearss, D. J., Conner, M. W., et al. (1998). A farnesyltransferase inhibitor induces tumor regression in transgenic mice harboring multiple oncogenic mutations by mediating alterations in both cell cycle control and apoptosis. *Mol Cell Biol 18*, 85–92.

Bergo, M. O., Leung, G. K., Ambroziak, P., Otto, J. C., Casey, P. J., Gomes, A. Q., Seabra, M. C., and Young, S. G. (2001). Isoprenylcysteine carboxyl methyltransferase deficiency in mice. *J Biol Chem 276*, 5841–5845.

Bergo, M. O., Ambroziak, P., Gregory, C., George, A., Otto, J. C., Kim, E., Nagase, H., Casey, P. J., Balmain, A., and Young, S. G. (2002). Absence of the CAAX endoprotease Rce1: Effects on cell growth and transformation. *Mol Cell Biol 22*, 171–181.

Bernhard, E. J., Kao, G., Cox, A. D., Sebti, S. M., Hamilton, A. D., Muschel, R. J., and McKenna, W. G. (1996). The farnesyltransferase inhibitor FTI-277 radiosensitizes H-ras-transformed rat embryo fibroblasts. *Cancer Res 56*, 1727–1730.

Bernhard, E. J., McKenna, W. G., Hamilton, A. D., Sebti, S. M., Qian, Y., Wu, J. M., and Muschel, R. J. (1998). Inhibiting Ras prenylation increases the radiosensitivity of human tumor cell lines with activating mutations of Ras oncogenes. *Cancer Res 58*, 1754–1761.

Bishop, W. R., Bond, R., Petrin, J., Wang, L., Patton, R., Doll, R., Njoroge, G., Catino, J., Schwartz, J., Windsor, W., et al. (1995). Novel tricyclic inhibitors of farnesyl protein transferase: Biochemical characterization and inhibition of Ras modification in trasfected COS cells. *J Biol Chem 270*, 30611–30618.

Bollag, G., and McCormick, F. (1991). Regulators and effectors of *Ras* proteins. *Ann Rev Cell Biol 7*, 601–632.

Bos, J. L. (1990). *Ras* gene mutations and human cancer. In *Molecular Genetics in Cancer Diagnosis*, J. Cossman (ed.). Amsterdam, Netherlands: Elsevier Scientific Publishing, pp. 273–287.

Chardin, P., Camonis, J. H., Gale, N. W., van Alest, L., Schlessinger, J., Wigler, M. H., and Bar-Sagi, D. (1993). Human SOS1: A guanine nucleotide exchange factor for Ras that binds to GRB2. *Science 260*, 1338–1343.

Chen, W.-J., Andres, D. A., Goldstein, J. L., Russell, D. W., and Brown, M. S. (1991). cDNA cloning and expression of the peptide-binding ß subunit of rat p21ras farnesyltransferase, the counterpart of yeast DPR1/RAM1. *Cell 66*, 327–334.

Chen, Z., Otto, J. C., Bergo, M. O., Young, S. G., and Casey, P. J. (2000). The C-terminal polylysine region and methylation of K-Ras are critical for the interaction between K-Ras and microtubules. *J Biol Chem 275*, 41251–41257.

Chin, L. ,A. ,T., Pomerantz, J., Wong, M., Holash, J., Bardeesy, N., Shen, Q., O'Hagan, R., Pantginis, J., Zhou, H., et al. (1999). Essential role for oncogenic Ras in tumour maintenance. *Nature 400*, 468–472.

Clarke, G. J., and Der, C. J. (1995). Ras proto-oncogene activation in human malignancy. In *Cellular Cancer Markers*, C. T. Garrett and S. Sell (ed.). Totowa, NJ: Humana, pp. 17–52.

Cox, A. D. (2001). Farnesyltransferase inhibitors: Potential role in the treatment of cancer. *Drugs 61*, 723–732.

Cox, A. D., Hisaka, M. M., Buss, J. E., and Der, C. J. (1992). Specific isoprenoid modification is required for function of normal, but not oncogenic, Ras function. *Mol Cell Biol 12*, 2606–2615.

Crespo, N. C., Ohkanda, J., Yen, T. J., Hamilton, A. D., and Sebti, S. M. (2001). The farnesyltransferase inhibitor, FTI-2153, blocks bipolar spindle formation and chromosome alignment and causes prometaphase accumulation during mitosis of human lung cancer cells. *J Biol Chem 276*, 16161–16167.

deSolms, S. J., Giuliani, E. A., Graham, S. L., Koblan, K. S., Kohl, N. E., Mosser, S. D., Oliff, A., Pompliano, D. L., Rands, B., Scholz, T. H., et al. (1998). N-arylalkyl pseudopeptide inhibitors of farnesyl-transferase. *J Med Chem 41*, 2651–2656.

DeVita, V., Hellman, S., and Rosenberg, S. (1997). *Cancer Principles and Practice of Oncology*, 5th ed. Philadelphia: Lippincott Raven Press.

Dolence, E. K., Dolence, J. M., and Poulter, C. D. (2000). Solid-phase synthesis of a farnesylated CaaX peptide library: Inhibitors of the Ras CaaX endoprotease. *J Comb Chem 2*, 522–536.

Donaldson, J. G., Finazzi, D., and Klausner, R. D. (1992). Brefeldin A inhibits Golgi membrane–catalyzed exchange of guanine nucleotide onto ARF protein. *Nature 360*, 350–352.

Du, W., and Prendergast, G. C. (1999). Geranylgeranylated RhoB mediates inhibition of human tumor cell growth by farnesyltransferase inhibitors. *Cancer Res 59*, 5924–5928.

Du, W., Lebowitz, P., and Prendergast, G. C. (1999a). Cell growth inhibition by farnesyltransferase inhibitors is mediated by gain of geranylgeranylated RhoB. *Mol Cell Biol 19*, 1831–1840.

Du, W., Lebowitz, P. F., and Prendergast, G. C. (1999b). Elevation of α2(I) collagen, a suppressor of Ras transformation, is required for stable phenotypic reversion by farnesyltransferase inhibitors. *Cancer Res 59*, 2059–2063.

Du, W., Liu, A., and Prendergast, G. C. (1999c). Activation of the PI3'K-AKT pathway masks the proapoptotic effect of farnesyltransferase inhibitors. *Cancer Res 59*, 4808–4812.

Dunten, P., Kammlott, U., Crowther, R., Weber, D., Palermo, R., and Birktoft, J. (1998). Protein farnesyltransferase: Structure and implications for substrate binding. *Biochemistry 37*, 7907–7912.

Egozi, Y., Weisz, B., Gana-Weisz, M., Ben-Baruch, G., and Kloog, Y. (1999). Growth inhibition of Ras-dependent tumors in nude mice by a potent Ras-dislodging antagonist. *Int J Cancer 80*, 911–918.

Elad, G., Paz, A., Haklai, R., Marciano, D., Cox, A., and Kloog, Y. (1999). Targeting of K-Ras 4B by S-trans, trans-farnesyl thiosalicylic acid. *Biochim Biophys Acta 1452*, 228–242.

End, D. W. (1999). Farnesyl protein transferase inhibitors and other therapies targeting the Ras signal transduction pathway. *Invest New Drugs 17*, 241–258.

Feldkamp, M. M., Lau, N., Roncari, L., and Guha, A. (2001). Isotype-specific Ras.GTP-levels predict the efficacy of farnesyl transferase inhibitors against human astrocytomas regardless of Ras mutational status. *Cancer Res 61*, 4425–4431.

Gampel, A., Parker, P. J., and Mellor, H. (1999). Regulation of epidermal growth factor receptor traffic by the small GTPase RhoB. *Curr Biol 9*, 955–958.

Gibbs, J. B., and Oliff, A. (1994). Pharmaceutical research in molecular oncology. *Cell 79*, 193–198.

Gibbs, J. B., and Oliff, A. (1997). The potential of farnesyltransferase inhibitors as cancer chemotherapeutics. *Ann Rev Pharm Toxicol 37*, 143–166.

Gibbs, J. B., Pompliano, D. L., Mosser, S. D., Rands, B., Lingham, R. B., Singh, S. B., Scolnick, E. M., Kohl, N. E., and Oliff, A. (1993). Selective inhibition of farnesyl-protein transferase blocks Ras processing in vivo. *J Biol Chem 268*, 7617–7620.

Gibbs, J., Oliff, A., and Kohl, N. E. (1994). Farnesyltransferase inhibitors: Ras research yields a potential cancer therapeutic. *Cell 77*, 175–178.

Graham, S. L., deSolms, S. J., Giuliani, E. A., Kohl, N. E., Mosser, S. D., Oliff, A., Pompliano, D. L., Rands, E., Breslin, M., Deana, A. A., et al. (1994). Pseudopeptide inhibitors of Ras farnesyl-protein transferase. *J Med Chem 37*, 725–732.

Hara, M., Akasaka, K., Akinaga, S., Okabe, M., Nakano, H., Gomez, R., Wood, D., Uh, M., and Tamanoi, F. (1993). Identification of Ras farnesyltransferase inhibitors by microbial screening. *Proc Natl Acad Sci USA 90*, 2281–2285.

Helms, J. B., and Rothman, J. E. (1992). Inhibition by brefeldin A of a Golgi membrane enzyme that catalyses exchange of guanine nucleotide bound to ARF. *Nature 360*, 352–354.

Ise, K., Nakamura, K., Nakao, K., Shimizu, S., Harada, H., Ichise, T., Miyoshi, J., Gondo, Y., Ishikawa, T., Aiba, A., and Katsuki, M. (2000). Targeted deletion of the H-ras gene decreases tumor formation in mouse skin carcinogenesis. *Oncogene 19*, 2151–2156.

Itoh, K., Yoshioka, K., Akedo, H., Uegata, M., Ishizaki, T., and Narumiya, S. (1999). An essential part for Rho-associated kinase in the transcellular invasion of tumor cells. *Nat Med 5*, 221–225.

Jahner, D., and Hunter, T. (1991). The *Ras*-related gene *rhoB* is an immediate-early gene inducible by v-Fps, epidermal growth factor, and platelet-derived growth factor in rat fibroblasts. *Mol Cell Biol 11*, 3682–3690.

James, G. L., Goldstein, J. L., Brown, M. S., Rawson, T. E., Somers, T. C., McDowell, R. S., Crowley, C. W., Lucas, B. K., Levinson, A. D., and Marsters, J. C. (1993). Benzodiazepine peptidomimetics: Potent inhibitors of Ras farnesylation in animal cells. *Science 260*, 1937–1942.

Jansen, B., Schlagbauer-Wadl, H., Kahr, H., Heere-Ress, E., Mayer, B. X., Eichler, H., Pehamberger, H., Gana-Weisz, M., Ben-David, E., Kloog, Y., and Wolff, K. (1999). Novel Ras antagonist blocks human melanoma growth. *Proc Natl Acad Sci USA 96*, 14019–14024.

Jiang, K., Coppola, D., Crespo, N. C., Nicosia, S. V., Hamilton, A. D., Sebti, S. M., and Cheng, J. Q. (2000). The phosphoinositide 3-OH kinase/AKT2 pathway as a critical target for farnesyltransferase inhibitor–induced apoptosis. *Mol Cell Biol 20*, 139–148.

Kainuma, O., Asano, T., Hasegawa, M., and Isono, K. (1996). Growth inhibition of human pancreatic cancer by farnesyl transferase inhibitor. *Gan To Kaguku Ryoho 23*, 1657–1659.

Karp, J. E., Kaufmann, S. H., Adjei, A. A., Lancet, J. E., Wright, J. J., and End, D. W. (2001). Current status of clinical trials of farnesyltransferase inhibitors. *Curr Opin Oncol 13*, 470–476.

Kato, K., Cox, A. D., Hisaka, M. M., Graham, S. M., Buss, J. E., and Der, C. J. (1992). Isoprenoid addition to Ras protein is the critical modification for its membrane association and transforming activity. *Proc Natl Acad Sci USA 89*, 6403–6407.

Katzav, A., Kloog, Y., Korczyn, A. D., Niv, H., Karussis, D. M., Wang, N., Rabinowitz, R., Blank, M., Shoenfeld, Y., and Chapman, J. (2001). Treatment of MRL/lpr mice, a genetic autoimmune model, with the Ras inhibitor, farnesylthiosalicylate (FTS). *Clin Exp Immunol 126*, 570–577.

Kim, E., Ambroziak, P., Otto, J. C., Taylor, B., Ashby, M., Shannon, K., Casey, P. J., and Young, S. G. (1999). Disruption of the mouse Rce1 gene results in defective Ras processing and mislocalization of Ras within cells. *J Biol Chem 274*, 8383–8390.

Kloog, Y., and Cox, A. D. (2000). RAS inhibitors: Potential for cancer therapeutics. *Mol Med Today 6*, 398–402.

Kloog, Y., Cox, A. D., and Sinensky, M. (1999). Concepts in Ras-directed therapy. *Expert Opin Investig Drugs 8*, 2121–2140.

Koblan, K. S., Culberson, J. C., deSolms, S. J., Giuliani, E. A., Mosser, S. D., Omer, C. A., Pitzenberger, S. M., and Bogusky, M. J. (1995). NMR studies of novel inhibitors bound to farnesyl-protein transferase. *Protein Sci 4*, 681–688.

Kohl, N. E., Mosser, S. D., deSolms, S. J., Giuliani, E. A., Pompliano, D. L., Graham, S. L., Smith, R. L., Scolnick, E. M., Oliff, A., and Gibbs, J. B. (1993). Selective inhibition of *Ras*-dependent transformation by a farnesyltransferase inhibitor. *Science 260*, 1934–1937.

Kohl, N. E., Redner, F., Mosser, S., Guiliani, E. A., deSolms, S. J., Conner, M. W., Anthony, N. J., Holtz, W. J., Gomez, R. P., Lee, T.-J., et al. (1994). Protein farnesyltransferase inhibitors block the growth of Ras-dependent tumors in nude mice. *Proc Natl Acad Sci USA 91*, 9141–9145.

Kohl, N. E., Omer, C. A., Conner, M. W., Anthony, N. J., Davide, J. P., deSolms, S. J., Giuliani, E. A., Gomez, R. P., Graham, S. L., Hamilton, K., et al. (1995). Inhibition of farnesyltransferase induces regression of mammary and salivary carcinomas in *Ras* transgenic mice. *Nat Med 1*, 792–797.

Koo, H. M., McWilliams, M. J., Alvord, W. G., and Vande Woude, G. F. (2000). Ras oncogene-induced sensitization to 1-beta-D-arabinofuranosylcytosine. *Cancer Res 59*, 6057–6062.

Lebowitz, P. F., Davide, J. P., and Prendergast, G. C. (1995). Evidence that farnesyl transferase inhibitors suppress Ras transformation by interfering with Rho activity. *Mol Cell Biol 15*, 6613–6622.

Lebowitz, P., Casey, P. J., Prendergast, G. C., and Thissen, J. (1997a). Farnesyltransferase inhibitors alter the prenylation and growth-stimulating function of RhoB. *J Biol Chem 272*, 15591–15594.

Lebowitz, P. F., Sakamuro, D., and Prendergast, G. C. (1997b). Farnesyltransferase inhibitors induce apoptosis in Ras-transformed cells denied substratum attachment. *Cancer Res 57*, 708–713.

Lebowitz, P. F., and Prendergast, G. C. (1998). Non-Ras targets for farnesyltransferase inhibitors: Focus on Rho. *Oncogene 17*, 1439–1447.

Leonard, D. M. (1997). Ras farnesyltransferase: A new therapeutic target. *J Med Chem 40*, 2971–2990.

Lerner, E. C., Zhang, T. T., Knowles, D. B., Qian, Y. M., Hamilton, A. D., and Sebti, S. M. (1997). Inhibition of the prenylation of K-Ras, but not H- or N-Ras, is highly resistant to CAAX peptidomimetics and requires both a farnesyltransferase and a geranylgeranyltransferase-I inhibitor in human tumor cell lines. *Oncogene 15*, 1283–1288.

Lingham, R. B., Silverman, K. C., Bills, G. F., Cascales, C., Sanchez, M., Jenkins, R. G., Gartner, S. E., Martin, I., Diez, M. R., and Pelaez, F. (1993). *Chaetomella acutiseta* produces chaetomellic acids A and B which are reversible inhibitors of farnesyl-protein transferase. *Appl Microbiol Biotechnol 40*, 370–374.

Liu, A.-X., Du, W., Liu, J.-P., Jessell, T. M., and Prendergast, G. C. (2000). RhoB alteration is required for the apoptotic and antineoplastic responses to farnesyltransferase inhibitors. *Mol Cell Biol 20*, 6105–6113.

Liu, A.-X., Cerniglia, G. J., Bernhard, E. J., and Prendergast, G. C. (2001a). RhoB is required for the apoptotic response of neoplastically transformed cells to DNA damage. *Proc Natl Acad Sci USA 98*, 6192–6197.

Liu, A.-X., Rane, N., Liu, J.-P., and Prendergast, G. C. (2001b). RhoB is dispensable for mouse development, but it modifies susceptibility to tumor formation as well as cell adhesion and growth factor signaling in transformed cells. *Mol Cell Biol 21*, 6906–6912.

Liu, M., Bryant, M. S., Chen, J., Lee, S., Yaremko, B., Lipari, P., Malkowski, M., Ferrari, E., Nielsen, L., Prioli, N., et al. (1998). Antitumor activity of SCH 6636, an orally bioavailable tricyclic inhibitor of farnesyl protein transferase, in human tumor xenograft models and wap-ras transgenic mice. *Cancer Res 58*, 4947–4956.

Long, S. B., Casey, P. J., and Beese, L. S. (1998). Cocrystal structure of protein farnesltransferase complexed with a farnesyl di-phosphate substrate. *Biochemistry 37*, 9612–9618.

Lowy, D., and Willumsen, B. (1993). Function and regulation of Ras. *Ann Rev Biochem 62*, 851–891.

Mangues, R., Seidman, I., Pellicer, A., and Gordon, J. W. (1990). Tumorigenesis and male sterility in transgenic mice expressing a MMTV/N-ras oncogene. *Oncogene 5*, 1491–1497.

Mangues, R., Corral, T., Kohl, N. E., Symmans, W. F., Lu, S., Malumbres, M., Gibbs, J. B., Oliff, A., and Pellicer, A. (1998). Antitumor effect of a farnesyl protein transferase inhibitor in mammary and lymphoid tumors overexpressing N-ras in transgenic mice. *Cancer Res 58*, 1253–1259.

Marom, M., Haklai, R., Ben-Baruch, G., Marciano, D., Egozi, Y., and Kloog, Y. (1995). Selective inhibition of Ras-dependent cell growth by farnesylthiosalisylic acid, *J Biol Chem 270*, 22263–22270.

Miquel, K., Pradines, A., Sun, J., Qian, Y., Hamilton, A. D., Sebti, S. M., and Favre, G. (1997). GGTI-298 induces G0-G1 block and apoptosis whereas FTI-277 causes G2-M enrichment in A549 cells. *Cancer Res 57*, 1846–1850.

Moasser, M. M., Sepp-Lorenzino, L., Kohl, N. E., Oliff, A., Balog, A., Su, D. S., Danishefsky, S. J., and Rosen, N. (1998). Farnesyl transferase inhibitors cause enhanced mitotic sensitivity to taxol and epothilones. *Proc Natl Acad Sci USA 95*, 1369–1374.

Moores, S. L., Schaber, M. D., Mosser, S. D., Rands, E., O'Hara, M. B., Garsky, V. M., Marshall, M. S., Pompliano, D. L., and Gibbs, J. B. (1991). Sequence dependence of protein isoprenylation. *J Biol Chem 266*, 14603–14610.

Nagasu, T., Yoshimatsu, K., Rowell, C., Lewis, M. D., and Garcia, A. M. (1995). Inhibition of human tumor xenograft growth by treatment with the farnesyltransferase inhibitor B956. *Cancer Res 55*, 5310–5314.

Omer, C. A., Kral, A. M., Diehl, R. E., Prendergast, G. C., Powers, S., Allen, C. M., Gibbs, J. B., and Kohl, N. E. (1993). Characterization of recombinant human farnesyl-protein transferase: Cloning, expression, farnesyl diphosphate binding and functional homology with yeast prenyl-protein transferases. *Biochemistry 32*, 5167–5176.

Omer, C. A., Chen, Z., Diehl, R. E., Conner, M. W., Chen, H. Y., Trumbauer, M. E., Gopal-Truter, S., Seeburger, G., Bhimnathwala, H., Abrams, M. T., et al. (2000). Mouse mammary tumor virus-Ki-RasB transgenic mice develop mammary carcinomas that can be growth-inhibited by a farnesyl:protein transferase inhibitor. *Cancer Res 60*, 2680–2688.

Park, H. W., Boduluri, S. R., Moomaw, J. F., Casey, P. J., and Beese, L. S. (1997). Crystal structure of protein farnesyltransferase at 2.25 angstrom resolution. *Science 275*, 1800–1804.

Paz, A., Haklai, R., Elad-Sfadia, G., Ballan, E., and Kloog, Y. (2001). Galectin-1 binds oncogenic H-Ras to mediate Ras membrane anchorage and cell transformation. *Oncogene 20*, 7486–7493.

Prendergast, G. C. (2000). Farnesyltransferase inhibitors: Antineoplastic mechanism and clinical prospects. *Curr Opin Cell Biol 12*, 166–173.

Prendergast, G. C. (2001a). Actin' up: RhoB in cancer and apoptosis. *Nature Rev Cancer 1*, 162–168.

Prendergast, G. C. (2001b). Knockout drug screens. *Nature Biotechnol 19*, 919–920.

Prendergast, G. C., and Du, W. (1999). Targeting farnesyltransferase: Is Ras relevant? *Drug Resist Updates 2*, 81–84.

Prendergast, G. C., and Rane, N. (2001). Farnesyltransferase inhibitors: Mechanisms and applications. *Expert Opin Investig Drugs 10*, 2105–2116.

Prendergast, G. C., Davide, J. P., deSolms, S. J., Giuliani, E., Graham, S., Gibbs, J. B., Oliff, A., and Kohl, N. E. (1994). Farnesyltransferase inhibition causes morphological reversion of *Ras*-transformed cells by a complex mechanism that involves regulation of the actin cytoskeleton. *Mol Cell Biol 14*, 4193–4202.

Purcell, W. T., and Donehower, R. C. (2002). Evolving therapies: Farnesyltransferase inhibitors. *Curr Oncol Rep 4*, 29–36.

Qiu, R. G., Chen, J., McCormick, F., and Symons, M. (1995). A role for Rho in Ras transformation. *Proc Natl Acad Sci USA 92*, 11781–11785.

Rabinovich, G. A., Rubinstein, N., and Fainboim, L. (2002). Unlocking the secrets of galectins: A challenge at the frontier of glyco-immunology. *J Leukocyte Biol 71*, 741–752.

Rees, J. (2002). Complex disease and the new clinical sciences. *Science 296*, 698–700.

Reiss, Y., Goldstein, J. L., Seabra, M. C., Casey, P. J., and Brown, M. S. (1990). Inhibition of purified p21^{ras} farnesyl:protein transferase by Cys-AAX tetrapeptides. *Cell 62*, 81–88.

Rose, W. C., Lee, F. Y., Fairchild, C. R., Lynch, M., Monticello, T., Kramer, R. A., and Manne, V. (2001). Preclinical antitumor activity of BMS-214662, a highly apoptotic and novel farnesyltransferase inhibitor. *Cancer Res 61*, 7507–7517.

Rowell, C. A., Kowalczyk, J. J., Lewis, M. D., and Garcia, A. M. (1997). Direct demonstration of geranylgeranylation and farnesylation of Ki-Ras in vivo. *J Biol Chem 272*, 14093–14097.

Rowinsky, E. K. (2000). The pursuit of optimal outcomes in Cancer therapy in a new age of rationally designed target-based anticancer agents. *Drugs 60*, 1–14.

Sahai, E., Ishizaki, T., Narumiya, S., and Treisman, R. (1999). Transformation mediated by RhoA requires activity of ROCK kinases. *Curr Biol 9*, 136–145.

Schlitzer, M., Winter-Vann, A., and Casey, P. J. (2001). Non-peptidic, non-prenylic inhibitors of the prenyl protein-specific protease Rce1. *Bioorg Med Chem Lett 11*, 425–427.

Sebti, S. M., and Hamilton, A. D. (2000). Farnesyltransferase and geranylgeranyltransferase I inhibitors in cancer therapy: Important mechanistic and bench to bedside issues. *Exp Opin Invest Drugs 9*, 2767–2782.

Sepp-Lorenzino, L., and Rosen, N. (1998). A farnesyl:protein transferase inhibitor induces p21 expression and G1 block in p53 wild type tumor cells. *J Biol Chem 273*, 20243–20251.

Sepp-Lorenzino, L., Ma, Z., Rands, E., Kohl, N. E., Gibbs, J. B., Oliff, A., and Rosen, N. (1995). A peptidomimetic inhibitor of farnesyl:protein transferase blocks the anchorage-dependent and -independent growth of human tumor cell lines. *Cancer Res 55*, 5302–5309.

Shih, T. Y., Papageorge, A. G., Stokes, P. E., Weeks, M. O., and Scolnick, E. M. (1980). Guanine nucleotide-binding and autophosphorylating activities associated with the p21src protein of Harvey murine sarcoma virus. *Nature 287*, 686–691.

Shih, T. Y., Stokes, P. E., Smythers, G. W., Dhar, R., and Oroszlan, S. (1982). Characterization of the phosphorylation sites and the surrounding amino acid sequences of the p21 transforming proteins coded for by the Harvey and Kirsten strains of murine sarcoma viruses. *J Biol Chem 257*, 11767–11773.

Shirasawa, S., Furuse, M., Yokoyama, N., and Sasazuki, T. (1993). Altered growth of human colon cancer cell lines disrupted at activated Ki-Ras. *Science 260*, 85–88.

Sinn, E., Muller, W., Pattengale, P., Tepler, I., Wallace, R., and Leder, P. (1987). Coexpression of MMTV/v-Ha-ras and MMTV/c-myc genes in transgenic mice: Synergistic action of oncogenes in vivo. *Cell 49*, 465–475.

Sun, J., Qian, Y., Hamilton, A. D., and Sebti, S. M. (1995). Ras CAAX peptidomimetic FTI 276 selectively blocks tumor growth in nude mice of a human lung carcinoma with K-Ras mutation and p53 deletion. *Cancer Res 55*, 4243–4247.

Sun, J., Qian, Y., Hamilton, A. D., and Sebti, S. M. (1998). Both farnesyltransferase and geranylgeranyltransferase I inhibitors are required for inhibition of oncogenic K-Ras prenylation but each alone is sufficient to suppress human tumor growth in nude mouse xenografts. *Oncogene 16*, 1467–1473.

Sun, J., Blaskovich, M. A., Knowles, D., Qian, Y., Ohkanda, J., Bailey, R. D., Hamilton, A. D., and Sebti, S. M. (1999). Antitumor efficacy of a novel class of non-thiol-containing peptidomimetic inhibitors of farnesyltransferase and geranylgeranyltransferase I: Combination therapy with the cytotoxic agents cisplatin, Taxol, and gemcitabine. *Cancer Res 59*, 4919–4926.

Suzuki, N., Urano, J., and Tamanoi, F. (1998). Farnesyltransferase inhibitors induce cytochrome c release and caspase 3 activation preferentially in transformed cells. *Proc Natl Acad Sci USA 95*, 15356–15361.

Torrance, C. J., Agrawal, V., Vogelstein, B., and Kinzler, K. W. (2001). Use of isogenic human cancer cells for high-throughput screening and drug discovery. *Nature Biotech 19*, 940–945.

Travers, H., French, N. S., and Norton, J. D. (1996). Suppression of tumorigenicity in Ras-transformed fibroblasts by alpha 2(I) collagen. *Cell Growth Diff 7*, 1353–1360.

Tsuchida, T., Kijima, H., Oshika, Y., Tokunaga, T., Abe, Y., Yamazaki, H., Tamaoki, N., Ueyama, Y., Scanlon, K. J., and Nakamura, M. (1998). Hammerhead ribozyme specifically inhibits mutant K-ras mRNA of human pancreatic cancer cells. *Biochem Biophys Res Commun 253*, 368–373.

Ura, H., Obara, T., Shuda, R., Itoh, A., Tanno, S., Fujii, T., Nishino, N., and Kohgo, Y. (1998). Selective cytotoxicity of farnesylamine to pancreatic carcinoma cells and Ki-ras-transformed fibroblasts. *Mol Carcinogen 21*, 93–99.

van Golen, K. L., Davies, S., Wu, Z. F., Wnag, Y., Bucana, C. D., Root, H., Chandrasekharappa, S., Strawderman, M., Ethier, S. P., and Merajver, S. D. (1999). A novel putative low-affinity insulin-like growth factor–binding protein, LIBC (lost in inflammatory breast cancer), and RhoC GTPase correlate with the inflammatory breast cancer phenotype. *Clin Cancer Res 5*, 2511–2519.

van Golen, K. L., Bao, L. W., DeVito, M. M., Wu, Z.-F., Prendergast, G. C., and Merajver, S. D. (2002). Reversion of RhoC GTPase-induced transformation in inflammatory breast cancer cells by treatment with a farnesyl transferase inhibitor. *Molec Cancer Therapeutics 1*, 575–583.

Weisz, B., Giehl, K., Gana-Weisz, M., Egozi, Y., Ben-Baruch, G., Marciano, D., Gierschik, P., and Kloog, Y. (1999). A new functional Ras antagonist inhibits human pancreatic tumor growth in nude mice. *Oncogene 18*, 2579–2588.

Whyte, D. B., Kirschmeier, P., Hockenberry, T. N., Nunez-Olivia, I., James, L., Catino, J. J., Bishop, W. R., and Pai, J. K. (1997). K- and N-ras geranylgeranylated in cells treated with farnesyl protein transferase inhibitors. *J Biol Chem 272*, 14459–14464.

Williams, T. M., Ciccarone, T. M., MacTough, S. C., Bock, R. L., Conner, M. W., Davide, J. P., Hamilton, K., Koblan, K. S., Kohl, N. E., Kral, A. M., et al. (1996). 2-substituted piperazines as constrained amino acids: Application to the synthesis of potent, non-carboxylic acid inhibitors of farnesyltransferase. *J Med Chem 39*, 1345–1348.

Zeng, P.-Y., Rane, N., Du, W., Chintapalli, J., and Prendergast, G. C. (2003). Role of RhoB and PRK in the suppression of epithelial cell transformation by farnesyltransferase inhibitors. *Oncogene 22*, 1124–1134.

Zhang, F. L., Kirschmeier, P., Carr, D., James, L., Bond, R. W., Wang, L., Patton, R., Windsor, W. T., Syto, R., Zhang, R., and Bishop, W. R. (1997). Characterization of Ha-ras, N-ras, Ki-Ras4A, Ki-Ras4B as in vitro substrates for farnesyl protein transferase and geranylgeranyl protein transferase type I. *J Biol Chem 272*, 10232–10239.

15

CLINOMICS: POSTGENOMIC CANCER CARE

Daniel D. Von Hoff, Haiyong Han, and David Bearss

INTRODUCTION

Clinomics, the application of oncogenomics to cancer care, would appear to be a straightforward application of genomic technologies to help obtain a prognosis for a patient or to select an effective and less toxic regimen for patients. However, as will be seen in this chapter, something that would seem straightforward to bring from the bench to the bedside presents many challenges that begin with access to the patient's tissue. The surgical procedures necessary to obtain tissue for genomics will not be advocated by the physician or accepted by the patient unless there is a clear benefit-to-risk ratio. There are currently several measurements made in the clinic to individualize patient therapy such as measurement of estrogen receptor (ER), progesterone receptor (PgR), HER2/*neu*, CD20, and CD52. Such assays are performed immunohistochemically except in assays of HER2/*neu* gene amplification by FISH to determine whether a patient is a candidate to receive Herceptin. While immunohistochemistry is commonly performed in pathology laboratories, genomic techniques have yet to make their ways into hospital laboratories. Although a genomic technique (i.e., microarray) has been applied to breast, lymphoma, and other types of tumors, these studies have only been retrospective in nature. Ongoing prospective clinical trials are needed to evaluate the utility of genomics in the area of prognostication for patients. As the reader will see,

Oncogenomics: Molecular Approaches to Cancer, Edited by Charles Brenner and David Duggan
ISBN 0-471-22592-4 © 2004 John Wiley & Sons, Inc.

there are already a tremendous number of agents approved that are supposed to attack specific targets. However, there have been surprisingly few attempts to approve new agents against tumors with the specific target of interest. Possible reasons for this are discussed in detail. Our major conclusion is that unless the diagnostic test for likely efficacy is included in the development of the new agent from the beginning of clinical trials, there is little likelihood that it will ever be utilized to determine who should or should not receive the agent. Finally, in the clinical trial arena, to convince clinicians that genomics may provide a better way to treat patients, clinical trials are needed that are difficult to design and implement. Several possibilities for design of clinical trials are offered that could provide convincing evidence. However, we do not feel it is likely that any of these clinical trial designs will be easily conducted except for the "3 versus 1" trial, herein proposed. In summary, we argue that genomics will continue to provide great new targets for development of new therapies. For reasons that we will make clear, it may be difficult for clinical trials to prove rigorously that genotypic selections can improve the likelihood that a patient will benefit from a particular therapy against that target. However, utilizing patterns of gene expression to predict prognosis or response to therapy may be easier for clinicians to adopt as we have endorsed other patterns such as CAT and PET scans.

There is no doubt that oncogenomics will some day have a tremendous impact on the way we practice the medicine of oncology. However, before clinicians adopt genomics to give prognoses to patients, to design treatment regimens for patients, or to help in any of the aspects of caring for patients, there are many challenges to face and many steps to take. To signify those challenges and issues, we have coined the term *clinomics*, meaning application of genomics to patient care. The critical issues of clinomics, addressed in this chapter, are listed in Box 15-1.

CURRENT PRACTICE OF INDIVIDUALIZING THERAPIES

Over the years there have been a large number of attempts to individualize patients' therapies using a variety of techniques. Some of these techniques were introduced and are now obsolete, but several are being utilized on a daily basis. Table 15-1 outlines certain targets, the therapeutics used to hit those targets, and the techniques used to detect those targets. As can be seen in Table 15-1, there are several ways in which we are already individualizing therapies. The principal tool is immunohistochemistry, though fluorescent in situ hybridization (FISH) is used to detect amplification of HER2/*neu*. This technique appears preferable to immunohistochemistry techniques, although it is still a matter of continuous debate and controversy (Vogel et al., 2002). For a few types of tumors in which there are target-directed therapies, clinicians in academic medical centers can advocate testing the patient's tumor prior to the onset of therapy (see Table 15-1). The testing is usually done on the original diagnostic material that remains embedded in paraffin. Newly obtained tumor specimens are not used, because at the time of presentation with metastatic disease, it is often difficult to secure large quantities of tumor sample.

It is of major interest that even with a positive result on immunohistochemistry, the likelihood that a patient will respond to the targeted therapy is really quite low, e.g., from 11–14% for HER2/*neu*-positive patients responding to Herceptin to a high of 67% of patients whose tumors are ER+ responding to hormonal therapies such as tamoxifen.

- How clinicians are already individualizing therapies using currently available tools

- How clinicians are already determining prognoses for patients but still need more definitive data

- Attempts at individualizing therapies and prognoses (not yet adopted by the oncology community)

- Therapeutics already available to hit specific targets should clinicians choose to test such targets

- Challenges in acquiring tumors from patients to perform genomic measurements and possible methods of bypassing those challenges

- Examples of specific clinical trial situations and designs that would help convince clinical oncologists and regulatory bodies that genomics could lead to a way to approve new agents not based on tumor histology but rather on tumor genotype

Box 15-1.

TABLE 15-1. Current Examples of Individualized Patient Therapy

Target	Therapeutics Against the Target	Technique(s) Used to Assay for the Target	References
Estrogen receptor	Tamoxifen, toremifene, megace, aromatase inhibitors	Largely immunohisto-chemistry; occasional biochemical or radioimmunoassay	Osborne, 1998
Progesterone receptor	Same as above	Same as above	Osborne, 1998 Ravdin et al., 1992
CD20	(Rituxan), Rituximab; (Zevalin) radiolabeled ibritumomab	Immunohistochemistry, with or without flow cytometry	McLaughlin et al., 1998
CD52	(Campath) Alemtuzumab	Same as above	Keating et al., 2002
HER2neu	(Herceptin) Trastuzumab	Immunohistochemistry; fluorescent in situ hybridization (FISH)	Pegram et al., 1998
C117 (c-kit)	(Gleevec) Imatinib mesylate	Immunohistochemistry	Demetri, et al., 2002
CD33	(Mylotarg) Gemtuzumab ozogamicin	Immunohistochemistry	Voutsadakis, 2002 Bross, et al., 2001

These relatively low response rates even with highly positive targets are obvious clues that the strategy of targeting therapies, as practiced in 2003, is not a panacea.

CURRENT PRACTICE OF DETERMINING PATIENT PROGNOSIS

The most important tools that clinicians currently have to determine a patient's prognosis are, of course, staging of the patient's tumor (e.g., degree of spread), degree of differentiation for some types of tumors, and other scales such as depth of invasion of the primary tumor (e.g., in melanoma). ER, PgR, and HER2/*neu* have all been employed to predict whether a patient would respond well (ER+ or PgR+) or not respond well (ER−, PgR−, or HER2/*neu* positive) to treatments (Elledge et al., 1992; Fisher et al., 1988). As discussed in Chapter 5, there has been some tantalizing information reported on several types of malignancies in which microarray information has led to placing patients in unfavorable or favorable prognostic categories (Table 15-2). All of these studies have created a great deal of excitement in the oncology community. This is largely because the genomics information provided by the microarray approach is generating *patterns* of information rather than looking at only individual genes (e.g., Her2/*neu*). This makes sense to physicians who are accustomed to patterns of information in most of their diagnostic tests (e.g., CAT scans, PET scans, bone scans, etc.). Unfortunately, to date, all of these studies have been done retrospectively. In general, data on clinical correlations with preclinical work are not accepted as the standard of care unless clinical trials are done prospectively.

TABLE 15-2. Studies Utilizing Genomics for Prognostication

Tumor Type	Findings	References
Breast	There is a gene expression pattern (profile) that predicts a short interval to distant metastases. The gene expression pattern outperforms all currently used clinical parameters for predicting disease outcome.	Van't Veer, et al., 2002
Diffuse large B-cell lymphoma	Diffuse large B-cell lymphoma placed in more aggressive and in less aggressive categories.	Alizadeh et al., 2000
Breast (hereditary)	Heritable mutations influence gene expression profiles.	Hedenfalk et al., 2001
Melanoma	Molecular classification defines a different subset of melanoma.	Bittner et al., 2000
Alveolar rhabdomyosarcoma	Ability to classify small round-cell tumors.	Khan et al., 1998
Acute leukemia	Ability to distinguish between AML and ALL.	Golub et al., 1999
Diffuse B cell lymphoma	Gene expression profiles predict survival after chemotherapy.	Rosenwald et al., 2002

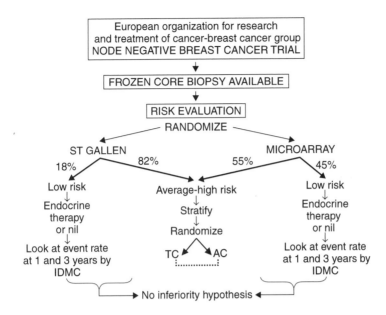

Figure 15-1. The use of microarray for predicting patient prognosis: a prospective clinical trial study design.

Fortunately, the European Organization for Research and Treatment of Cancer is performing a prospective clinical trial on the use of microarray for predicting patient prognosis. It is very important that several more prospective studies, outlined in Figure 15-1, are done to determine the real role of genomics in prognostication for individual patients.

PAST ATTEMPTS AT INDIVIDUALIZING THERAPIES

A major concern for some investigators hoping to apply genomics to selecting the most appropriate therapy for individual patients with cancer is the history of a previously developed system widely known as a human tumor cloning assay (HTCA; Salmon and Hamburger, 1978; Hamburger and Salmon, 1977). The system was widely studied and used to select the most appropriate chemotherapy for an individual patient. A patient's tumor was biopsied and the tumor cells were exposed to various concentrations of possible therapeutic agents. The cells were then plated in soft agar. After 14 days, colonies in drug-treated and non-drug-treated plates were counted. The patients were then treated with the drug or drugs that decreased the colony formation by $\geq 50\%$.

There were thousands of patients' tumor specimens collected and tested in this system. The percent true negatives for these assays were between 84% and 96% (i.e., the assay correctly indicates an agent would not work) while the percent true positives (i.e., the assay correctly indicates an agent would work) were between 67% and 80%. (Von Hoff, 1990). This is as reliable as other assays used in oncology (e.g., estrogen receptor assays) or microbiology (e.g., disc sensitivity techniques). However, there were very few prospective clinical trials of the cloning assay and other predictive assays performed (Von Hoff, 1990). One prospective randomized clinical trial of the human tumor cloning assay was conducted in patients who had progressed despite all prior therapies. The patient's therapy was chosen based on the HTCA versus the clinician's selection. The study clearly demonstrated that the HTCA gave an increase in response rate but no improvement in survival (Von Hoff et al., 1990).

It is of interest that the HTCA and other in vitro predictive assays such as the extreme drug resistance (EDR) assay (Kern and Weisenthal, 1990) were never completely adopted (although EDR is offered commercially). The reasons include the following:

- There was never a high enough number of tumor cells available to test the number of agents that researchers wanted to test (testing multiple agents increased the likelihood of finding one that worked).
- Not all patients could have a biopsy of their tumor. Some patients and their physicians were also not willing to risk the procedure, as results could be mortal.
- Over 40% of the assay results were unsuitable for evaluation (not enough growth of colonies in the assay, tumor cells not viable, etc.). This is in contrast to techniques such as EDR where results are approximately 90% suitable for evaluation (Orr et al., 1999).
- For the most part, only single agents were tested in vitro and physicians were reluctant to treat the patient with single agents.

Dwelling on the history of a seemingly antiquated technique such as HTCA would not seem imperative given the excitement over new genomic methods. However, it is important to remember some of the shortcomings of those prior in vitro assays because there are many concerns that the same issues may arise as we attempt to apply genomic methods to the selection of therapies for individual patients.

AVAILABLE TARGET-DIRECTED THERAPEUTICS

Table 15-3 provides a list of the targets that can currently be measured in patients' tumors and the available therapeutic agents that hit those targets. Despite knowing the targets for these agents, the target is rarely assayed in patients' specimens. There are likely several reasons, including the following:

- Patients and physicians are reluctant to rebiopsy the patient because biopsies carry risks of discomfort and occasionally death.
- There have been no prospective trials for the majority of these agents (even Herceptin) that test the agent in separate individuals whose tumors do and do not overexpress or possess the target.
- Retrospective studies to compare presence of target versus response to therapies are difficult because of informed consent issues (e.g., researchers cannot retrospectively correlate results without patient consent if patient identifiers are used).
- Given the limited options for cancer care, physicians and patients will try an agent if it is considered that the tumor *might* possess the target.

TABLE 15-3. Standard Agents Available Clinically or Soon to Be Available Designed to Hit Specific Targets

Target	Agent(s)
Estrogen receptor	Tamoxifen (Novaldex), toremifene (Fareston), aromatase inhibitors: anastrozole (Armidex), exemestane (Aromasin), letrozole (Femara)
HER2/*neu*	Trastuzumab (Herceptin)
CD20	Rituxamab (Rituxan), radiolabeled ibritumomab (tiuxetan, Zevalin)
CD52	Alemtuzumab (Campath)
Progesterone receptors	Megestrol acetate (Megace)
Androgen receptor	Bicalutamide (Casodex), flutamide (Eulexin)
Asparagine synthase (low levels cause sensitivity)	l-asparaginase (Elspar), pegaspargase (Oncaspar)
Thymidylate synthase (low levels cause sensitivity)	5-fluorouracil
Dihydrofolate reductase (low levels cause sensitivity)	Methotrexate
GAR transformylase	Pemetrexed, LY231514 (Alimta)
Mismatch repair of abnormal cells	Gemcitabine, LY188011 (Gemzar)
Thymidine phosphorylase (high levels cause activation of the agent)	Capecitabine (Xeloda)
CD117	Imatinib mesylate, STI 571 (Gleevec)
Adenosine deaminase	Pentostatin sodium (Nipent), cladribine (Leustatin)
Somatostatin receptor	Octreotide (Sandostatin; Sandostatin LAR Depot)
Topoisomerase I	Irinotecan, CPT-11 (Camptosar), topotecan (Hycamptin)
Topoisomerase II	Etoposide (VePesid)
RAR	All-trans-retinoic acid: tretinoin (Vesanoid)
COX-2	Celecoxib (Celebrex)
DNA polymerase	Cytosine arabinoside, ara-c (Cytosar)
RXR	Bexarotene (Targretin)
IL2 receptor	IL-2
Ribonucleotide reductase	Hydroxyurea (Hydrea), gemcitabine, (Gemzar)

An excellent example of how genomic information might be used is with the agent capecitabine. Capecitabine has been found empirically to have clinical activity against pancreatic cancer, and is approved for treating patients with breast cancer and colorectal cancer. (O'Shaughnessy et al., 2002; Van Cutsem et al., 2001; Cartwright et al., 2002). As noted in Figure 15-2, capecitabine is initially activated by the enzyme thymidine phosphorylase, which is upregulated in certain tumors (particularly liver metastases from GI cancer; Schüller et al., 1997, 2002). The response rate to capecitabine is very low when devoid of prior measurement of thymidine phosphorylase protein expression in an individual patient's tumor: 15% in patients with refractory breast cancer, 12% in patients with primary untreated colorectal cancer, and 2% in patients with previously

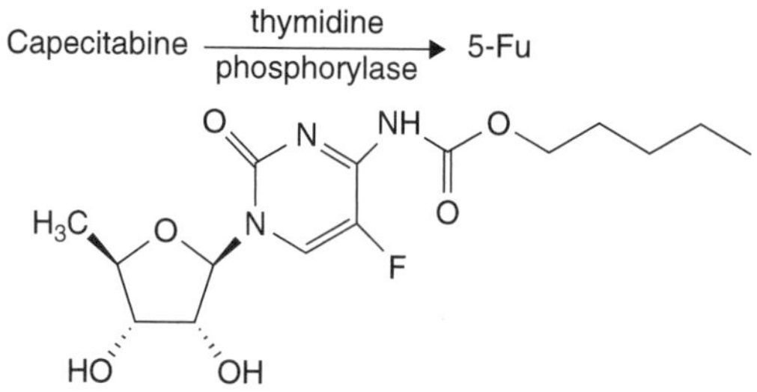

Figure 15-2. Activation of capecitabine by thymidine phosphorylase.

TABLE 15-4. New Agents and Their Targets in Clinical Development

Agent	Target	Sponsor
SAHA	Histone deacetylase	Aton
PX-12	Thioredoxin reductase	ProLx
2C4	HER2/*neu*	Genentech
AG2037	GAR transformylase	Pfizer
HMN214	Polo kinase	Nippon Shinyaku/IDEC
Brostallicin	GST (activated by)	Pharmacia
ABT 510	Thrombospondin mimetic	Abbott
NM-3	VEGF inhibitor	Ilex
NB1011	TS agent (activated by)	NewBiotics
SGN-15	cBR96 doxorubicin immunoconjugate	Seattle Genetics
TLK286	GST (activated by)	Telik
G17DT	Gastrin	Aphton
Ab EGFR	EGFR	Abgenix
Alanosine	MTAP-deficient tumors	Salmedix
Aplidine	Palmityl thioesterase	PharmaMar
CEP751	NGF/TRK A	Cephalon
CEP701	NGF/TRK A	Cephalon
AGN195183	RAR antagonist	Allergan
Ab TRAIL 1&2	TRAIL	Hum Genome
C1033	EGFR	Pfizer
G3139	Bcl-2	Genta
HIF inhibitor	HIFα	ProLx
Oncophage	HSP-vaccine	Antigenics
Apomine	FXR interactive	Ilex
SKB40875	Maytansine Mo Ab conjugate	GSK
MB-8	Methylase	MethyGene/MGI
LY293111 (MEPM)	Leukotriene B4 antagonist	Lilly
Velcade	Proteosome	Millennium
CI779	mTDR	Am Home Prod
ISIS3521	Protein kinase C	ISIS
Flavopiridol	Cyclin D1	Aventis

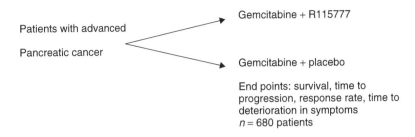

Figure 15-3. Design for a randomized trial of a farnesyltransferase inhibitor in patients with advanced pancreatic cancer.

treated pancreatic cancer. It would seem unproblematic to do a clinical trial to determine whether there is merit to treating only those patients whose tumors have upregulated thymidine phosphorylase activity; however, it has not yet been prospectively tested in the clinic.

There are almost certainly some important lessons here. Despite having a major hypothesis as to why a patient's tumor may or may not respond to a particular anticancer agent, these hypotheses are seldom tested. Perhaps this is because the assays to measure targets are not widely available, the patients have no additional options, individuals are troubled by negative results, or there is no support available to conduct a prospective trial of the hypothesis. A funding agency may specify that the sponsor should conduct the trial. The sponsor, however, might not necessarily want to know the responses to an agent, since it may decrease the number of patient recipients. Essentially, unless a diagnostic marker for response or lack of response is placed in the beginning of development of the agent (as was the case for Herceptin), it is extremely unlikely that one will ever be utilized.

Table 15-4 lists some of the new agents, currently in development. As can be seen in this table, there are multiple new agents with many new mechanisms of action, yet most are not being developed on a genotype-specific basis. The recent news of the negative result of a farnesyltransferase inhibitor for patients with advanced pancreatic cancer may offer an explanation. Figure 15-3 details the design of a prospective clinical trial of the farnesyltransferase inhibitor R115777 designed to hit tumor cells with mutated *ras* in phase I clinical trials (Patnaik, et al., 2000). Despite the fact that mutated *ras* is found in the vast majority of patients with pancreatic cancer, the trial outlined in Figure 15-3 showed no difference in survival, time to tumor progression, response rate, or time to deterioration in symptoms (Van Cutsem, et al., 2002). Why did R115777 fail? First, as we learned in Chapter 14, the mechanism of action of FTIs is more complicated than we initially thought. Second, the patients' mutation status of *ras* was not known or used as a criterion for study entry. Nonetheless, the negative conclusion of such a large study conducted on a well-studied genomic target is discouraging.

THE CHALLENGE OF OBTAINING A TUMOR SAMPLE

While it may seem simplistic to obtain a tumor sample from patients with widely metastatic cancer, it turns out that this is a formidable challenge. Obviously, to make an initial diagnosis, oncologists have to be aggressive, even if it takes major surgery, to determine whether the patient has cancer and to ascertain the histology. Usually, biopsy yields a reasonable sample on which to perform histological as well as genomic studies. Currently, most of the tissue is immediately preserved by dropping it in formalyn with portions of interest embedded in paraffin. An exception is breast cancer specimens, which are sometimes frozen in liquid nitrogen to allow for determination of estrogen receptor status via a biochemical assay.

Estrogen and progesterone receptor studies are now routinely determined by immuno-histochemistry such that tumors are now frozen in liquid nitrogen only for determination of percent S-phase cells by flow cytometry. Essentially, all other tissues harvested at surgery are placed in formalyn with only selected portions put into paraffin. As discussed in Chapter 8 on tissue microanalysis, this type of fixation is generally incompatible for analysis of nucleic acids or proteins, except for immunohistochemistry. Thus, necessary changes may include technique-specific collection of tumor samples or adaptations of genomics techniques to specimens retrieved from paraffin. The latter approach would also be useful for retrieving archival specimens (in which a clinical history has already been documented) to investigate correlations with prognosis, response to treatment, etc. Unfortunately, there are very few fully annotated, archived specimen banks available at this time.

A major challenge for collecting tissues for genomic studies is that currently there is such a necessity to be invasive for cancer diagnosis. Two advances are allowing for less invasive diagnostics: (1) spiral CT scanning and PET scans, which allow for biopsies in more accessible areas; and (2) thin needles coupled with CT guidance to obtain enough material for a diagnosis (see Fig. 15-4).

However, the relatively few tumor cells (usually $<10^5$) obtained with a needle biopsy present problems for genomic-proteomic assays because the pathologist needs to look at a certain number of slides. Obviously, the amplification steps involved in immunological and nucleic acid–based assays will need further enhancements in order to molecularly diagnose a variety of markers simultaneously. According to Chapter 8, microanalysis techniques and fixation in 70% ethanol are making strides toward successful profiling of limited patient samples.

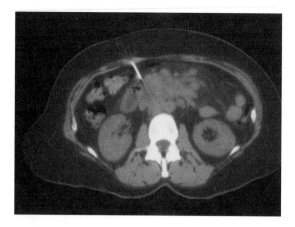

Figure 15-4. Skinny needle with CT scan guidance. Notice the needle going directly into the pancreas.

There are some major ongoing efforts to try to optimize needle biopsies so that tumor cells might be obtained threefold above the now possible 10% of patients on a clinical trial. A group at Case Western Reserve has devised a technique that appears to be safer than conventional needle biopsy methods, which can result in a collapsed lung in a lesion biopsied in the lung or can cause severe bleeding if the liver is biopsied. Dowlati and colleagues at Case Western utilized a technique whereby they injected matrigel (a collagen gel) to seal the biopsy areas (Dowlati et al., 2001) following needle biopsy of the tumor cells.

There are multiple investigators working on a less complicated way to obtain tumor cells from patients: acquiring circulating tumor cells. At least two techniques are being used to collect the circulating tumor cells. The first technique, termed *onco-pheresis* (see Fig. 15-5), is performed via leukopheresis on a patient (a cell separation technique using 12-gauge needles whereby the patient's blood is circulated through a machine that can be programmed to collect mononuclear cells). To separate the circulating tumor cells from normal cells, the cells are treated with keratin 8, 18, and 19 antibodies that are bound to magnetic beads. The bound and unbound beads are then passed through a magnet to collect the mononuclear cells (Krüger et al., 2000).

Other investigators are utilizing about 40 cc of peripheral blood and performing similar cell separation techniques to pull out the mononuclear "tumor" cells. Once again, however, the yield of this technique is rather meager (about 100–1000 cells). Our team has demonstrated that these cells can easily be displayed via laser scanning techniques. As described in Chapter 8, cells on the laser scanner can easily be utilized for immunohistochemistry studies. However, there are so few cells that amplification would be required to perform any genomic studies. As described in Chapter 5, amplification is common in microarray analysis. In proteomic analysis, as described in Chapter 9, when antibodies are available, 2D-PAGE Western analysis can be done for limited numbers of samples. Thus, we may be able to screen for particular

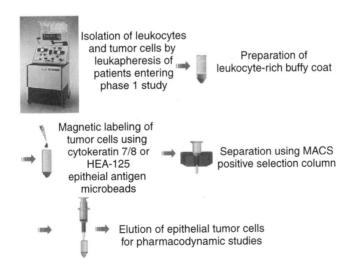

Figure 15-5. Isolation of circulating tumor cells from patients' blood using leukopheresis and magnetic bead positive selection.

biomarkers but we probably cannot screen for global protein patterns unencumbered by hypothesis.

Another major question is whether the circulating tumor cells are representative of all of the cells in the primary or metastatic tumor compartments. Some investigators feel that these shed cells may not be representative and may be more apoptotic than an aggressive cell population.

At present, it seems that the best way to obtain tumor cells from a patient for genomic studies is to obtain a large biopsy. However, before this can be done routinely (e.g., for a clinician to recommend this level of aggressiveness), there will have to be some evidence that such an aggressive procedure would actually lead to an improvement in treatment for the patient or would help avoid giving the patient ineffective and/or toxic therapies. A randomized trial (as is outlined below) is needed to build confidence as to whether genomics can be of help to an individual patient.

CLINICAL TRIAL DESIGNS REGARDING THE USE OF GENOMICS TO INDIVIDUALIZE PATIENT THERAPIES

Figure 15-6 details a clinical trial design that has the potential to convince most oncologists of the value of genomics. If a patient is going to undergo an aggressive biopsy procedure, he or she would subsequently expect to receive the agent that the genomic study predicts will be successful rather than the standard of care. To help with patient accrual, the study has a 2-to-1 randomization so that patients have twice the chance for receiving a selection of an agent based on genomic information. We are proposing time-to-tumor progression as an end point for the study. If patients in either arm of the study are doing better than patients in the other arm, crossover could be allowed to the other method of choosing an agent. Superior data would be obtained if survival were the primary end point without allowing for crossover. An alternative end point would be response rate (e.g., the percentage of patients who have shrinkage of their tumors). The trial design in Figure 15-6 is solid, but it is a design that would make it difficult to recruit patients.

An alternative randomized trial design is outlined in Figure 15-7. We call it the "3 vs. 1" trial design. In this design, the patient has an equal chance of receiving three (one plus two additional) agents selected by a genomics method versus one agent selected by a genomics method. Because both arms of the trial receive the best available agent, we believe that such a design will increase patient and physician participation. It still leaves the fundamental question unanswered as to whether aggressive biopsy can be justified for targeted therapy, but it does answer the question of whether more

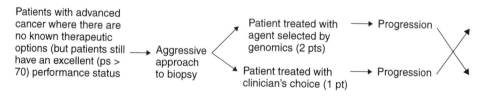

Figure 15-6. A potentially convincing genomics clinical trial into which recruitment would be difficult.

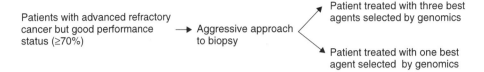

Figure 15-7. The "3 vs. 1" clinical trial method.

targets (and therapies) selected by genomics provide a benefit versus one target (and one therapy) selected by genomics. Obviously, the interaction of drugs (and patients) is a complicated matter such that successes and failures in 3 vs. 1 trials will be drug specific. However, if a best available agent leaves room for improvement, such trials may do much to validate additional target-directed strategies.

A final trial design is inspired by a patient with pancreatic cancer who had a remarkable response to the new and durable DNA interactive agent, irofulvene (Eckhardt et al., 2000). Unfortunately, in a follow-up phase II study, there were only two responses (an overall 4% response rate; Von Hoff et al., 2000). What distinguished the responders versus the nonresponders is unknown, but there have been clues from preclinical studies that tumors that have a defect in the nucleotide excision repair gene, ERCC3, are more sensitive to irofulvene (Kelner et al. 1994, 1995). Based on that finding, Dr. Raymond Nagle at the Arizona Cancer Center has worked to develop an antibody against ERCC3 and tested it against 11 pancreatic cancer cell lines (with 3 having ERCC3 deficiencies by Western blotting) as well as 38 pancreatic cancers taken directly from patients. As shown in Figure 15-8, 7 of the 38 tumors demonstrated a lack of this repair enzyme by immunohistochemistry. This finding inspires a final trial design in which genotype can be utilized as shown in Figure 15-9.

In the above trial design, patients with advanced pancreatic cancer, all of whom have the deletion/mutation in ERCC3, receive treatment with irofulvene. We already

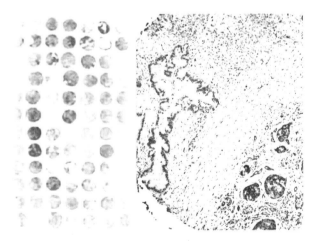

Figure 15-8. ERCC immunohistochemistry. A tissue array of tumors taken directly from patients. Higher magnification shows islet cells positive for ERCC3, which serves as a nice internal control for positivity of normal cells versus negativity of pancreatic cancer cells. See insert for color representation of this figure.

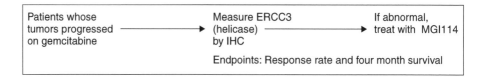

Figure 15-9. Proposed study to test the hypothesis that patients whose tumors have abnormalities in ERCC3 will be sensitive to Irofulvene.

know that in an unselected population the response rate is 4% with a 6-month survival of 15%. In the trial design in Figure 15-9, we are expecting a response rate considerably higher than that. The sample size for this trial is relatively small (35 patients to document a response rate of 50% ± 20% and a 6-month survival of 30% ± 10%). If the response goal is met, this trial would clearly document whether the measurement of deletions or mutations of ERCC3 will improve a patient's chance for response. We believe this type of trial design could be convincing to fellow clinicians that genotyping can participate in a greater patient response rate and survival. The trial design could also be quickly adopted for other agents that have intrinsically low response rates and inherent toxicities.

The astute reader will note that these trials are easier when they are hypothesis-based with respect to the target population because the genotyping does not have to be done on a truly genomic scale. If we lacked a hypothesis regarding the target genotype and had to score thousands of genes or proteins by microarray or proteomic methods, we would need a great deal more tissue and have to justify larger biopsies for treatments that have overall low response rates. Thus, the pure discovery aspects of genomics—that basic scientists can uncover new mechanisms without a preexisting hypothesis in genome-wide studies—do not translate directly to the clinic in prospective studies. We are strongly in agreement with the arguments in Chapter 1 that clinical studies must be firmly based on all preclinical information. We can and must burn money on assays and low-probability experiments at every stage up to the clinic, but we can never treat patients or patient materials as commodities.

USES OF GENOMICS IN DRUG DEVELOPMENT

Whereas prospective trials involving large amounts of primary biopsy material may be difficult to conduct, it is clear from all of the preceding chapters that genomic studies have a major role in identifying cancer genes and targets, classifying different types of disease, and performing mechanistic studies on the nature of different neoplastic diseases. In our own work on pancreatic cancer, we have used microarrays to identify genes that are overexpressed in pancreatic cancer cell lines versus normal pancreas (Han et al., 2002). As explained in Chapter 1 and elsewhere, those enzymes that are upregulated are considered candidate drug targets for genotype (or expression-phenotype)-specific elimination. However, targeting tumor cells with deleted/mutated genes is a more difficult, less "drug-able" situation. We believe this is where genomics may have the greatest appeal to drug developers and clinicians—i.e., what to do for patients with a deleted/mutated gene. It is very difficult to replace the function of a deleted/mutated gene, although there are several ongoing attempts (e.g., gene therapy studies) to do so.

As discussed by Hartwell, Friend, and their co-workers (Hartwell et al., 1997; Friend and Oliff, 1998) and in Chapters 10 an appealing approach to find targets for tumors with missing genetic information is to utilize a synthetic lethal screen in a model organism. If a second mutation is identified that renders a first cancer-associated mutation to be lethal, then the protein product of the second gene would be considered a candidate drug target to kill that cancer genotype. Additionally, as discussed in Chapter 12, modifier screens in mice can potentially identify targets that would reduce cancer incidence if inhibited.

THE FUTURE OF CLINOMICS

One of the things that will become clear in future years is to what degree particular oncogenomic markers dominate a tumor's or a patient's responses to therapy. If it could be shown that the levels of only five different gene products determined which protocol a patient should be put on, the tissue needs for such assays would eliminate the invasive biopsy problem. For some types of agents and tumors, this may be true, such that patients can get the full benefit of genotype-specific treatments without the amount of tissue, cost, and technology of genome-wide analyses. For other types of tumors and agents, a handful of markers will not suffice and we may need microarray or proteomic studies to provide more extensive patterns of up- and downregulated genes to rule in or rule out particular treatments. Prospectively designed trials (like the ongoing EORTC trial) will be essential to convince clinicians of the value of these approaches. In summary, the use of genomics for patient care presents substantial challenges to both basic scientists and clinical investigators. A large amount of additional work is needed to accelerate the move of genomics to improve patient care.

REFERENCES

Alizadeh, A. A., Eosem, N., David, R. E., Ma, C., Lossos, I. S., Rosenwald, A., et al. (2000). Distinct types of diffuse large B-cell lymphoma identified by gene expression profiling. *Nature 403*, 503–511.

Bittner, M., Meltzer, P., Chen, Y., Jiang, Y., Seftor, E., Hendrix, M., et al. (2000). Molecular classification of cutaneous malignant melanoma by gene expression profiling. *Nature 406*, 536–540.

Bross, P. F., Beitz, J., Chen, G., Chen, X. H., Duffy, E., Kieffer, L., et al. (2001). Approval summary: Gemtuzumab Ozogamicin in relapsed acute myeloid leukemia. *Clin Cancer 7*, 1490–1496.

Cartwright, T. H., Cohn, A., Varkey, J. A., Chen, Y.-M., Szaltrowski, T. P., Cox, J. V., et al. (2002). Phase II study of oral capecitabine in patients with advanced or metastatic pancreatic cancer. *J Clin Oncol 20* (1), 160–164.

Demetri, G., Von Mehren, M., Blanke, C. D., Van Den Abbeele, A. D., Eisenberg, B., Roberts, P. J., et al. (2002). Efficacy and safety of imatinib mesylate in advanced gastrointestinal stromal tumors. *N Engl J Med 347* (7), 472–480.

Dowlati, A., Haaga, J., Remick, S. C., Spiro, T. P., Gerson, S. L., Liu, L., et al. (2001). Sequential tumor biopsies in early phase clinical trials of anticancer agents for pharmacodynamic evaluation. *Clin Cancer Res 7*, 2971–2976.

Eckhardt, S. G., Baker, S. D., Britten, C. D., Hidalgo, M., Siu, L., Hammond, L. A., et al. (2000). Phase I and pharmacokinetic study of irofulven, a novel mushroom-derived cytotoxin, administered for five consecutive days every four weeks in patients with advanced solid malignancies. *J Clin Oncol 18* (24), 4086–4097.

Elledge, R. M., McGuire, W. L., and Osborne, C. K. (1992). Prognostic factors in breast cancer. *Semin Oncol 19*, 244–253.

Fisher, B., Redmond, C., Fisher, E., and Caplan, R. (1988). Relative work of estrogen or progesterone receptors and pathologic characteristics of differentiation as indicators of prognosis in node negative breast cancer patients: Findings from National Surgical Adjuvant Breast and Bowel Protocol B-06. *J Clin Oncol 6* (7), 1076–1087.

Friend, S. H., and Oliff, A. (1998). Emerging uses for genomic information in drug discovery. *N Engl J Med 338* (2), 125–126.

Golub, T., Sionim, D., Tamayo, P., Huard, C., Gaasenbeek, M., Mesirov, J. P., et al. (1999). Molecular classification of cancer: Class discovery and class prediction by gene expression monitoring. *Science 286*, 531–537.

Hamburger, A. W., and Salmon, S. E. (1977). Primary bioassay of human tumor stem cells. *Science 197*, 461–463.

Han, H., Bearss, D. J., Browne, L. W., Calaluce, R., Nagle, R. B., and Von Hoff, D. D. (2002). Identification of differentially expressed genes in pancreatic cancer cells using cDNA microarray. [Erratum appears in *Cancer Res* (2002) Aug. *62* (15), 4532]. *Cancer Res 62* (10), 2890–2896.

Hartwell, L. H., Szankasi, P., Roberts, C. J., Murray, A. W., and Friend, S. H. (1997). Integrating genetic approaches into the discovery of anticancer drugs. *Science 278*, 1064–1068.

Hedenfalk, I., Duggan, D., Chen, Y., Radmacher, M., Bittner, M., Simon, R., et al. (2001). Gene-expression profiles in hereditary breast cancer. *N Engl J Med 344* (8), 539–548.

Keating, M. J., Flinn, I., Jain, V., Binet, J. L., Hillmen, P., Byrd, J., et al. (2002). Therapeutic role of alemtuzumab (Campath-1H) in patients who have failed fludarabine: Results of a large international study. *Blood 99*, 3554–3661.

Kelner, M. J., McMorris, T. C., Estes, L., Rutherford, M., Montoya, M., Goldstein, J., et al. (1994). Characterization of illudin S sensitivity in DNA repair–deficient Chinese hamster cells. Unusually high sensitivity of ERCC2 and ERCC3 DNA helicase-deficient mutants in comparison to other chemotherapeutic agents. *Biochem Pharmacol 48* (2), 403–409.

Kelner, M. J., McMorris, T. C., Estes, L., Starr, R. J., Rutherford, M., Montoya, M., et al. (1995). Efficacy of acylfulvene illudin analogues against a metastatic lung carcinoma MV522 xenograft nonresponsive to traditional anticancer agents: Retention of activity against various mdr phenotypes and unusual cytotoxicity against ERCC2 and ERCC3 DNA helicase-deficient cells. *Cancer Res 55* (21), 4936–4940.

Kern, D. H., and Weisenthal, L. M. (1990). Highly specific prediction of antineoplastic drug resistance with an in vitro assay using suprapharmacologic drug exposures. *J Natl Cancer Inst 82* (7), 582–588.

Khan, J., Simon, R., Bittner, M., Chen, Y., Leighton, S. B., Pohida, T., et al. (1998). Gene expression profiling of alveolar rhabdomyosarcoma with cDNA microarrays. *Cancer Res 58* (22), 5009–5013.

Kruger, W., Datta, C., Badbaran, A., Togel, F., Gutensohn, K., Carrero, I., et al. (2000). Immuno-magnetic tumor cell selection—implications for the detection of disseminated cancer cells. *Transfusion 40* (12), 1489–1493.

McLaughlin, P., Grillo-Lopez, A. J., Link, B. K., Levy, R., Czuczman, M. S., Williams, M. E., et al. (1998). Rituximab chimeric anti-CD20 monoclonal antibody therapy for relapsed indolent lymphoma: Half of patients respond to a four-dose treatment program. *J Clin Oncol 16*, 2825–2833.

Orr, J. W., Jr., Orr, P., and Kern, D. H. (1999). Cost-effective treatment of women with advanced ovarian cancer by cytoreductive surgery and chemotherapy directed by an in vitro assay for drug resistance. *Cancer J Sci Am 5* (3), 174–178.

Osborne, C. K. (1998). Steroid hormone receptors in breast cancer management. *Breast Cancer Res Treat 51* (3), 227–238.

O'Shaughnessy, J., Miles, D., Vukelja, S., Moiseyenko, V., Ayoub, J. -P., Cervantes, G., et al. (2002). Superior survival with capecitabine plus docetaxel combination therapy in anthracycline-pretreated patients with advanced breast cancer: Phase III trial results. *J Clin Oncol 20*, 2812–2823.

Patnaik, A., Eckhardt, S. G., Izbicka, E., Rybak, M., McCreery, H., Davidson, K., et al. (2000). Administration of biologically and clinically relevant doses of the farnesyl transferase inhibitor R115777 and gemcitabine are feasible without pharmacokinetic (PK) interactions: A phase I and PK study *(Proceedings of the 11th NCI-EORTC Symposium on New Drugs in Cancer Therapy). Clin Cancer Res 6* (supplement), 4517S. Abstract 255.

Pegram, M. D., Pauletti, G., and Slamon, D. J. (1998). Her-2/neu as a predictive marker of response to breast cancer therapy. *Breast Cancer Res Treat 52* (1–3), 65–77.

Ravdin, P. M., Green, S., Dorr, T. M., McGuire, W. L., Fabian, C., Pugh, R. P., et al. (1992). Prognostic significance of progesterone receptor levels in estrogen receptor–positive patients with metastatic breast cancer treated with tamoxifen: Results of a prospective Southwest Oncology Group study. *J Clin Oncol 10*, 1284–1291.

Rosenwald, A., Wright, G., Chan, W. C., Connors, J. M., Campo, E., Fisher, R. I., et al. (2002). The use of molecular profiling to predict survival after chemotherapy for diffuse large-B-cell lymphoma. *N Engl J Med 346* (25), 1937–1947.

Salmon, S. E, and Hamburger, A. W. (1978). Quantitation of differential sensitivity of human tumor stem cells to anticancer drugs. *N Engl J Med 298*, 1321–1327.

Schüller, J., Cassidy, J., Reigner, B. G., Durston, S., Roos, B., Ishitsuka, H., et al. (1997). Tumor selectivity of Xeloda™ in colorectal cancer patients. *Proc Annu Meet Am Soc Clin Oncol 16*, 227a. Abstract 797.

Schüller, J., Cassodu, K., Dumont, E., Roos, B., Durston, S., Banken, L., et al. (2000). Preferential activation of capecitabine in tumor following oral administration to colorectal cancer patients. *Cancer Chemother Pharmacol 45* (4), 291–297.

Van Cutsem, E., Twelves, C., Cassidy, J., Allman, D., Bajetta, E., Boyer, M., Bugat, R., et al. (2001). Oral capecitabine compared with intravenous fluorouracil plus leucovorin in patients with metastatic colorectal cancer: Results of a large phase III study. *J Clin Oncol 19* (21), 4097–4106.

Van Cutsem, E., Karasek, P., Oettle, H., Vervenne, W., Azawlowski, P., Schoffski, P., et al. (2002). Phase III trial comparing gemcitabine + R115777 (Zarnestra) versus gemcitabine + placebo in advanced pancreatic cancer (PC). *Proc Annu Meet Am Soc Clin Oncol 21*, 130a. Abstract 517

Van't Veer, L. J., Da, H., Van de Vijver, M. J., He, Y. D., Hart, A. A.M., Mao, M., et al. (2002). Gene expression profiling predicts clinical outcome of breast cancer. *Nature 415*, 530–536.

Vogel, C. L., Cobleigh, M. A., Tripathy, D., Gutheil, J. C., Harris, L. N., Fehrenbacher, L., et al. (2002). Efficacy and safety of trastuzumab as a single agent in first-line treatment of HER2-overexpressing metastatic breast cancer. *J Clin Oncol 20* (3), 719–726.

Von Hoff, D. (1990). He's not going to talk about *in vitro* predictive assays again, is he? *J Natl Cancer Inst 82*, 96–101.

Von Hoff, D. D., Sandbach, J., Clark, G., Turner, J., Forseth, B., Piccart, M., et al. (1990). Selection of cancer chemotherapy for a patient by an *in vitro* assay versus a clinician. *J Natl Cancer Inst 82*, 110–116.

Von Hoff, D. D., Cox, J. V., Tempero, M. A., Eder, Jr., J. P., Eckhardt, S. G., Rowinsky, E. K., et al. (2000). Phase II trial of irofulven (MGI114) in patients with advanced pancreatic cancer who have progressed on gemcitabine. *Proc Annu Meet Am Soc Clin Oncol 19*, 309a. Abstract 1219

Voutsadakis, I. A. (2002). Gemtuzumab Ozogamicin (CMA-676, Mylotarg) for the treatment of CD33+ acute myeloid leukemia (review). *Anti-Cancer Drugs 13*, 685–692.

Section V

CONCLUSION

16

ONCOGENOMICS AND THE NCI DIRECTOR'S VISION FOR 2015

Andrew C. von Eschenbach

We stand at an inflection point in our nation's effort to conquer cancer. Remarkable advances in biomedical research and the emergence of powerful new technologies over the past decades have allowed us to develop a profound understanding of the molecular underpinnings of cancer. We now know cancer to be both a genetic disease and a cell-signaling failure, and we know that specific processes are required for its development and progression. This understanding is allowing us to develop target-specific interventions that "hit" a cancer at vulnerable points in its growth process and preempt its progression to a lethal phenotype. From this solid foundation, we now have the unprecedented opportunity to strategically harness emerging advances and technologies and use them to confront the challenges of cancer today and tomorrow.

Cancer research is a national priority. Approximately 1.4 million U.S. citizens will be newly diagnosed and 560,000 of us will die of cancer this year. These are daunting statistics, and the aging of the baby-boomer population and shifting demographics of America during the next 15–20 years represent enormous healthcare and economic challenges that we must begin to prepare for now.

At the same time, as this book wonderfully illustrates, we are now making unprecedented progress in conquering our most debilitating diseases—especially cancer. Our nation's investment in basic research has fueled the engine of discovery, thereby enabling unparalleled advances in illuminating the genetic changes and molecular

Oncogenomics: Molecular Approaches to Cancer, Edited by Charles Brenner and David Duggan
ISBN 0-471-22592-4 © 2004 John Wiley & Sons, Inc.

mechanisms that ultimately produce cancer. The sequencing of the human genome and associated progress in new areas such as functional genomics and proteomics provide us with a clearer picture of the mechanisms by which cancer develops and ravages the human body. For the first time, we have within our grasp the ability to design target-specific interventions to preempt this process. We must enrich these extraordinary advances in basic science with equally extraordinary efforts to develop new agents and technologies to actualize these interventions at key steps in cancer progression. We now understand that cancer is a process—a process with multiple opportunities to develop new, more effective interventions to prevent, detect, and treat cancer.

To capitalize on this knowledge, we must significantly accelerate the pace of progress across the entire research continuum. The pathway begins with discovery of knowledge that underpins the development of new molecules and tools and ends with the delivery of diagnostics and therapeutics to all people who need them. Discovery, development, and delivery must be made seamless, therefore it is crucial that we take the steps needed to ensure that all phases of the research enterprise are functioning together optimally.

THE CHALLENGE

We now envision a time when the suffering and the death that are caused by cancer will be eliminated; and we believe that it is realistic to set ourselves a challenge goal to achieve this vision by the year 2015. We are not saying that all cancer will be cured. What we are saying is that in this 11-year time-frame, some cancers will be cured, but many more will be transformed into chronic, manageable diseases that patients can live with—not die from. There is precedent for this paradigm shift. In a single generation, we made enormous strides in reducing deaths from coronary artery disease and converting this disorder into a condition that people live with and manage. Likewise, using our knowledge of the AIDS virus, molecular biology, and skills in developing target-based therapy, we have developed treatments for AIDS patients that both save lives and preserve quality of life. We can do the same for cancer.

This vision presents new challenges for the NCI and for everyone working to conquer this devastating disease. We will meet those challenges by further strengthening basic research, especially in advancing our understandings about the mechanisms of cancer progression. In parallel, we will intensify our focus on clinical research, and on translating these advances into effective cancer prevention, screening, and when necessary, diagnosis and treatment for all our citizens.

ACCELERATING RESEARCH AND DEVELOPMENT ACROSS THE ENTIRE CONTINUUM

In discovery, we will lead a national integrative cancer biology effort to unravel the critical events of cancer biology, and the tumor microenvironment and macroenvironment. This systems biology approach will allow us to dissect the complex and redundant reactions and interactions within cells and their environments, and will enhance our technical capabilities to identify molecular targets and create new therapies. We will also focus on harnessing new technologies in areas such as molecular imaging, proteomics and genomics, and nanotechnology. These new technologies offer the promise of developing new platforms to monitor cells, identifying intricate molecular changes, and delivering therapeutics to specific targets within the cell. The application of these advanced technologies is no longer a dream. Advances in positron emission tomography, coupled with new molecular imaging agents, now make functional monitoring possible, permitting clinicians to visualize the biologic progress of cancer. Scientists and engineers are working to achieve this goal through the NCI's unique programs that foster the development of innovative technologies for cancer diagnosis and treatment.

The NCI will also place new emphasis on the development process—the translation of basic research advances into new products that are ultimately delivered to cancer patients. This is especially true in the area of cancer therapeutics. It currently takes 15–20 years for a promising new molecule to reach patients, a rate that is unacceptable if we are to meet the challenge goal. Genomics and proteomics are providing us with hundreds, potentially thousands, of new therapeutic targets for cancer; but the enterprise is not optimized to develop and deliver these "new paradigm" drugs. This is a systems problem and it can be solved. In collaboration with the National Institutes of Health (NIH), the Food and Drug Administration (FDA), and other partners in the public and private sectors, we will work to streamline the development of chemoprevention and cancer drugs and speed their delivery to patients. In all that we do, we will encourage the removal of barriers that separate us by creating a new environment that encourages and rewards multidisciplinary research and collaboration.

The NCI will also undertake programs to optimize the process of developing new drugs by validating new cancer targets. The emerging field of proteomics provides us with unimagined opportunities to apply these new targeted therapies and preventive strategies by detecting cancer early enough to stop, slow, or possibly reverse disease progression. Novel disease biomarkers are finally providing us with new screening tools to detect early-stage cancer in populations and individuals; and the NCI will utilize its enormous strength in molecular epidemiology to provide rational strategies for cancer prevention and disruption of progression within populations. Underpinning all these initiatives will be the deployment of a bioinformatics infrastructure that will allow us to integrate data from multiple fields of research and make them broadly accessible to the cancer research community.

All these tactics will be directed at reducing suffering and death from cancer. That does not mean that we will lessen our emphasis on someday eliminating cancer—quite the opposite—but in the near-term, we will focus on changing the course of cancer by reducing its morbidity and mortality.

We stand at a pivotal crossroad, a defining moment in the history of this nation's effort to prevent and cure cancer. An ever-increasing body of scientific knowledge and an array of advanced technologies provide us with the opportunity to detect cancer early and preempt the progression of the disease. We now embark on a new course that will prevent as many cancers as possible, and enable patients to live with cancer as a chronic, nondebilitating disease that doesn't threaten their vitality, careers, and families. We have within our grasp the power to eliminate the suffering and death from cancer—and we will succeed.

INDEX

Oncogenomics: Molecular Approaches to Cancer, Edited by Charles Brenner and David Duggan
ISBN 0-471-22592-4 © 2004 John Wiley & Sons, Inc.